T0354723

HEALTH
Is Your
Birthright

HEALTH
Is Your
Birthright

How to Create the
Health You Deserve

Ellen Tart-Jensen, PhD, DSc

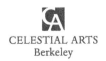

CELESTIAL ARTS
Berkeley

DEDICATION

This book is dedicated to the health and happiness of every man,
woman, and child on this beautiful blue-green planet we call Earth.
It is dedicated to the divine physician within us all, who,
when called upon earnestly with faith, can heal perfectly.

Copyright © 2006 by Ellen Tart-Jensen

Published in the United States by Celestial Arts, an imprint of the Crown Publishing Group,
a division of Random House LLC, a Penguin Random House Company, New York.
www.crownpublishing.com
www.tenspeed.com

Celestial Arts and the Celestial Arts colophon are registered trademarks of Random House, LLC.

The lyrics on page x from "Walk in Balance" by Denean are used with permission
courtesy of Variena Music ©. "Walk in Balance" is on the CD Fire Prayer which is
available at www.ethereanmusic.com.

Library of Congress Cataloging-in-Publication Data
   Tart-Jensen, Ellen.
      Health is your birthright : how to create the health you deserve / Ellen Tart-Jensen.
         p. cm.
      Includes bibliographical references.
      1. Self-care, Health—Popular works. I. Title.
   RA776.95.T37 2006
   613—dc22
                              2006027982
ISBN: 978-1-58761-273-2

Cover design by Nancy Austin and Chloe Rawlins
Text design by Chloe Rawlins
Text production by Tasha Hall

First Edition

The information contained in this book is based on the experience and research of the author.
It is not intended as a substitute for consulting with your physician or other health-care provider.
Any attempt to diagnose and treat an illness should be done under the direction of a health-care
professional. The publisher and author are not responsible for any adverse effects or consequences
resulting from the use of any of the suggestions, preparations, or procedures discussed in this book.

Contents

PART 2: CASE STUDIES

Preface

SOME PEOPLE WHO READ the title of this book may become angry, especially if someone they love is severely disabled and perhaps has been that way since birth. They may feel this title is a mockery to those who have never been healthy and seemingly never will be. I understand these feelings. I was genetically handicapped with scoliosis and spent a large part of my childhood in and out of hospitals that were hundreds of miles from my family, enduring excruciating physical and emotional pain. To treat my severely curved spine, the doctors used a thousand pounds of pressure to straighten it two inches, and they placed a sixteen-inch stainless steel rod inside the vertebrae. I wore a brace for a year and a body cast for a year. Then, at age twenty-four, I was in an accident that caused the rod to damage tissue and bone. It had to be removed from my spine. The pain was so unbearable, not even morphine brought relief. For years after that surgery I suffered from exhaustion, chronic fatigue, fibromyalgia, and unspeakable pain in every muscle, nerve, tendon, and ligament of my body. Because of the intense pain and exhaustion, I also struggled each day with deep depression. I was angry, too. Why had this happened to me? Where was the God I had been raised to believe in? I spent hours crying and shouting, "Why me?!" It seemed at times that death would be a blessed escape. I felt as if I were a burden to my family and useless in the world. I couldn't work, I needed help to dress myself, and worst of all, my bowels would not function without a daily enema. At my lowest point, a friend left a poem by my bed called "Don't Quit," by Jill Wolf. It went like this:

> *Don't quit when the tide is lowest,*
> *For it's just about to turn,*
> *Don't quit over doubts and questions,*
> *For there's something you may learn.*
>
> *Don't quit when the night is darkest,*
> *For it's just a while till dawn;*

Don't quit when you've run the farthest,
For the race is almost won.

I read it and I read it again. I took a deep breath and said a deep, but simple prayer, "Dear God, show me the path to health and help me have the courage to follow it. Help me to be as well as I can be!" After saying the prayer, I heard the Beatles singing on the radio: "When I find myself in times of trouble, Mother Mary comes to me, speaking words of wisdom, let it be . . . there will be an answer, let it be." I was determined to find those answers.

Now I feel healthier than I ever have before. I feel strong and free from pain. My spine is still fused from my shoulders to the end of my lumbar vertebrae, but I am well because of the natural health laws I discovered and have followed to this day. My mind is clear and I am wonderfully happy.

This book is the culmination of fifty years of a life spent searching for answers about why some people are healthy and others are ill, why some people are happy and others are sad, why some people are rich and others are poor. After healing myself and moving from a life of constant pain, depression, and poverty because I wasn't able to work into a life of health, joy, and abundance; and after coaching hundreds of others to do the same, I have come to truly believe that health is our birthright! There are specific laws in nature, laws that God gave to us to follow in order to be healthy and happy. Sadly, over the generations, many people have abandoned these laws and created sickness and disease. Even our beautiful blue-green planet Earth is out of balance and "ill" because mankind has polluted the air, water, and soil. I believe that most of the illnesses we suffer from today were created through some misuse or abuse of the laws of nature at some point in the history of human life on earth.

From a broad, holistic perspective, we see health as our birthright; from a personal perspective, however, we may feel that neither we nor our severely handicapped loved ones can be healed. I believe there is always a way to better ourselves and be the best we can be, no matter what our current position in life. Instead of thinking of ourselves as victims and telling ourselves there is no hope, we can take charge of our lives and fight one more round. The first step is to begin following the principles in this book with a positive attitude; you may be surprised by how well you become or how well you help your loved one to become.

A mother brought her disabled son to see me because he was suffering with constant colds and flu. The boy was in a wheelchair. Due to a high fever the mother had experienced while her son was in the womb, his brain had been damaged. He was unable to speak or move and was fed through a feeding tube in his stomach. I asked the mother what she was putting in the feeding tube, and she said, "Cake icing." She felt this was easy to give him and would provide him with quick energy. She had no idea that the cake icing provided no nutrition and was weakening his immune system. I suggested that she feed her son lightly steamed vegetables blended with almond milk made from soaked nuts, along with raw vegetable juice. The following month she reported that her son was healthier than he had ever been. His body was growing stronger, and he was no longer ill with colds and flu. His eyes were becoming clear and alert, and he was even looking at her. This is a rather extreme case, but I use it as an illustration that there is always hope. Where there is life, there is hope.

Most people who read this book will not be in such a challenging position. However, if you are a handicapped person due to genetics, illness, or injury or a chronically ill person, you can take steps to improve your life. You can learn from your illness and grow into a better person because of it.

I have been very inspired by Mattie J. T. Stepanek, an eleven-year-old boy, who had a rare form of muscular dystrophy. I never met Mattie in person, but the courage and wisdom he expressed in his poems have moved me to tears. In spite of his pain and illness, Mattie wrote poetry of hope in his beautiful books, *Heartsongs* and *Journey through Heartsongs*. He took a life of extreme difficulty and made it into a life that was special.

When I was disabled, I was sad for a long time and, because of the severe pain, wondered whether I would ever have the energy or ability simply to make it from the bed to the closet to dress myself. However, after the day I prayed for health and strength, I made a deep inner commitment and covenant with myself that somehow, no matter how long the road or how difficult the path, I would find a way to heal my body. Before the healing could begin, I had to shift from a victim frame of mind to an "I can make it!" frame of mind. I had to put my anger, sadness, and "poor me" syndrome aside so healing could take place. I now know all our thoughts are like prayers. Whatever we are holding onto in our minds will multiply in our lives. In my case, I have grown tremendously and learned a great deal because of the pain I endured. I do not believe we have to endure pain in order to learn and grow, but I do feel that if we have an affliction, we can choose to learn from it. Today, I have a busy practice coaching people about health and lecturing throughout the world on natural health care and nutrition.

Based on the laws of nature, my own experience, and clinical evidence, I provide practical, simple-to-understand tools that anyone may follow. Some readers of this book may be very sick, while others may be looking for preventative suggestions or may want to learn how to live a healthy, balanced lifestyle in order to feel stronger and more vibrant each day. I have purposefully avoided being too technical so any reader can understand how to create a healthy body and lifestyle. Following the principles in this book will help you take your power back, maximize your ability to heal yourself, and give you the knowledge of what is needed to be the healthiest you can be. In doing so, you will necessarily contribute to the planet's health too. If we all bought organic foods, rather than foods that have been heavily sprayed with chemicals, our demand would force farmers to stop spraying their crops. Chemicals would stop filling our rivers and damaging our soil. Our planet could once again become the healthy home it was divinely designed to be. Practicing the laws of health will help to create peaceful bodies, and practicing peace will create healthier bodies, bringing us more peace on Earth.

By healing our bodies and our planet, we also will strengthen our genetic pool and pass to our children a legacy of health and peace, rather than illness and war. We will restore the earth, her soil, her waters, and her atmosphere. By taking responsibility for how we live our lives and what we consume, we can reestablish health as our birthright for the generations to come!

When we learn to walk in balance
The healing will take place
The healing of this earth our mother
The healing of the human race

—Denean

Acknowledgments

I AM THANKFUL TO MY FATHER, Rayford Tart, my mother, Janice Tart, my sister, Donna Dyer, her husband Allen Dyer, and my two beautiful nieces, Laura and Carmen Dyer, as well as my grandparents and extended family for the unconditional love and kindness they have given me throughout my life.

I would like to thank my dear husband, Art Jensen, for his daily support of my work in natural healing and in the writing of this book. I am grateful to my late father-in-law, Dr. Jorgan Bernard Jensen, for all that he taught me in the field of nutrition and iridology.

I am grateful to my editor at Celestial Arts, Meghan Keeffe, and the many other hands there for editing and formatting my manuscript: Chloe Rawlins, Tasha Hall, Shirley Coe, Kim Catanzarite, and Ken DellaPenta. Thanks to Nancy Austin for the lovely cover design. I would also like to credit Dr. Kimberly Balas for her contributions to the herbal tea section.

I would like to thank my book agents, David Knight and Rickey Berkowitz, of Book Talk Literary Group. I am most grateful to Jo Ann Deck, publisher at Celestial Arts, for being attuned to my desire to help others so that the finished book might convey the essence of my spirit.

To all the beautiful angels who have been bright lights in supporting the writing of this book—you know who you are and I thank you all! I thank all my colleagues in the International Iridology Practitioners Association for being part of my dream to see iridology and nutrition take their proper place in the world of health care.

Introduction

WE LIVE IN A FAST-PACED WORLD, with all the modern conveniences of cell phones, email, websites, microwaves, television, radio, airplane travel, multilane highways, traffic jams, condominiums without yards, air conditioning, fast-food restaurants, TV dinners, and packaged foods. Many of us have lost all connection with nature. We have conveniences galore at our fingertips, but we are more rushed and hurried than we have ever been. Because of this, more people than ever before are suffering from anxiety, stress, panic attacks, chronic fatigue, chronic pain, migraines, ulcers, obesity, high blood pressure, high cholesterol, heart attacks, stroke, arthritis, and myriad other health problems. Diabetes is becoming more and more prominent throughout the United States—and even in Third World countries, where soft drinks have become readily available.

The incidence of cancer is rising too. In 1928, J. Ellis Barker wrote in *Cancer: The Surgeon and the Researcher*, "Cancer is a disease of over-civilization or faulty civilization, and is caused by chronic poisoning in almost any form, and it cannot be doubted that much disease is caused by our being bombarded with chemicals and poisons in minute quantities at all meals." Statistics show that at that time, one out of every nine people in the United States died of cancer. In 1957, Alexander Berglas, in *Cancer: Nature, Cause and Cure*, stated that one out of every four persons in the United States would contract cancer during his or her lifetime. Current statistics show that one of every three Americans develops this dreaded disease. To counteract their problems, people are consuming billions of dollars worth of aspirins, antacids, sleeping pills, antibiotics, analgesics, diuretics, laxatives, caffeine, nicotine, and alcohol each year as quick fixes to make it through each day. I believe that if these are used in large quantities on a regular basis, they will weaken the body and the immune system over time so that it becomes much more susceptible to all sorts of illnesses including cancer.

The time has come for us to take a look at how we are living our lives. People usually begin to search for answers to their health problems when a crisis occurs or when they are tired of feeling tired and sick of feeling sick. The wise person can learn from the mistakes of others and begin to take better care of himself or herself right now. But how does one go about being healthy? The market is full of self-help books and shelves of vitamins. We must begin by introducing more whole, natural, organic foods into our diets and eliminating foods that have been processed, refined, packaged, overcooked, salted, sugared, deep-fried, chemically preserved, and artificially colored. Our bodies are made of the earth's natural elements and remain healthy when nourished with fresh fruits, vegetables, whole grains, beans, nuts, and seeds. In remote areas of the world where people eat foods straight from earth that has not been tampered with, diseases that we experience are virtually unknown.

❧ PART 1 ☙

Creating
a Healthy
Body

I BELIEVE WE ARE ALL cocreators with God. We are not victims, tossed about with no say-so over what happens in our lives. We create our lives through thought, word, and deed. If we want a stone removed from our garden, we must bend over, pick it up and move it. First we see the stone, then we decide that it needs to be moved, make the choice to move it, and actually move it. If we deny that the stone is there and do nothing about it, the stone will remain there indefinitely. The same is true for any health problem we may have. We must first face or acknowledge our problem. Then we embrace it by choosing to do something about it and beginning to look for help. It may seem overwhelming at first, but remember: "Ask and ye shall receive, seek and ye shall find, knock and the door will be opened unto you." You may gain information and inspiration from a book a friend gave you or from the message on a billboard or in a magazine advertisement. Continue to seek until you have the knowledge you need to get well. Then you can begin to erase the problem—you can begin to follow a course of action for healing. Whatever course you choose, commit to it! Doubt and hesitation will keep you from getting well. Patience, courage, determination, and persistence will bring you renewed strength, energy, and well-being. Remember, your illness was not created overnight, and it will take some time to heal. While you take the first steps of replacing worn-out thoughts with new thoughts of courage, faith, and trust, your body will gradually be replacing worn-out cells with vibrant new cells.

Whatever your health problem, there are many tools you can use to get well. In this part, you will find tools to enhance your daily nutrition with beneficial foods and beverages, add healthy exercises and healing therapies to your life, learn about natural home remedies, understand the value of food supplements, and cleanse the body from within. Please don't think you have to use every health tool provided in this book right away! Instead, try to implement one health tool each week until they become part of your new life.

To help you stay focused and on track, purchase a beautiful journal. Not just any journal, but a special one, just for you, with colors and designs that bring you joy. Then write about what you have accomplished each day. If you were able to go for a walk outside in fresh air and sunshine, give yourself a gold star in your journal for that day!

When I was suffering from chronic pain and severe fatigue, it took every ounce of willpower I could muster to crawl out of bed and walk outside. Often, I fell asleep on the grass, exhausted, before going back home. Still I persevered, believing in the benefits of allowing sunshine to bathe me with warmth and vitamin D, fresh air to fill my lungs, and oxygen to circulate through my veins. I added good nutrition habits to further rebuild my body. Over time, these therapies paid off.

How does one keep going when the light at the end of the tunnel seems so far away or even nonexistent? Take baby steps. Let small accomplishments count. If you can read, read uplifting, inspiring stories. Put pictures of healthy people doing healthy things in your journal and on your wall. Visualize yourself well. Most of all, be committed and know that your day of health and peace will come!

I often read this poem when I was healing, and now I read it to my clients:

Until one is committed, there is
hesitancy, the chance to draw back,
Always ineffectiveness concerning all acts of initiative (and creation).
There is one elementary truth the
ignorance of which kills countless
Ideas and splendid plans; that the moment
one definitely commits Oneself,
then Providence moves too.
All sorts of things occur to help one that
would never otherwise have occurred.
A whole stream of events issues from the decision,

Raising in one's favor all manner of unforeseen incidents
and meetings and
Material assistance which no man or woman could have dreamed
Would have come his way.
Whatever you can do or dream
You can begin it.
Boldness has genius, power and magic in it.
Begin now.

—Johann Wolfgang von Goethe (1749–1832)

chapter 1 ༄

Good Nutrition

Let food be thy medicine and medicine be thy food.
—Hippocrates

IT IS SAD THAT OUR FOODS have become so processed and denatured. Many people have lost their innate ability to know what their bodies need to eat in order to be nourished. Our taste buds have become dull from eating too many sweet and salty foods. Some people are hungry all the time and never feel satisfied after a meal. Thousands of American citizens eat enormous amounts of food, yet are overweight and undernourished!

The Laws of Nature

We are creatures of nature, just as all animals are. However, we have lost our understanding of the laws of nature. Animals know what to consume in order to be healthy. They know how to feed their young to ensure their strength and vitality. Many animals know how to store food for the winter. They avoid crops that have been heavily sprayed with chemicals—crops that humans eat. When insects get into our cupboards, they will go after the natural organic foods over their processed and highly preserved counterparts—whole grain over refined white flour, for example, or real sugar over artificial sweeteners—though they have never read a book on nutrition!

I believe in an overall divine plan, and I believe that if people had always followed the laws of nature, health would be our birthright today. Early peoples once lived very close to nature. They knew how to hunt and fish and gather the herbs, nuts, and seeds of the land. Some planted crops and knew how to rotate them so the soil's minerals were preserved. They knew how to use healing herbs, whether in teas, salves, ointments, or poultices, and they drank pure water. They moved and worked in harmony, with the seasons and with nature.

When I was teaching in the Philippines a few years ago, I found that a large number of the people there were suffering from diabetes and decaying teeth due to the introduction of soda pop in their country. Everywhere I looked, people were drinking soft drinks!

It might have seemed wonderful at first, in the United States in the early 1900s, to have soda fountains and soft drinks. It might have seemed marvelous and wonderfully convenient when TV dinners became readily available and fast-food restaurants opened everywhere, but we need to wake up and take a close look at what we have created. We have more cancer and heart disease than ever before. Our children are suffering from obesity and attention deficit hyperactivity disorder (ADHD), both of which are exacerbated by foods high in sugar and empty calories. We need to become responsible consumers and follow the laws of nature.

After my surgery as a child of twelve, I began to crave those easily available sweets. I had not cared much for sweets before the operation. In retrospect, I realize the tremendous stress that surgery caused my adrenal glands and therefore my pancreas. If my mother made a cake, I was unable to concentrate on my homework for thinking about that cake sitting in the cupboard. What was worse, the more I ate, the more I wanted! I never felt satisfied. As a teenager in high school, I was twenty pounds overweight. This disturbed me terribly. I couldn't understand why my willpower was weak in regard to foods when it seemed so strong in every other area of my life. I tried to eat less, but soon the hunger or craving for sweets took over and I would find myself eating more than I should. It took many years for me to learn about hypoglycemia and the types of foods I needed to eat to remain healthy and balanced.

In my practice, I have seen hundreds of people try to follow some sort of diet. Some of these diets are extreme. There are all-fruit diets, high-protein diets, low-carb diets, low-fat diets, low-cholesterol diets, low-sodium diets, starvation diets, and low-calorie diets to name just a few. People, in general, are confused by all the diets touted in the bookstores. I tried them all. I tried with all my might to stick to whatever diet I was on. If it wasn't on my diet, I ignored my instinct whispering that my body needed a specific food. When I was on the fruitarian diet, I started losing hair and feeling lethargic. When I was on the all-protein diet, I was constipated and tired. When I was on the low-fat diet, my skin and scalp became very dry and I felt hungry and wanted to eat something every hour. Now, after reading hundreds of books on nutrition, studying nutrition formally, and working with thousands of clients, I deeply believe that maintaining a balanced diet of fresh, natural foods is the key to good nutrition. I love Richard Simmons' philosophy that we should let go of the word *diet* because it has the word *die* in it! We want to eat nutritious, whole, beautifully prepared foods that promote life, health, and joy.

If you are rigidly following an extreme diet and you feel healthy, happy, and balanced and are truly listening to your inner instincts, it may be right for you; just be open to change if you begin to feel out of balance. I respect whatever works for each individual. Raw foods and fruits may be eaten for a time in order to cleanse the body, but the body may require more variety after a while. Diets may vary regionally. People living in hot climates, such as India, are more suited to fruit and vegetable diets since their bodies don't have to shield them from freezing temperatures. People from colder climates, such as Norway and Switzerland, usually require more protein and some warm, cooked grains.

The nutritional plan I offer here has helped hundreds of people drop excess pounds, maintain their normal weight, feel energetic, and heal a majority of the health problems they were experiencing. Thin people have gained weight, and specific programs have helped people heal specific problems.

We want to adopt a way of eating that we can follow throughout life. We need some initial discipline to train ourselves to eat foods that are pure, fresh, and whole. However, we don't want to feel cheated out of the foods we like. I had a client recently who said she likes to plan a cheat day. She is very strict with her diet during the week, and on Saturday she eats whatever and as much as she wants—including ice cream, soda, pie, and candy. I asked her if this plan had accomplished what she wanted, which was weight loss, and she said no.

For years, I pondered how to maintain my weight through balanced eating. One night in the middle of the winter when I was studying natural therapies in Switzerland, I awoke in the early morning hours while it was still dark. I looked outside and saw snow falling gently on the Alps. At that moment, I heard a clear statement in my mind, "Eat and enjoy whatever you want, but pay attention to what your body truly wants. Eat only when you're hungry, and stop when you're full." Those words were very powerful for me. I wrote them down and worked with them for over a year in order to change my indulging-and-then-starving pattern. It took lots of practice to pay attention to what my body really wanted.

People who are on diets may think they want coffee and doughnuts all the time, but they really don't. My late father-in-law, Dr. Bernard Jensen, used to tell this story: A woman came to him as a patient and told him she could live on coffee and doughnuts as long as she said a prayer to bless them before she ate them. Dr. Jensen told her he would like for her to consume only coffee and doughnuts for one week and then call him. After a day and a half of coffee and doughnuts, the lady called Dr. Jensen and told him she was very sick to her stomach and felt severe nausea. He then asked her what she would like to eat and she replied, "Homemade vegetable soup!" We need to trust that our bodies will let us know exactly what they need. The great thing is that when you do choose only nutritious foods, you start feeling better and lose the desire for junk foods.

Humbert "Smokey" Santillo, ND, writes in *Intuitive Eating: Everybody's Natural Guide to Total Health and Lifegiving Vitality through Food*:

> Imagine being so sensitized to your body's genuine needs that you naturally gravitate towards the foods and the eating style that will work best for your system. This is no fantasy, however. It is a very real possibility for you, and one that I have lived and shared with thousands of people.

Making Healthy Food Choices Based on the Laws of Nature

Eat foods that are pure, whole, fresh, and natural (not processed). Choose foods that are organic and unsprayed. Chemicals used on crops to kill insects are harmful to our bodies. In 1962, Rachel L. Carson's book *Silent Spring* shocked many slumbering citizens and awakened them to the vast threat that the toxic chemicals on our foods pose. The book was dedicated to Albert Schweitzer, who wrote, "Man has lost the capacity to foresee and to forestall. He will end by destroying the earth." The title, *Silent Spring*, vividly conjures the possibility of a spring without the beautiful songs of birds. She wrote about toxic chemicals such as DDT that are sprayed on crops to rid them of insects but infect and kill birds as well. DDT has been found in the livers of ocean fish thousands of miles from where the chemical was used. The United

States has since banned DDT, but it is still sold to Third World countries, from which we buy food. Half a million chemicals are now in use, and pesticide use has more than doubled since 1962.

Artificial chemical fertilizers are manufactured from petrochemicals and have very few of the trace minerals vital to our health. Soil exposed to artificial fertilizers produces poor plants, which therefore attract lots of insects, causing the farmers to use more chemical sprays, resulting in a vicious cycle. Organic foods are grown without pesticides and harmful artificial fertilizers. I know a wonderful Amish farmer named Jacob Miller who grows beautiful, large healthy crops of vegetables and herbs. He said to me, "The plants are healthy and free from bugs because the soil is healthy. The human body is much the same and will be able to resist disease and be free from 'bugs' [germs, viruses, or parasites] when it is healthy." He tests his soil each year to see which nutrients are deficient, then replenishes those nutrients with organic compost and minerals. We need to give our bodies whole foods rich in vitamins and minerals to keep them strong. We are literally made from the dust of the earth.

It is also important to choose foods that have not been preserved with artificial chemicals or dyed with food colorings. Read labels! If the words on a label are too long to understand, leave the product on the shelf. Chemicals are not natural and can harm our bodies. Dr. Ben Feingold researched children with ADHD and found that artificial preservatives and food colorings had definite detrimental effects on their behavior. He has written a very informative book called *Why Your Child Is Hyperactive*.

Choose foods that have not been irradiated. Irradiation is sometimes used as an alternative to chemical preservatives. Sadly, food irradiation is done with gamma rays from cobalt, which can cause genetic mutation, just like radioactive elements.

Don't choose foods that were cooked in a microwave oven. Research now shows that microwaved food is dangerous to our health. For example, according to a 1993 study by Dr. Bernard H. Blanc, Swiss Federal Institute of Technology and University, and Dr. Hans U. Hertel, Environmental-Biological Research and Consultation,

> *Eight test persons—all on a macrobiotic diet—volunteered for this study. They committed themselves to a very strict regimen. All food, which was heated, defrosted or cooked in the microwave oven, caused*

significant changes in the blood of the test persons. These changes included: Decrease of all hemoglobin values, increase of the hematocrit, leukocytes and cholesterol values. Lymphocytes showed a more distinct short-term decrease after the intake of food from the microwave oven than after the intake of other variants.

The measured effects of microwave-irradiated food—as opposed to non-irradiated food—showed changes in the blood of test persons, indicative of an early pathogenic process, similar to the actual start of cancer.

According to Hertel, interviewed by Tom Valentine, "Common scientific belief states that cholesterol values usually alter slowly over longer periods of time. In this study the markers increased rapidly after the consumption of the microwaved vegetables." Also, the lymphocytes, which are a major part of our immune system, were decreased, and there were anemic tendencies in the subjects. In addition, blood changes were shown similar to those in the beginning stages of cancer.

According to a 1992 study by Richard Quan, MD, of Dallas, Texas, and John A. Kerner, MD, of Stanford University, microwaving breast milk is also unhealthy:

Women who work outside the home can express and store breast milk for feedings when they are away. But parents and caregivers should be careful how they warm this milk. A new study shows that microwaving human milk—even at a low setting—can destroy some of its important disease-fighting capabilities and "compared to heated breast milk, microwaved milk lost lysozyme activity, lost antibodies and fostered the growth of more potentially pathogenic bacteria."

Don't choose foods that have been packaged in aluminum cans, and don't cook your food in aluminum cookware or wrap it in aluminum foil. Also avoid baking powder that contains alum or aluminum. Many studies have shown that people with Alzheimer's disease have high amounts of aluminum in their brains. While the aluminum/Alzheimer's link remains unproven, lots of reports show that high levels of aluminum can be toxic to the body. According to the Agency for Toxic Substances and Disease Registry, people may have respiratory problems and coughing when exposed to high levels of aluminum in the air. They have also found that children and adults who have received aluminum in certain medical treatments developed bone diseases. Others that have used deodorants containing aluminum have developed serious skin rashes. The international science journal, *Neurotoxicology*, reported in April 1995 on a critical study that was conducted in Sydney, Australia, showing a direct pathway from tap water carrying aluminum through the intestinal tract, into the bloodstream and to the brain. Rats were given water treated with alum. Two weeks later, aluminum was found in their brains. Judy Walton, the scientist that performed the study, noted the worldwide increase in Alzheimer's over the past seventy years and stated, "We really should look seriously at revisiting this possibility that aluminum addition to foods and drinking water is a health hazard." I believe that waiting for definitive proof that aluminum can cause Alzheimer's before taking some measures of precaution is unwise. Foods should be cooked in stainless steel or glass cookware; clay pots and stainless steel waterless cookware are also wonderful choices.

When cooking your food, do not cook it to death with large amounts of water. Steam your vegetables in a stainless steel steamer and keep them up out of the water or use waterless cookware. Do not fry foods in deep grease; sauté them in a small amount of olive oil, grape seed oil, or coconut oil instead.

Tool Kit for Making Healthy Food Choices

Choose foods and substances that are pure, whole, fresh, and natural. Avoid denatured, preserved, processed foods; these can be harmful to our bodies. It is much easier to let go of foods that do not abide by the laws of nature if we have delicious foods to replace them with. This tool kit offers wonderful choices for eating healthfully.

BEANS

Avoid:

Canned, salted pork and beans

Replace with:

Dried beans that have been grown organically and have been soaked before cooking so they are easier to digest, or bean sprouts

DAIRY PRODUCTS

Avoid:

Pasteurized milk

Ice cream that is high in preservatives and sugar or artificial sweeteners

Yogurt that is high in sugar and lacks friendly bacteria

Cheese that is made from pasteurized milk contains dyes, preservatives, and hormones

Margarine

Eggs that have been fried in grease or overcooked

Eggs that have been salted and pickled

Replace with:

Certified raw goat's milk that is organic and hormone free

Certified raw cow's milk that is organic and hormone free

Almond milk that is organic and hormone free

Rice milk that is organic and hormone free

Oat milk that is organic and hormone free

Ice cream that is made from certified raw cow's or goat's milk, frozen bananas, or rice milk and is sweetened with maple syrup, raw honey, or stevia (a sweet, noncaloric herb)

Yogurt that is made from organic goat's or cow's milk and has live bacteria

Cheese made from certified raw cow's or goat's milk, almonds, or seeds

Unsalted butter, preferably organic Ghee (clarified butter)

Organic coconut oil

Organic olive oil

Eggs that are organic, hormone free, and fertile

FRIED FOODS

Avoid:

Foods fried in deep grease

Replace with:

Foods sautéed in a small amount of organic olive oil, grape seed oil, or coconut oil

FRUITS AND VEGETABLES

Avoid:

Canned fruits with sugar and preservatives
Canned vegetables with salt and preservatives
Iceburg lettuce

Replace with:

Fresh fruits
Fresh vegetables
Romaine, butter, endive, green leaf and red leaf lettuces

GRAINS

Avoid:

Flour-based bread, especially white-flour bread
Crackers made from white flour
White-flour pasta
Cream of wheat and packaged cereals with sugar, salt, and preservatives

Replace with:

Breads made from sprouted whole grains
If sprouted-grain breads are not available, breads made from whole-grain
    flour such as barley, kamut, millet, quinoa, rice, or spelt
Crackers made from rice flour or rye flour
Rice cakes
Rice, corn, or quinoa pasta
Spaghetti squash (cooks up much like spaghetti)
Whole-grain cereals made from amaranth, brown rice, buckwheat, millet,
    quinoa, rolled oats, rye, or wild rice
Packaged cereals that are wheat-free and made from organic-grain without
    added sugar, salt, or preservatives

I usually recommend that people who are ill avoid all wheat. If you are
not ill and are not suffering from sinus congestion, gas and bloating, or
celiac disease (an inability to absorb gluten), you may eat whole wheat in
moderation. More than a couple slices of whole wheat bread per day may
cause weight gain or lead to gluten intolerance. Grinding your own wheat
and making flour is of course the healthiest of all.

A Note about Grains and Allergies

Dr. Dan Kalish has done some research at his health clinic, The Natural Path. He has found, as I have, that many people have a subclinical, or hidden, gluten intolerance. Symptoms may include suffering from sinus congestion, gas and bloating after a meal, chronic fatigue, environmental illness, and lowered immunity. A highly specialized salivary test for subclinical gluten intolerance has accurately tested thousands of people with this disorder, making it easier to discover and treat the problem. Dr. Kalish explains:

> *Sub-clinical gluten intolerance refers to exposure to the gliadin molecule and to a specific inflammatory reaction, taking place in the small intestine of afflicted individuals. . . . To clarify, gliadin, the molecule that causes the problem, is present in some, but not all gluten containing foods. People with this problem must avoid glutens from the grains of wheat, rye, barley, oats, kamut, spelt, quinoa, amaranth, teff and couscous. Rice, corn, buckwheat and millet have glutens, but the glutens in these foods do not contain the gliadin molecule that can provoke the inflammatory reaction, therefore they are usually safe. In some cases people are allergic to rice, corn, buckwheat or millet, independent of the reaction to gluten/gliadin.*

If you suspect you have a gluten intolerance, avoid wheat for a week. If you don't feel better, additionally avoid all grains containing gliadin including rye, barley, oats, kamut, spelt, quinoa, amaranth, teff, soy, and couscous for a second week and thereafter. It may take up to nine months to reduce inflammation in the small intestine and heal irritated tissue. Many who are gliadin intolerant also have corn allergies. If you don't feel well after two weeks of avoiding gliadin, omit corn for a week. If you have a corn allergy, you should feel better soon. Soaking grains overnight and cooking in a Crock-Pot is the best way to prepare grains. Hawthorne berry tea and flax seed tea may soothe the inflamed intestinal lining. Colon and tissue cleansing as described in chapter 7, is a remarkable way to help heal this disorder more quickly.

MEATS

Avoid:

Pork, especially sausage and bacon

Processed meats, especially lunch meat and hot dogs containing nitrates, and nitrites in general

Replace with:

Veggie burgers

Veggie sausage

Turkey sausage and turkey bacon (60 percent less fat than regular pork bacon)

Lunch meats that have been sliced from freshly cooked chicken, turkey, and roast beef that contain no nitrates

NUT AND SEED BUTTERS

Avoid:

Peanut butter that is high in sugar and canola oil

Roasted nut and seed butters

Replace with:

Aflatoxin-free peanut butter (such as peanut butter made from sun-dried organic peanuts)

Raw, organic almond, sesame, or sunflower seed butter, which are much healthier than peanut butter

Soaked, blended nuts and seeds

Nuts and seeds can be soaked while they are sprouting, making them easier to digest. Soaking nuts and seeds also reduces the quantity of fat by half. Soaked nuts and seeds can be dried in a dehydrator or blended into creams. (To learn how to make delicious almond creams, see the recipe later in this chapter.) I believe that every day we should also eat a few nuts and seeds that have not been soaked. Either grind them or chew them well. We can eat more of the soaked nuts and seeds daily because they are so easily digested. If a person is ill or has a digestive disorder, soaked nuts and seeds are better for them. Soaked, blended nuts and seeds can be kept in a quart jar in the refrigerator and used as a snack between meals to help balance the blood sugar. Nut and seed creams are also wonderful for nursing mothers to help keep their milk from drying up.

NUTS AND SEEDS

Avoid:

Roasted, salted nuts and seeds
Peanuts

Peanuts are not really a nut, but a legume. Most people think of them as nuts, so they are listed here. Peanuts are high in calcium, magnesium, phosphorus, potassium, and protein. However, nonorganic peanuts are saturated with pesticides, and organic peanuts often contain a mold called aflatoxin, which is carcinogenic.

Replace with:

A wide variety of raw, unsalted nuts and seeds

Raw nuts and seeds are high in beneficial oils (high-density lipoproteins), which help keep our arteries clean and skin glowing. Nuts and seeds contain lignans, which are believed to protect against hormone-sensitive cancers, such as those of the breast and prostate. Dr. Bernard Jensen used to say, "Think of the nuts and seeds as the 'glands' of the plants that can help to feed and nourish the glands of the body." The healthiest nut choices are almonds, Brazil nuts, and walnuts, which are very high in protein, calcium, magnesium, phosphorus, potassium, iron, selenium, zinc, and vitamin E. Calcium, magnesium, and potassium help prevent muscle cramping. Young people, who are growing rapidly and using their muscles a great deal, are often deficient in these three minerals and get leg cramps. These three minerals are also important in calming the nervous system. Iron is necessary for preventing anemia, and the bones need calcium and phosphorus to be strong. The heart is a muscle and needs potassium to be healthy. Selenium, zinc, and vitamin E help to strengthen the immune system and fight free radicals in the body, and they are well-known for helping prevent cancer. Black walnuts are high in all the minerals mentioned with the exception of selenium. Black walnuts also contain manganese, which is excellent for the memory.

Sesame, sunflower, and pumpkin seeds contain high amounts of calcium, magnesium, iron, phosphorus, potassium, and zinc. Pumpkin seeds are among the highest in zinc of all the nuts and seeds, and they are excellent for the prostate gland. Pumpkin seeds also kill parasites in the body.

Ground flaxseeds are so beneficial everyone should include them in their daily nutritional plan. Flaxseeds are high in fiber and help keep the colon working smoothly. You must grind the flaxseeds, however, in order to receive their healthy benefits. The oil in the flaxseeds is high in lignans, which protect against several types of cancer. Many people take flaxseed oil, which, when fresh, is very good but lacks the soluble fiber so beneficial to the colon. According to research from Tufts University, even refrigerated flaxseed oil has a shelf life of only six weeks before it becomes rancid.

OILS

Avoid:

    Canola oil

    Cottonseed oil, which comes from heavily sprayed cotton crops

    Foods containing partially hydrogenated oils, such as nondairy creamers or packaged baked goods and crackers

    Oils that have been extracted by heat and processed to preserve them

    Partially hydrogenated oils or fats, including margarine and shortening

Canola oil comes from rapeseed, a food we do not eat because it is highly toxic. According to John Thomas in *Young Again: How to Reverse the Aging Process*, "Rape is the MOST toxic of all food plants. Insects will not eat rape. It is deadly poisonous." He goes on to say that "canola oil . . . forms latex-like substances that form agglutination of the red corpuscles. . . . Rape oil (canola oil) antagonizes the central and peripheral nervous systems. Deterioration may take years to manifest." *Canola* is not the name of a natural plant. It is called *canola* because it was developed in Canada and it is short for *Canada oil*. Some documents state that it was developed by the genetic engineering of the rapeseed plant. Other authorities say it was developed by hybrid propagation techniques. It's confusing and it's controversial, and it comes down to this: Not enough long-term research has been done on this oil to consider it safe for consumption.

The hydrogen used to harden margarine also can harden bodily tissues. Trans-fatty acids occur when polyunsaturated oils are hardened into margarine through hydrogenation. According to James Balch, MD, and Phyllis Balch, CNC, in *Prescription for Nutritional Healing:* "One recent study found that trans-monounsaturated fatty acids raise LDL (bad) cholesterol levels. Simultaneously, the trans-fatty acids reduced the HDL (good) cholesterol readings." Some people think that eating margarine will help lower their cholesterol, but they are misinformed. Michael T. Murray, ND, and Jade Beutler, RRT, RCP, stated in *Understanding Fats and Oils: Your Guide to Healing with Essential Fatty Acids*, "Trans-fatty acids and hydrogenated oils have been linked to low birth weight in infants, low quality and volume of breast milk, abnormal sperm production and decreased testosterone in men, heart disease, increased levels of harmful cholesterol in humans, prostate disease, obesity, suppression of the immune system and essential fatty acid deficiency."

Replace with:
   Organic, cold-pressed oils such as extra-virgin olive oil or grape seed, sesame, avocado, coconut, and sunflower oils

Olive oil is a wonderful oil because it helps balance the body's pH. If your pH is too acidic, it can damage the central and peripheral nervous systems. You may cook with grape seed, olive, or coconut oil because they can withstand high temperatures and retain their nutritional value. Never heat other oils to high temperatures; they will become rancid and toxic to the body. Keep all oils in the refrigerator.

Even a little real organic butter occasionally is better for you than margarine. Butter is high in vitamins A and D, which are very good for the eyes. Be sure to use organic, hormone-free butter, though. The hormones in dairy and beef products create all sorts of problems with women's menstrual cycles, including premenstrual syndrome (PMS) and menopausal imbalances.

SALT

Avoid:
   Table salt and salted foods

Using too much salt has become a problem in our country. According to *The Supermarket Handbook*, by Nikki and David Goldbeck, "The most common form of salt on the supermarket shelf is a product referred to as 'table salt.' In [its] purifying process, iodine is added, plus dextrose to stabilize it, sodium bicarbonate to keep it white and chemical anticaking agents to keep it free flowing." Avoid using table salt and use caution when purchasing sea salt. When buying sea salt, look for unrefined sea salt; it will be light gray in color. Most sea salt is heated to extreme temperatures, thereby changing its molecular structure and robbing it of all essential minerals, then other chemicals are often added to iodize it, whiten it, and make it easy to pour. Unrefined sea salt is much better for us because it contains ninety-two essential minerals and trace minerals, while refined sea salt may contain only sodium and chloride. Almost all packaged foods contain an excessive amount of salt. Most people's taste buds have become so accustomed to added salt, they have lost the ability to taste the delightful flavors of foods. Each cell of our body contains a sodium-potassium pump that helps move fluids in and out of the cells. Eating too much salt upsets this system, causing our cells to retain too much sodium. When that happens, water is held within the cells, swelling occurs, and our heart has to pump harder, often causing high blood pressure. Our kidneys become overworked and do not release the fluids they should. High blood pressure is directly related to stress, poor kidney functioning, and/or an imbalance in the body's fluids and minerals. Avoid using table salt as much as possible. If you are ill, avoid using it altogether.

Replace with:
    Salt-free powdered vegetable broths and seasonings
    Liquid amino acids
    Granular seaweed, such as dulse and kelp
    Unrefined sea salt, in small amounts

If you have ever tasted your tears, you noticed they were salty. Lymph fluid needs natural sodium to lubricate the cellular membranes and hold calcium in solution. Sodium chloride in table salt has been isolated and refined from other nutrients that might help the body utilize it. When we take minerals into the body in plant form, we utilize the whole food. The body easily assimilates sodium from vegetables. Look for vegetable seasonings that are salt free. Add dried, organic herbal seasonings such as thyme, oregano, basil, rosemary, dill, garlic, onion, or sage to your food. Dr. Jensen called natural sodium the youth element because of its ability to keep the joints limber. The stomach also needs natural sodium for proper digestion. Under stress, sodium is depleted rapidly, causing digestive disorders, gout, and arthritic conditions. Organic sodium is found in celery, green leafy vegetables, okra, strawberries, goat's milk, and mineral whey drink. If you have digestive disorders, gout, or arthritis, try the recipe for mineral whey drink found later in this chapter. Mineral whey is the clear fluid that comes from the goat's milk while separating it from the solids in order to make cheese. It is naturally high in minerals and organic sodium. The juice from celery and green leafy vegetables helps to heal and prevent arthritis because the sodium aids in dissolving calcium deposits.

Seaweed is a wonderful source of natural sodium, calcium, trace minerals, and iodine. Dulse, kelp, and kombu can be purchased in powdered form and used to season salads, soups, and vegetables; nori's the ideal "sushi" wrap for brown rice and vegetables; and hijiki, which looks like noodles when soaked, is crunchy and delicious in salads. Seaweed is a delicious way to fortify the body with minerals and to strengthen the thyroid gland with iodine. People in Japan do not often get goiter (an enlargement of the thyroid gland) because they eat lots of fish and seaweed, which are high in natural iodine. People in Switzerland have a tendency for goiter because they live in the Alps and do not get enough iodine in their diets. Salt from the sea that has been allowed to dry in the wind and the sun and is not highly treated or refined is rich in native minerals and may be used in small amounts.

SUGAR AND SWEETENERS

A Note about Sugar

Glazed doughnuts, rich chocolates, chunky ice cream, creamy puddings, cakes, candies, pies, cookies: Many people think of these sweets with joy and anticipation. They may remind us of happy times from childhood such as birthday parties or holidays. Many people have been rewarded for a job well done with a sweet treat. In the old days sweets were truly a treat and were few and far between. They were often made with real maple syrup taken from a tree or honey pulled from a beehive. It took time to churn a freezer of ice cream by hand or make a cake from scratch. Today, ready-made sweet foods are everywhere. In addition to the myriad desserts available in the United States, as well as in a rapidly growing number of other countries, sugar is now in virtually every packaged food on the shelf. One 12-ounce soft drink contains the equivalent of thirteen teaspoons of sugar! Soft drinks were once sweetened with sugar derived from sugarcane or sugar beets, but now they are sweetened with high fructose corn syrup which is sweeter than sugar and costs the soft drink industry less. However, according to Sharon Elliott and other researchers in an article published by the *American Journal of Clinical Nutrition* (November, 2002), high fructose corn syrup is metabolized differently in our bodies than sugar or glucose. While glucose can be metabolized by every cell of the body, all fructose must be metabolized by the liver. *Washington Post* writer Sally Squires reported on March 11, 2003 some very important information presented by George A. Bray, former director of Louisiana State University's Pennington Biomedical Research Center. Bray explained that when eating glucose, the body increases insulin production, which enables sugar to be carried into the cells to be used as energy. It also causes the body to produce a hormone called leptin that helps store fat and regulate the appetite. It suppresses production of another hormone the stomach makes that helps regulate food uptake, called ghrelin. She goes on to say that according to Peter Havel, associate professor of nutrition at University of California Davis that "Fructose doesn't stimulate insulin secretion. It doesn't increase leptin production or suppress production of ghrelin. That suggests that consuming a lot of fructose, like consuming too much fat, could contribute to weight gain." Meanwhile, a team of researchers led by Dr. Meira Fields of the U.S. Department of Agriculture found that when fructose was given to rats that were deficient in copper, they developed high cholesterol, enlarged hearts, and anemia. Their livers were cirrhotic and filled with fat. Rats that were fed glucose were unaffected. (Fields, M. *Proceedings of the Society of Experimental Biology and Medicine,* 1984, 175:530–537.) Even peanut butter and ketchup are 30 to 40 percent sugar, mostly in the form of high fructose corn syrup! High fructose corn syrup has replaced sugar in almost every food product on the market. It can be found in yogurt, bread, applesauce, fruit juices, cookies, crackers, and many other things. Read labels and avoid anything that contains it.

What has this sugar craze done to our bodies? Growing numbers of people throughout the United States and worldwide are suffering from diabetes, obesity, hypoglycemia, gum infections, yeast infections, tooth decay, and hyperactivity—all traced to the ingestion of excessive amounts of sugar.

When sugar enters the body, it feeds harmful bacteria that dwell in the mouth. Within minutes after eating a sugary dessert, tooth decay begins. Extensive ingestion of sugar without brushing the teeth creates gum diseases such as gingivitis and periodontitis.

Refined white sugar contains no nutrients, so the body has to draw from its storehouse of enzymes and nutrients to digest it. All of the

B vitamins, which are vital to nerve health, and vitamin C, which is important to keeping the immune system active and to repairing connective tissue, are required. Excessive amounts of sugar can even leach calcium and other minerals from the bones to help process it. Place a chicken bone in a cup of pop for one week and watch how soft it becomes! Nor does white sugar give any nutrition back to the body. When one eats an apple, the apple contains sugar, but it also contains enzymes, vitamins, and minerals that help the body process the sugar.

A Note about Aspartame

Artificial sweeteners containing aspartame are two hundred times sweeter than sugar. Because it contains very few calories, aspartame has been tremendously popular with dieters and diabetics. It is in soft drinks, instant coffees and teas, sugar-free gum, breath mints, juice drinks, puddings, yogurt, laxatives, and even multivitamins. It is served in packets along with the sugar on tables in restaurants.

H. J. Roberts, in *Aspartame (NutraSweet): Is It Safe?*, writes about a significant number of people who used aspartame and reported having nausea and diarrhea, headaches, trouble with memory, problems sleeping, changes in their vision, moodiness, and confusion. Some even reported having convulsions.

There are three components in aspartame: phenylalanine and aspartic acid, which are both amino acids; and methanol, known as methyl alcohol or wood alcohol. Aspartame should not be used by persons with PKU (phenylketonuria). These people lack the enzyme necessary to digest phenylalanine, and if taken into their bodies, it can cause brain damage. A warning for phenylketonurics is found on aspartame products. Methanol can be poisonous and toxic in anyone. It can cause inflammation, swelling, and even blindness.

A Note about Splenda

Another artificial sweetener that has become most popular is sucralose, a synthetic compound known by its trade name, Splenda. It is four times sweeter than aspartame, twice as sweet as saccharin, and five to six hundred times sweeter than sugar. It is a chlorocarbon manufactured by the selective chlorination of sucrose. Short-term studies done by the manufacturer on rats revealed that sucralose caused shrunken thymus glands and swelling of the kidneys and liver. The FDA decided that because the studies were not done on humans they were not substantial and inconclusive. However, many people have given testimonials that report rashes, intestinal cramping, diarrhea, headaches, weight gain, disruption of sleep patterns, numbness, and dizziness. In Dr. Janet Hull's new book, *Splenda: Is It Safe Or Not?*, she gives scientific evidence that suggests that sucralose may be dangerous for human consumption. I suggest avoiding it completely!

A Note about Saccharin

Saccharin has mostly been replaced by better-tasting products that contain aspartame. While aspartame is more toxic than saccharin, research has shown that saccharin caused bladder cancer in rats. Many researchers believe that it could be carcinogenic in humans when taken in sufficient dosages.

All artificial sweeteners are chemicals and are potentially toxic to the body. They are not food so they don't give the body the boost of energy it is calling for when one craves sweets. Therefore, when the body doesn't feel energized, it craves the carbohydrates. Often those who eat artificial sweeteners end up gaining more weight than those who eat sweeteners from natural sources. These natural sweeteners give the body the energy it craves so the person doesn't keep going back to the refrigerator for more food.

Avoid:
All products containing aspartame
Splenda and all products containing Splenda
Saccharin
Refined white sugar
Desserts made from white flour and white sugar

Replace with:
Stevia, a natural herb with few calories that can balance the pancreas and reduce cravings for sweets
Agave
Blackstrap molasses, which is high in minerals and B vitamins
Certified raw organic honey (except for children under two, who have not developed the ability to digest it)
Pure Grade B maple syrup, which is less refined and contains more nutrients than Grade A syrup

Rice bran syrup, which is high in minerals including silicon as well
as B vitamins

Unrefined cane sugar, for special occasions only

Carob candy, a nutritious substitute for chocolate

Organic chocolate, preferably raw, in small quantities for special
occasions

Stevia is the best sweetener for someone who is watching his weight or has diabetes or hypoglycemia. Stevia is a sweet, noncaloric herb native to Paraguay that has been used to sweeten foods and beverages for centuries. It is two to three hundred times sweeter than sugar but has very little effect on blood glucose and does not cause cavities. It is sold in health food stores as a dietary supplement and comes in powdered or liquid form.

Organic blue agave nectar is a delicious and nutritious sweetener to use. The best, most natural agave nectar comes from the pineapple-shaped core of the blue agave plant, which is a desert succulent that grows in the mineral rich volcanic soil of Mexico. The nectar, or syrup, is light in color and thinner than honey. Research done by the Glycemic Research Institute in Washington, DC, has shown that the blue agave nectar is safe for non-insulin dependent (type 2) diabetics because it has a low glycemic level. It is also great for hypoglycemics, those trying to lose weight, or anyone watching their carbohydrate intake. In recipes, three-fourths cup of agave nectar will equal one cup of table sugar. When purchasing agave nectar, make sure it has the Glycemic Research Institute (GRI) seal of approval on it.

Xylitol is a safe natural sweetener that comes from the bark of the birch tree, fibrous vegetables, and fruits and corncobs. It is also produced naturally in normally metabolising bodies. Xylitol looks and tastes almost exactly like sugar, but while sugar causes havoc in the body, xylitol helps heal and repair. Xylitol also helps prevent tooth decay and fights bacteria. It has 75 percent fewer carbohydrates than sugar, 40 percent less calories, and causes very little change in insulin levels. Xylitol is available in crystalline form and can be used in place of sugar to sweeten beverages, or in baking. Make sure xylitol is from the bark of the birch tree or other natural plant source before purchasing.

For healthy desserts, look for delicious cookies made from rice flour rather than wheat flour and sweetened with maple syrup, stevia, agave nectar, xylitol, or fruit juice. Practice making your own cookies with oat flour, spelt flour, or rice flour, and use maple syrup, stevia, or agave to sweeten them. Carob brownies and cakes can be made with rice, spelt, or whole-wheat flour and maple syrup. Shop at health food stores for wonderful ice creams made from rice milk and popsicles made from fruit juice. You can make your own tapioca pudding with rice milk.

ADDICTIVE SUBSTANCES

Avoid:

Tobacco, nicotine, and social drugs

Organic tobacco is available, as are organic cigarettes free from pesticides and chemicals. However, tobacco smoke is very irritating to the lungs and arteries. It disturbs the blood sugar balance. In addition, nicotine is very hard on the adrenal glands and heart. If you are a smoker, ask yourself why you smoke. Is it for emotional reasons? Follow therapeutic remedies that will help you stop smoking. Any type of addiction enslaves us and keeps us from being free.

AVOID FREE RADICALS

Free radicals are highly reactive molecules or fragments of molecules that wreak havoc in our bodies. They have electrons that are unpaired in their outer orbits. Because of this imbalance, they are unstable and very aggressive with other molecules.

When a cell has been damaged by free radicals, the cell is less able to import oxygen and nutrients or excrete cellular wastes. Cells then begin to rupture and spill their damaging contents into the surrounding tissues. Free radicals can even alter genetic codes by damaging nucleic acids (RNA and DNA), causing abnormal cell growth. This destruction leads to rapid aging, the growth of malignancies, impaired immune function, arteriosclerosis, and damage to joint linings, which leads to arthritis and many other major health problems.

Air pollution, tobacco smoke, polyunsaturated fats, rancid fats, and processed foods are sources of free radicals. By avoiding these harmful substances and replacing them with wholesome, life-giving foods and juices, you will effectively decrease free-radical damage in your body. Antioxidants bind to and neutralize free radicals in the body. They are abundant in fresh fruits and vegetables. Several vitamins and minerals act as antioxidants as well. These include vitamin A, beta-carotene, vitamin E, and vitamin C. Selenium, zinc, copper, and manganese combine with enzymes and help fight free radicals.

COMBINE FOODS PROPERLY

Food combinations have many wonderful benefits that help improve health, though some restrictions do apply. Some people have become so paranoid about food combinations that they eat only one food at each meal. Also, I have had clients who were so concerned about proper food combining that they were afraid to eat and enjoy their meals, and they became malnourished. These responses are unnecessarily extreme. However, if you are extremely ill or have severe allergies, strict food combining is very important for optimal digestion and absorption.

It's best to eat fruits alone. Fruits digest very rapidly, and if they are eaten with grains, for example, they begin to ferment while the grains are still digesting. This causes gas. Too much gas over long periods of time can cause hiatal hernias because of the continuous pressure imposed on the cardiac sphincter muscle. So if you like fruit in the morning, have it at least ten to twenty minutes before your meal. Fruits can be combined with vegetables more easily than with grains because vegetables digest quickly. Our ancestors often ate vegetables from the earth and fruit from trees at the same time. Avocados combine well with all foods. Melons should definitely be eaten alone.

We should also separate starches from proteins. However, the body can tolerate the combination if the starch is a natural whole grain and not a white-flour product. Try the meal plans provided in the following tool kit, and notice whether you are having gas or burping. If so, you should eat fruits alone and even separate whole grains and natural starches, such as potatoes, from proteins. For example, have vegetables and a grain at a meal or vegetables and a protein at a meal.

Soaked nuts and seeds combine well with all foods except melons because they are digested and absorbed quite easily. It is important to soak all grains or beans for twelve to twenty-four hours before cooking them. They will digest easier and cause less gas. Beans contain enzyme inhibitors that are removed through soaking. You may want to take an enzyme supplement with your meal to aid digestion. Most Americans over the age of forty are deficient in natural digestive enzymes and should supplement them with their meals.

EAT A VARIETY OF FOODS

Nature has provided us with a multitude of beautiful, delicious foods of all colors to choose from. Different foods contain different nutrients. We should eat a variety of foods each day in order to provide our bodies with the vitamins and minerals they need to be well. Remember, our bodies are made up of the earth's elements. Our bones need calcium, our skin needs silicon, and our thyroid gland needs iodine to function properly. Each part of our body requires specific nutrients. If you are accustomed to living on sodas and chips, coffee and doughnuts, TV dinners, or all fruit or all meat, you are not getting the wide variety of nutrients your body requires on a daily basis. Deficient organs become sick organs and will not function properly. Follow the menu plans in this book to get a variety of foods in your diet each day.

ADD FIBER TO YOUR NUTRITIONAL PROGRAM

Constipation, colon cancer, Crohn's disease, colitis, and diverticulitis have become too common in our modern world. The intestinal tract needs fiber to keep it clean and healthy. Fiber also promotes good peristalsis (healthy muscle contractions that keep food and waste matter moving through the body), and it helps lower high levels of cholesterol. According to a study published in the *Journal of the American Medical Association*, oat bran was shown to lower blood cholesterol levels. Choose foods high in fiber from: fruits; vegetables; legumes; nuts; seeds, including ground flaxseeds; and whole grains such as brown rice, barley, millet, rye, quinoa, amaranth, and oats. A diet that is high in fiber can greatly regulate blood sugar levels and help manage both hypoglycemia and diabetes.

EAT RAW VEGETABLES WITH YOUR MEALS

When we eat raw vegetables, we are eating foods as Mother Nature provided them. Raw vegetables are so good for us because they provide living enzymes, electrolytes, vitamins, minerals, and phytonutrients.

Phytonutrients, also called phytochemicals, are the elements in most fruits and vegetables that help give them their color. Scientists have found that these valuable nutrients are potent antioxidants that help neutralize free radical damage and help the body fight disease by mobilizing natural killer cells and helper T-cells. They help to fight cancer and protect the heart. While some phytonutrients remain intact during cooking, such as those in broccoli, many are destroyed when exposed to high heat. Raw vegetables are also high in fiber. The enzymes help digest our meals better. If you have difficulty digesting raw vegetables, use a food processor or blender to chop and grind the vegetables, making them easier to chew and digest. Finely grind cabbage for coleslaw and carrots for carrot salad. Grind beets, zucchini, yellow squash, carrots, cucumbers, and jicama, and place them on a bed of lettuce. (See salad recipes later in this chapter.) Blended vegetables make good salads and cold soups.

Be sure to wash all raw vegetables well to remove any eggs, worms, or parasites. Soak them in raw apple cider vinegar and water for five minutes (see page 56). Then scrub them with a good vegetable brush.

CHOOSE 80 PERCENT ALKALINE-FORMING FOODS AND 20 PERCENT ACID-FORMING FOODS

Ripe fruits, including organic lemons and limes, that were ripened on the vine, raw apple cider vinegar, vegetables, and soaked sprouted grains, nuts, seeds, and beans are alkaline-forming foods. Meats, cheeses, eggs, beans that have not been soaked, white flour, soft drinks, coffee, and black tea are acid-forming foods. Oranges and grapefruits that were not ripened on the vine produce acids in the body.

Dr. Bernard Jensen recommended eating two fruits and six vegetables per day to achieve the 80 percent of alkaline-forming foods. He recommended 10 percent protein and 10 percent starch per day to make up the 20 percent of acid-forming foods.

Fruits are alkaline-forming; however, they are high in fruit sugar, so I recommend no more than two fruits per day. If a person is ill, I recommend avoiding fruits altogether for a while. People with arthritis may have increased pain from eating too many fruits. People who want to lose weight should have no more than one fruit a day because the fruit sugar can turn to body fat. Of course, if it comes down to fruit or chocolate cake, fruit would be a nice substitute!

Vegetables are excellent for us, and we should eat a wide variety each day. Eating six different kinds of vegetables each day would be great. Consider having this many varieties in a salad.

We do need some protein. A large part of our body is made up of proteins, including our cell walls, digestive enzymes, and hair. Our brain and nervous system cannot function without protein. However, most Americans eat far too much meat. Dr. Samuel West, in *The Golden Seven Plus One*, shows how proteins can become trapped within the blood, causing pain, swelling, or inflammation in the body. The important thing is that protein come from natural organic sources and that it be digested well and absorbed. The balanced nutritional plans provided in this book improve health and well-being.

UNDERSTAND YOUR PH BALANCE

Biochemist Carey Reams did a great deal of research on the importance of pH, which stands for "potential of hydrogen," a measure of the acid and alkaline balance in our bodies. We cannot be healthy if our bodies are too acidic or too alkaline. This balance is almost as important as breathing or the heart beating. When the pH within our bodies is balanced, it maintains healthy metabolism and allows the body to function optimally.

Dr. Robert Young has done extensive research on the pH of urine and saliva, and in his comprehensive book *The pH Miracle*, he suggests the following normal pH ranges.

Saliva: 6.8 to 7.2 throughout the entire day, 6.8 to 8.4 right after meals
Urine: 6.8 to 7 before meals, 6.8 to 8.4 right after meals

Acidosis, or Overacidity

Most Americans are overacidic because their diet includes processed foods and too much meat, sugar, salt, caffeine, and alcohol. According to Richard Anderson, ND, NMD, in *Cleanse and Purify Thyself*:

The further we deplete our minerals and move towards greater acidity, the more our bodies lose control over pH, and the more the liver and all organs are impaired. From this depletion of minerals and development of acidity, our immune systems become depressed. We also can lose the ability to create hydrochloric acid, the bile turns acid, our normal friendly bacteria mutates and we then become susceptible to infiltration

of "germs"—various bacteria, viruses, fungus, yeast and perhaps proto-
zoa. Both minerals and harmonious feelings are essential in maintain-
ing this delicate pH and metabolic balance.

An overacid environment can lead to serious health conditions. Some
of these include kidney stones, plaque in the arteries, osteoporosis, arthritis, cardiovascular deficiency, lowered immune function, free-radical damage, fatigue, weight gain, water retention, dry hard stools, burning tongue,
and bad breath. We must have sufficient alkaline reserves to buffer the acids
in our body. Calcium cannot stay in our bones if the body is overacidic.
Stress, as well as acidic foods, causes acidity in the body. We can stay
healthy by living a balanced life and consuming plenty of alkaline foods
that are pure, whole, fresh, and natural.

Alkalosis, or High Alkalinity

A less common condition in which the body is too alkaline can result from
the long-term use of alkaline drugs, such as those used for ulcers in the
stomach or intestinal tract. It can also result from excessive vomiting, diarrhea, and poor diet.

People suffering from alkalosis often have an intense, overexcitable
nervous system. They may even have anxiety or seizures. They may feel cold
or have sore muscles, cramps, allergies, sluggish digestion, constipation,
immune deficiency, and urinary tract weakness. They may also have calcium deposits, such as bone spurs.

TEST YOUR PH

If you sense that your body is overalkaline or overacidic, test your pH for six
days by following the pH test provided below, based on Dr. Robert Young's
research. You will need some pHydrion paper (pH paper strips), which can
be purchased at most pharmacies. You will need one strip for each time you
check your saliva and one strip for each time you check your urine.

Test Start Date: _____

Upon waking, test your saliva with pHydrion paper. Wet the end of a
pHydrion test strip with your saliva before brushing your teeth, drinking,
or eating. Note the color change and record the pH number. Optimally, the
pH should be between 6.8 and 7.2.

First Saliva Test:

Day 1 _____ Day 2 _____ Day 3 _____
Day 4 _____ Day 5 _____ Day 6 _____

Now test your first urine of the morning. This is urine that has been stored in your bladder during the night and is ready to be eliminated when you get up. Urinate on a strip of pHydrion paper, note the color change, and record the pH number. Optimally, the pH should be between 6.8 and 7.2.

First Urine Test:

Day 1 _____ Day 2 _____ Day 3 _____
Day 4 _____ Day 5 _____ Day 6 _____

Next, test your morning urine a second time before eating any food. You will have eliminated the acid load from the day before, and optimally your second urine pH should be around 6.8 to 7.2.

Second Urine Test:

Day 1 _____ Day 2 _____ Day 3 _____
Day 4 _____ Day 5 _____ Day 6 _____

Eat breakfast. Wait five minutes, then check both your urine and saliva again. Record your results.

Second Saliva Test:

Day 1 _____ Day 2 _____ Day 3 _____
Day 4 _____ Day 5 _____ Day 6 _____

Third Urine Test:

Day 1 _____ Day 2 _____ Day 3 _____
Day 4 _____ Day 5 _____ Day 6 _____

Now wait a couple of hours after breakfast and check your saliva and urine again and record your results below.

Third Saliva Test:

Day 1 _____ Day 2 _____ Day 3 _____
Day 4 _____ Day 5 _____ Day 6 _____

Fourth Urine Test:

    Day 1 _____ Day 2 _____ Day 3 _____

    Day 4 _____ Day 5 _____ Day 6 _____

Two to three hours after lunch, check your saliva and urine again and record your results below.

Fourth Saliva Test:

    Day 1 _____ Day 2 _____ Day 3 _____

    Day 4 _____ Day 5 _____ Day 6 _____

Fifth Urine Test:

    Day 1 _____ Day 2 _____ Day 3 _____

    Day 4 _____ Day 5 _____ Day 6 _____

If you have sufficient alkaline reserves to buffer the acids in your system, the pH numbers will go up (greater alkalinity) from the first to the second urine and saliva tests. If you do not have enough alkalinity, then the pH numbers will show very little change or even go down from the first to the second and third morning pH tests. Our pH should always be between 6.8 and 8.4 right after meals and between 6.8 and 7.2 a couple of hours after meals. I like for my clients to test for six days in order to see a pattern, but really one can test their saliva and urine on a daily basis or (after the six days) periodically at various times throughout the week. Continue testing until your pH falls within a healthy range on a regular basis. Then you may want to check once a week to make sure you are maintaining a good pH.

If Your Body Is Overacidic

- Eat lots of raw vegetables, salads, and steamed vegetables.
- Eat Avocado Pudding (see page 55) daily until your pH comes into normal range, then as often as you desire. It makes a great healthy morning breakfast or even dessert (see the recipe later in this chapter).
- Drink several glasses of raw organic vegetable juice throughout the day until your pH tests within range. Then continue with one glass of raw vegetable juice on a daily basis for maintenance and good health.
- Drink six to eight glasses of distilled water with ten drops of ionic liquid trace minerals added daily until proper pH is maintained.
- Take plant enzymes before each meal.

- Drink one to three liters of purified water with powdered green vegetables added. These green powders usually include a variety of all sorts of alkalinizing green vegetables such as celery, parsley, spinach, kale, collards, green kamut or wheat grass, alfalfa leaf, dandelion leaf, and barley grass. You may search for these in your local health store or call Bernard Jensen International listed in the resources section of this book.
- Eat seaweeds such as dulse, kelp, kombu, wakame, nori, and/or hijiki on a daily basis until pH comes into balance, then several times a week for maintenance.
- Take a liquid calcium-magnesium supplement daily until your pH comes into balance, then check with your health practitioner to see if you should continue.
- Drink potato peeling broth one to two times per day until your pH comes into balance, then once a week for maintenance; see the recipe later in this chapter.
- Drink mineral whey drink one to three times per day until your pH comes into balance, then daily or at least several times a week for maintenance; see the recipe later in this chapter.
- Drink one tablespoon of Dr. Jensen's Whole Life Food Blend (see resources) in eight ounces of water, one to three times daily until your pH comes into balance, then take it once daily for maintenance.
- Practice deep breathing and meditation.

If Your Body Is Too Alkaline

- Eat more acid-forming foods that are whole, fresh, and natural, such as whole-grain cereals, brown rice, beans, eggs, fish, chicken, and turkey.
- Take enzymes with each meal daily until your pH comes into balance, then check with your health practitioner to determine if you should continue. If you see whole bits of food in your stools it is likely that you need them.
- Include liquid calcium citrate and methylsulfonylmethane (MSM) in your diet daily until your pH comes into balance.
- Take vitamin B complex and vitamin C daily until your pH comes into balance.
- Use acidophilus and bifidus daily until your pH comes into balance.
- Add essential fatty acids to your nutritional program.
- Cook foods with a minimum of water. A steamer, Crock-Pot, or waterless cookware is preferable. Never fry foods in deep grease. Pan fry with a little

olive oil, coconut oil, grapeseed oil, ghee, or butter. Bake or broil rather than frying whenever possible.

EAT ESSENTIAL FATTY ACIDS, THE "GOOD" FATS

Not to be confused with trans-fatty acids, essential fatty acids (EFAs) are just that—essential. Christiane Northrup, MD, in her newsletter, *Health Wisdom for Women*, has reported that the following symptoms occur when people are deficient in essential fatty acids, the "good" fats:

- Dry "alligator" skin, cracked fingertips or cracked heels
- Bumpy "chicken" skin on backs of arms
- Brittle or soft nails
- Dry, unmanageable hair or dandruff
- Depression or moodiness
- Allergies, eczema, or psoriasis
- Hyperactivity
- Learning or memory problems
- Lowered immunity, frequent infections or poor wound healing
- Fatigue or weakness
- Excessive thirst or frequent urination

The good fats are terribly deficient in the American diet. These fats are the omega-3s and the omega-6s. Recent studies have shown that DHA, docosahexaenoic acid, an omega-3 fatty acid, is necessary for brain and nerve function, and is sorely lacking in the diets of those who are depressed, have learning disabilities, or have ADHD. Dr. Northrup states:

A deficiency in DHA is one of the main reasons individuals who've been on extremely low-fat diets for long periods of time become depressed. Several studies have shown a link between suicide or depression and following a very low-fat or fat-free diet. It's no wonder that the rise in the number of people on selective serotonin re-uptake inhibitor (SSRI) drugs such as Prozac and Zoloft seems to reflect the profusion of fat-free foods on the market.

She goes on to say:

The right kinds of fats are also important for the heart and cardiovascular system. Cardiovascular disease is the leading cause of premature death in the United States—for both men and women. . . In fact, research also suggests that deficiency of omega-3 fats is a factor in both Alzheimer's and Parkinson's disease.

Good fats are essential for our brain and nervous system, skin and nails, eyes, heart, and cardiovascular system, as well as the rest of our bodies. EFAs also are necessary to the development of a fetus's brain, nervous systems, and retinas, and they help to promote milk flow in nursing mothers. EFAs are an aid in losing weight since they help the body feel satisfied and keep it from feeling hungry for long periods of time. Plus EFAs help the body to release stored fat.

In people who have multiple sclerosis (MS), the myelin sheath that covers the nerves is destroyed. Michael T. Murray, ND, and Jade Beutler, RRT, RCP, in *Understanding Fats and Oils*, found that people with MS appear to have a defect in fatty acid absorption and transport, which would be a significant factor in their myelin deficiencies.

Essential fatty acids have been referred to as vitamin F, and they are the building blocks of oils and fats. Though they are vital to good health, the body cannot make them. Some of the best sources of DHA (an omega-3) are dark green leafy vegetables, organic eggs, and cold-water fish such as salmon, mackerel, rainbow trout, and sardines. Fish and fish oil can help heal psoriasis and dry skin disorders, high blood pressure, and arthritic inflammation. Good sources of other omega-3 EFAs, including linolenic and gamma-linolenic acids, are: eggs; free-range meat from animals that have consumed grass high in omega-3s; green leafy vegetables such as broccoli, collards, dandelion greens, and kale; legumes, raw nuts; seeds including ground flaxseeds; and oils such as fish oil, salmon, borage oil, primrose oil, sesame oil, and grape seed oil.

Good sources of omega-6 EFAs, which include alpha-linolenic and eicosapentaenoic acid (EPAs), are fresh deepwater fish, fish oil, walnut oil, and flaxseed oil. Essential fatty acids must be refrigerated and never heated in order to retain their beneficial properties. Heating oils to high temperatures changes the chemical bonds and creates dangerous free radicals.

INCORPORATE LECITHIN, ANOTHER GOOD FAT, INTO YOUR DIET

Every living cell in the human body needs lecithin in order to be healthy. Lecithin is a type of lipid that is partly soluble in water and acts as an emulsifying agent, enabling cholesterol and other fats to be dispersed in water and carried out of the body. This helps to cleanse fat from the arteries and protect the vital organs from fatty buildup.

The sheath covering the brain, nerve cells, muscles, and cell membranes that are responsible for nutrient absorption are composed of lecithin. Lecithin contains B vitamins, choline, inositol, and linolenic acid. It is found in grains, brewer's yeast, eggs, fish, legumes, and wheat germ. Most lecithin in the market is made from soybeans. James Balch, MD, and Phyllis Balch, CNC, in *Prescription for Nutritional Healing*, explain about lecithin derived from egg yolks:

> *Recently egg lecithin has become popular. This type of lecithin is extracted from the yolks of fresh eggs. Egg lecithin may hold promise for those suffering from AIDS, herpes, chronic fatigue syndrome and immune disorders associated with aging. Studies have shown that it works better for people with these disorders than soy lecithin does.*

RESPECT YOUR MEALS

Mealtimes should be pleasant, peaceful times during each day in which we sit down, relax, and enjoy our food. Observe your life. Are you allowing time and space to eat slowly and chew your food well? Or are you rushing through lunch, eating while driving and perhaps talking on a cell phone at the same time? Ask yourself if you are eating consciously, paying attention to the smell, taste, and texture of your food, or do you eat unconsciously without discernment about whether you are truly hungry or not? After you learn to make healthy food choices, it's just as important to learn when and how to eat the foods you have chosen. A bit of common sense can go a long way toward creating a healthy lifestyle. Read the following section and decide if you have healthy or unhealthy habits around eating. Write down the habits you have now and if they are not in alignment with creating good health, then write a new plan for change. Learn to make healthy food choices and also practice wholesome eating habits. Treat yourself well during meals.

Eat Only When You're Hungry, and Stop When You're Full

People eat for various reasons, many of which have little to do with hunger. Some people eat because they are sad, others eat because they are happy. Some people eat to satisfy deep-seated emotional needs. Adults who were rewarded with foods when they were children—often with sweets—may still look for love from these foods.

Nature intended us to feel hunger so we would nourish ourselves and feel satiated so we would stop eating. We need to discern between food hunger and emotional hunger. We also need to learn to stop eating when we feel full. Practice eating in moderation and noticing when you feel comfortably full (not stuffed!). This may take practice if you are used to overeating. The more you eat nutritious foods, the less you will feel the need to overeat. Studies have shown that those who practice eating moderately live longer, healthier lives.

If you eat for emotional reasons, practice bringing more joy into your life by doing the things you love, and you will find yourself to be less hungry.

Eat in Peace

When you are hungry and it's time to eat, place your food on your plate. Sit at a table in a relaxed position (not on the couch in front of the TV). Pause before you eat, and place your hands in your lap. Take a few deep breaths in and out through your nose and relax. Your body needs to be in a relaxed mode, governed by the parasympathetic nervous system, while you are eating in order to digest well. The parasympathetic nervous system is responsible for all internal responses including the digestion of food. It functions when we are in a relaxed state. The sympathetic nervous system is associated with fight-or-flight responses and functions during emergency situations. It inhibits digestion and accelerates breathing and heartbeat. Therefore, we don't want to be watching a scary movie while eating because it could actually put us into a sympathetic mode which can stop digestion. So calm yourself before going to the dinner table. Bless your food before you eat in whatever way is comfortable for you, and eat it with an attitude of gratitude. You might light a candle or put a flower in a pretty vase on your table. Eat peacefully with good company or alone. Soft, relaxing music in the background can help facilitate proper digestion, or you may choose to eat in silence. Eating in peace can help you get rid of annoying food allergies too. According to Phyllis and James Balch in *Prescription for*

Nutritional Healing, "particles of undigested food manage to enter the bloodstream and cause a reaction. Leaky gut syndrome is a term used to describe a condition in which the lining of the intestinal tract becomes perforated and irritated, and tiny particles of partially digested food enter the bloodstream, causing an allergic reaction." And Dr. Jeffrey Bland states in *Optimal Digestion*, "If food is poorly digested, it can produce ammonia, alcohol, and other chemicals in the body as a result of increased putrefaction. . . . The buildup of these toxins in the body can result in general toxicity. . . . Metabolic toxins may account for some cases of food sensitivity." Therefore, being in a relaxed state to allow the body to digest properly is crucial to the prevention of food allergies and poor health.

Food that is eaten in a hurry cannot be digested properly. Eating while you are walking around and talking on the phone severely compromises good digestion. Eating while driving through a fast-food restaurant or talking on a cell phone disturbs digestion. Too often, families watch the news while eating. It is no wonder people are suffering heartburn, gas, and ulcers!

I was very impressed when I was living in a small village in the Swiss Alps where, at noon each day, all the shops and businesses closed and everyone went home for lunch. Even the school children rode their bicycles home for lunch. Families spent time together between 12:00 and 2:00 each day. Eating food consciously is a step toward living lives consciously and with love.

Chew Your Food Well

Chew, chew, chew your food! Chew each bite of food at least twenty-five times. Digestion begins in the mouth. Food swallowed whole cannot be digested properly in the stomach. When we don't digest our food, we don't receive the vitamins and minerals it has to offer us. Undigested food can ferment and become food for parasites to live on and can create free radicals.

Never Consume Foods or Beverages That Are Too Hot or Too Cold

Ice-cold beverages and food or boiling-hot beverages and food can damage the delicate tissues in the mouth, esophagus, and stomach lining. Ice-cold or boiling-hot beverages taken with a meal can greatly impair digestion by paralyzing enzyme activity in the mouth and stomach. If you are accustomed to drinking really hot or cold beverages, try drinks that are a bit less extreme in temperature. Over time, you will prefer them and feel much better for drinking them!

Eat Your Evening Meal before 7:00 P.M.

It is important to eat your last meal of the day before 7:00 P.M. so your food will be fairly well digested when you go to bed. If you eat a heavy meal and then go to bed, your body will be digesting rather than relaxing. You may fall into a restless sleep, have bad dreams, and feel tired the next day. Quite often, people who eat late wake up between 1:00 and 3:00 A.M. because this is when the liver starts to cleanse. Eating late places a heavy burden on the liver, causing it to have to work harder. If you are hungry before going to bed, have a glass of raw vegetable juice, such as celery, parsley, cucumber, or carrot. The juice will help hold your blood sugar steady through the night and let you sleep.

Eating in Restaurants

Going out to eat can be relaxing and enjoyable. It allows you to spend time with friends and loved ones and have a night off from cooking. Others will serve you and wash the dishes afterward. However, many Americans have started eating out for breakfast, lunch, and dinner. This might be okay if they were eating at places that used organic foods and healthy recipes. But most of the time, this is not the case. People are eating in fast-food restaurants where food is prepared in deep grease that is saved and used again and again for days. Lots of white flour, white sugar, pasteurized milk, salt, and processed foods are used. I once saw a vial of blood that had been taken from a man who had just consumed a cheeseburger on a white-flour bun, french fries, and a milkshake. The vial was half full of creamy, thick fat thanks to that one meal! Fat clogs our arteries and veins, which causes our hearts to have to pump harder. This results in an enlarged heart, which is a tired heart and one that is much more likely to suffer a heart attack. Americans are among the most obese people in the world because of the types of foods they are eating coupled with a lack of exercise.

When you go out to eat, choose a restaurant that has a clean kitchen and prepares foods from scratch rather than using canned and packaged goods. Choose places that will cater to the customer and prepare foods with less salt and fat. Order seafood or chicken, and add salads made with

Romaine lettuce, green or red leaf lettuce or butter lettuce (you may have to make a special request for these, but it's worth it because they are more nutritious and contain more chlorophyll than iceberg lettuce), vegetables, baked potatoes, or brown rice. Try to avoid fried foods and foods with heavy sauces and creams. If you are normally healthy and want to have a dessert once in awhile, do so and enjoy it. Just don't make desserts and sweets a daily habit. Eat your meal in peace and joy. This can be more healing than eating a healthy meal in anger or sadness.

Tool Kit for Creating Healthy Meal Plans

Make a list of the foods you are accustomed to eating on the following meal plan work sheet. Then look at each food and, following the guide presented in the preceding tool kit on foods to avoid and foods to replace them with, create a new healthy meal plan work sheet with foods you will enjoy. I have provided an example for you of how to change average American meals into healthy ones, followed by more great ideas for delicious, healthy meal plans.

CURRENT MEAL PLAN WORK SHEET

List what you eat now. You may want to keep a journal for a week.

Breakfast:
Snack:
Lunch:
Snack:
Dinner:

Do you snack in the evening? If so, what do you eat? Write it down. A lot of people are in the habit of eating at night and then skipping breakfast, even lunch. This is a sure way to gain weight! If you go to sleep with a heavy meal in your stomach, it will most certainly turn to body fat. Start eating breakfast, and you will not be as hungry at night.

HEALTHY MEAL PLAN WORK SHEET

List healthy replacements for what you normally eat:

Breakfast:
Snack:

Lunch:

Snack:

Dinner:

SAMPLE MEAL PLANS BASED ON THE AVERAGE AMERICAN DIET

Breakfast

Average: Coffee and a bagel with margarine and jelly

Replace with: Herbal coffee such as Teecino, which can be purchased in all
health food stores, seven-grain sprouted bagel with organic butter and
jelly sweetened with fruit juice

Average: Orange juice, toast made of white-flour bread, and instant oatmeal with one or two teaspoons of sugar and milk

Replace with: Fresh-squeezed orange juice from organic oranges or apple
juice (have this about twenty minutes before meal), seven-grain
sprouted toast, and cooked whole rolled oats sweetened with six drops
of liquid stevia and rice milk. If you use vanilla rice or almond milk, you
may not need the stevia

Average: Coffee and sugar-coated dry cereal with milk

Replace with: Herbal coffee and millet or rice flakes sweetened with six
drops of stevia and vanilla rice milk

Average: Black tea with sugar, white-flour toast with margarine and jelly,
scrambled eggs, and bacon or sausage

Replace with: Herbal tea of your choice, seven-grain sprouted toast with
butter, fruit-sweetened jelly, poached eggs or soft-boiled eggs. and
turkey bacon or turkey sausage

Midmorning Snack

Average: Coffee and a doughnut

Replace with: Herbal coffee and two cookies made of rice flour—such as
buttered pecan, carob hazelnut, or macaroons—or a slice of raisin
pecan bread made from rice and millet flour, toasted, with a little
organic butter

Lunch

Average: Iced tea, french fries, and a hamburger or sandwich

Replace with: Cold herbal tea (no ice); baked "fries" (see the recipe later in this chapter); and a veggie burger, turkey burger, or organic hamburger, without a roll (or on a seven-grain sprouted roll), with healthy* mayonnaise, natural catsup, and mustard from your health food store, and with raw vegetables such as romaine lettuce, carrots, or celery

Average: Iced tea and a chicken sandwich on white-flour bread

Replace with: Cold herbal tea (no ice) and a sandwich made of chicken or turkey prepared from hormone-free fowl served on seven-grain sprouted bread with healthy* mayonnaise and/or mustard, and with raw vegetables such as romaine lettuce, butter lettuce, sliced tomatoes, carrots, celery, and coleslaw

Average: Iced tea and a hot dog

Replace with: Cold herbal tea (no ice) and a veggie, turkey, or chicken hot-dog with no bread (or on a seven-grain sprouted roll), with healthy* mayonnaise, mustard and catsup, and with raw vegetables such as carrot sticks or celery sticks

*Note on mayonnaise: It should be made without sugar, corn syrup, artificial preservatives, or canola oil.

Afternoon Snack

Average: Soft drink and a pack of peanuts or peanut butter and crackers

Replace with: Sparkling mineral water with lemon and stevia and rye crackers with organic almond, walnut, pecan or peanut butter

Dinner

Average: Spaghetti with white cream mushroom sauce and a salad made with iceberg lettuce and dressing

Replace with: Rice spaghetti or spaghetti squash with marinara sauce (vegetarian, made with grated zucchini, mushrooms, bell peppers, onions, and fresh basil or made with a little ground turkey or a little ground organic red meat); salad made from romaine lettuce and other raw vegetables such as grated carrots, jicama, and red bell pepper; dressing of olive oil and lemon juice or olive oil and raw organic apple cider vinegar with herbs such as basil, garlic, and thyme

Average: Pork chops, macaroni and cheese, and canned spinach

Replace with: Veggie burgers, lamb chops, or beef tenderloin; quinoa or
rice macaroni with just a little raw organic grated cheese or almond
cheese; steamed broccoli; and spinach salad with spinach, tomato,
cucumber, and mushrooms, with olive oil and lemon juice or raw
organic apple cider vinegar dressing

Average: Pork sausage, potato salad, and canned string beans

Replace with: Turkey sausage or grain sausage; potatoes dressed with
healthy mayonnaise, mustard, and pickles; steamed string beans;
and carrot sticks or celery sticks

Average: Fried chicken, mashed potatoes made from potato buds, and
frozen broccoli

Replace with: Chicken tossed in cornmeal with herbs such as basil, sage,
thyme, and paprika; baked tempeh seasoned with liquid aminos, basil,
thyme, and sage; baked, mashed potatoes made from organic freshly
steamed potatoes; fresh broccoli, steamed; followed an hour later by
apple pie made with spelt flour and sweetened with apple juice and
organic ice cream; or, better, a cored apple baked with cinnamon, nutmeg, walnuts, and maple syrup or stevia

A Note on Canned and Frozen Vegetables

It is best to use organic fresh foods, but in areas where it is difficult to get
these, you might try canned or frozen organic fruits or vegetables in your
health food store. Foods that have been picked at the height of ripeness and
quickly frozen or canned properly will retain lots of nutrients necessary for
good health. If you buy canned foods, look for cans that have an inner protective coating that protects the foods from the aluminum in the can. Read
labels on both canned and frozen foods and make sure they are not filled
with dyes, preservatives, sugar, high fructose corn syrup and salt. If you can
foods yourself, make sure you put them in sterile glass jars with a tight seal
to prevent spoilage. Also can with as little cooking time as possible and without salt and sugar. For excellent information on proper freezing and canning
techniques, have a look at the Food pages linked from the Ohio State
University website, www.ohioline.osu.edu. Here you'll find freezing and
canning fact sheets prepared by OSU's Human Nutrition Department.

MORE HEALTHY MEAL PLANS

Breakfast

Natural rice, millet, quinoa, amaranth, buckwheat, or oat cereal sweetened with rice or almond milk and topped with half a banana or a quarter cup of blueberries or a few raisins you poured boiling water over. Cereal can be crispy from the health store or cooked whole. Whole cereal that has been cooked on low heat in a Crock-Pot overnight or soaked overnight and then cooked is much better for you than processed crispy cereals out of the package. If you have any problems with gas, do not combine fruit with grains. Eat your fruit first, then have the cereal fifteen minutes to a half hour later.

Cereal, as above, topped with one to two tablespoons of a mixture of ground almonds, flaxseeds, pumpkin seeds, and sunflower seeds

Fruit salad made with noncitrus fruits, such as apple, banana, blueberries, mango, papaya, peaches, pears, or pineapple, topped with almond cream and a ground nut or seed mixture

One fruit followed by one or two poached, soft-boiled, or over-easy eggs with seven-grain sprouted toast or rye toast (may have grits, millet, or quinoa instead of toast with a half teaspoon organic unsalted butter or ghee).

One fruit followed by one or two poached, soft-boiled, or over-easy eggs with grits, millet, or quinoa with a half teaspoon organic unsalted butter

The Good Morning Health Shake (see page 54) served in a bowl with coarsely chopped almonds and black walnuts or a ground nut or seed mixture of almonds, flaxseeds, pumpkin seeds, sesame seeds, and sunflower seeds

Avocado Pudding (see page 55). This recipe tastes like vanilla or coconut cream and will not cause blood sugar imbalance.

Cornmeal pancakes, blue cornmeal pancakes, buckwheat pancakes, or whole-grain pancakes with blueberries, strawberries, or applesauce, a little butter or ghee, and a little pure, Grade B maple syrup. Wheat-free waffles are available in your health food store. If you have trouble with digestion, eat the fruit separately.

French toast made with organic eggs mixed with rice milk, cinnamon, and vanilla. Soak the sprouted bread in the egg mixture and cook in a little olive, grapeseed, or coconut oil on top of the stove until golden on each side. Serve with almond cream and pure, Grade B maple syrup, ghee, or organic butter.

Lunch

Rainbow salad made with romaine, endive, red and/or green leaf lettuces and lots of colorful vegetables. Add a natural dressing. Use lemon juice or apple cider vinegar and olive oil as a dressing or use a sesame and sunflower seed dressing. Top with soaked sunflower seeds (soaking the nuts and seeds removes half the fat).

Turkey, chicken, or tuna sandwich on rye bread, with healthy mayonnaise, lettuce, tomato, and buckwheat sprouts. Serve with carrots and celery.

Two rice cakes slightly toasted. Top with raw sesame butter, a slice of tomato, and lettuce. Serve with raw vegetables.

Tuna salad on lettuce with raw vegetables

Vegetable soup and raw vegetables and rice or rye crackers or cornbread

Egg salad on lettuce with raw vegetables

Tabouleh salad made with quinoa or millet rather than cracked wheat

Cold "soup" made with blended Romaine lettuce, avocado, cucumber, sprouts, tomato, carrots, garlic, and water. Season with vegetable seasoning, basil, and thyme. Serve in a bowl with pine nuts on top.

Dr. Bieler's potassium soup. (See the recipe later in this chapter.)

Dinner

Salad and stir-fry vegetables over brown rice or quinoa

Salad, baked potato, and broccoli

Steamed vegetable plate with beans and cornbread

Corn tacos with beans, ground turkey, or lean ground beef filling mixed with natural taco seasoning, chopped lettuce, tomatoes, onions, and celery

Baked or broiled chicken and string beans with salad

Broiled salmon patties, slaw, steamed vegetable, and cornbread

Spaghetti squash with vegetarian marinara sauce and salad

Steamed vegetable plate with string beans, beets, potatoes, black-eyed peas, and grated carrot salad. Top with ground sunflower, sesame and flaxseeds and a little olive oil.

Salad or coleslaw; baked or broiled organic fish, chicken, turkey, or lean organic red meat; and vegetables (steamed or baked)

Baked eggplant or zucchini "pizzas" topped with marinara vegetable sauce
and a small amount of grated organic cheese or almond cheese
Salad, steamed vegetables, and veggie or ground turkey burgers
Vegetable or split pea soup and salad
Salad and stir-fry vegetables over brown rice or quinoa
Salad and rice or amaranth pasta with marinara sauce

A Note on Drinks

It is better to drink before or after your meal than with it. If you feel like
drinking a beverage with your meal, take small sips of a beverage that is not
too hot or too cold. When you first get up in the morning, drink hot water
with fresh squeezed lemon, an herbal coffee substitute—such as Teecino—
green tea, or other herbal teas such as peppermint, apple/cinnamon, or oatstraw tea.

Tool Kit for Choosing Healthy Snacks

Choose foods for snacks from a wide variety of pure, whole, and natural
foods. If you eat snacks that are high in sugar and caffeine, such as a soft
drink and chocolate bar, you may feel satisfied and energetic for a short
time, but it won't be long before your blood sugar levels will crash and you
will be hungrier than ever. Whole foods, as nature provides them for us,
will balance your blood sugar and keep up your energy levels for hours. A
healthy snack can improve your metabolism, keep your weight balanced,
and help you think more clearly. Some snack suggestions follow.

Daytime Snacks

Snacks should be eaten between meals when you are hungry. If you are only
slightly hungry, you may still have a small snack; this will keep your blood
sugar balanced and even keep you from overeating when mealtime comes.
Then, when mealtime comes, you won't feel so starved that you need to
overeat.

Raw vegetables and hummus
Celery stuffed with raw nut butter, such as almond or sesame butter
One or two rice cakes, slightly toasted and spread with almond or sesame
butter
Toasted sprouted bread with organic goat, cow, or almond cheese

Raw vegetables with feta cheese, goat or cow cheese, sesame sauce, or
  sesame butter (see the recipe for sesame sauce later in this chapter)
Raw organic cottage cheese with carrots
One apple with twelve soaked almonds (soaked almonds are sprouted
  inside and will combine with fruit fairly well)
One-half papaya with a scoop of almond cream in the center (see the
  recipe for almond cream later in this chapter)
Sesame sauce dip with raw vegetables
A piece of fruit (if you do not have any problems with blood sugar)
Two-thirds cup of vegetable soup
One cup of organic yogurt
One glass of kefir (a beverage made of fermented cow's milk)
One-third cup of almond cream

EVENING SNACKS

If you are hungry in the evenings, have a light snack. You should never eat
a lot of heavy food and then go to bed. The food won't digest properly, will
probably keep you awake, and will likely turn to fat. The best food to have
in the evening is a glass of raw vegetable juice. Here are some other choices:

Rice pudding
Glass of rice milk or almond milk
4 to 6 ounces goat's milk yogurt (organic)
4 to 6 ounces cow's milk yogurt (organic), if you are not allergic to it
One papaya or banana
One-half cup almond cream
8 ounces raw vegetable juice

MAKE WISE FOOD CHOICES

Many people are not aware that there is a connection between their health
and the choices they make about eating. When we understand that some
foods are life-giving and healing while others are actually harmful to our
health, we can make more conscious choices about what we put into our
mouths. The following list of foods are those used often and those most
important to one's health. They are arranged starting with alkaline foods,
including fruits and vegetables that we should eat often, and progress into

more dense acidic foods such as bean, grains, and nuts, which we should eat less of.

Fruits
Eat one to three fruits per day, preferably not with other foods. When you are craving sweets, choose dates or figs stuffed with nuts, frozen banana ice cream (see the recipe later in this chapter), or other dessert choices in this book; when eating fruit as a dessert, have it at least a half hour after the meal.

Vegetables
Eat six different kinds of vegetables daily, raw, baked or steamed.

Potatoes
Potatoes can be eaten one to two times per week. Potatoes are best eaten baked or steamed with their skins on since most of the nutrients, especially potassium, is located there. Never boil or fry potatoes; these cooking methods destroy the nutrients. Cut out any eyes on the potatoes since they are toxic.

Beans
Lentils are probably the easiest bean to digest, but other beans are also good for you. Soak them overnight and then cook them. Eat beans several times per week with vegetables and salad. Beans are difficult for some people to digest. If this is the case for you, try the smaller beans such as adzuki, black, or navy beans.

Nuts
Nut butters and almonds are the best nut choices. However, walnuts, pecans, and Brazil nuts are also high in nutrients and good for us. Eat nuts in small portions, as they are high in fats. Soak almonds overnight. This starts the sprouting action inside the nut and reduces the fat content by half. Soaked almonds are delicious light snacks and much easier to digest than almonds that have not been soaked. Nuts are high in calcium, magnesium, and manganese.

Seeds
Seed butters, sesame seeds, and sunflower seeds or butter are best. Pumpkin seeds are also very nutritious because they are high in zinc and build the

male and female reproductive systems. They kill parasites, which we should always watch out for. Grinding seeds in a coffee or spice grinder ensures better digestion. Soaked seeds are also very good for you and are easier to digest and absorb than seeds that have not been soaked. They contain half the fat content of unsoaked seeds. See recipes for seed sauce, salad dressings, and dips later in this chapter.

Breakfast Cereals

Cooked cereals are best or cereals prepared with the thermos method. Amaranth, buckwheat, cornmeal mush, millet, quinoa, and whole rolled oats are all good choices. You may eat packaged cereals at times but make sure they are wheat free and sugar free. Also check that they are free from additives and preservatives and are low in salt.

Whole Grains

Whole grains may be used in soups, breads, and pancakes. Consider amaranth, barley, basmati rice, brown rice, buckwheat, millet, quinoa, rye, wild rice, or yellow cornmeal.

Bread and Crackers

Have one to two servings of bread or crackers per day. You can make your own bread with any of the whole grains listed above. Eat wheat-free crackers such as rice crackers or rice cakes.

Wheat has been overused in our country to the point that most people have allergies to it. Wheat is high in gluten, which makes it very gluey and hard to digest. It can cause sinus congestion, lung congestion, and constipation.

Buy the following types of bread: eleven-grain sprouted, kamut, pumpernickel rye, rice, rye, seven-grain sprouted, or spelt. Be sure to toast all bread; toasted bread is less gluey and easier to digest. If you are sensitive to gluten, stick to rice, millet, buckwheat, and corn breads. Buckwheat is actually a flower and not a grain.

Milk and Milk Substitutes

Cow's milk is very difficult for some people to digest. Clean, certified, raw cow's milk is better for us because it is high in enzymes and friendly bacteria that make it more digestible. Many people have allergies to cow's milk that cause sinus congestion and/or gas and bloating. Some people fear that if they don't drink milk, they will not get enough calcium, but there are many other sources of calcium. A glass of raw carrot or green juice made with beet tops, parsley, and kale contains the same amount of calcium as a glass of cow's milk, and it is easier to digest and absorb. Almonds, sesame seeds, and green leafy vegetables are also wonderful sources of calcium. The following are great substitutes for cow's milk: almond milk, oat milk, raw organic goat's milk, rice milk (try vanilla), and rice milk ice cream. Have one to three servings of nut, oat, rice, or goat's milk daily.

Eggs

Choose fertilized eggs from free-range hens. Most eggs come from chickens that live in cages their entire lives and never see the sun. They are fed chemical foods. Their egg yolks will be very pale yellow and taste very bland compared to the rich yellow yolks of healthy range-fed chickens that live outside in the fresh air and sunshine, eating bugs and grass. I recommend eating only range-fed eggs, which are fertilized. Fertilization makes the eggs more nutritious and better tasting. Eggs fertilized by a rooster have lecithin, which naturally lowers cholesterol. Shelton Farms and Alta Dena are two companies that carry fertilized eggs from healthy chickens grown outdoors. The color of an egg's shell does not make a difference in how healthy the egg is for you. The color is determined by the type of chicken that lays the egg.

A recent egg scare made people afraid to eat eggs for fear they would increase their cholesterol, but this has now been proved to be untrue. Also, real eggs provide much more nutritional value than egg substitutes. An egg contains all the amino acids necessary for human life. Soft-boiled eggs are best for you because the lecithin is still intact; cooking eggs at high temperatures for a long period of time destroys the lecithin. Lecithin helps to lower elevated cholesterol. And if you eat eggs from healthy chickens and gently wash the shells with soap and warm water right before use, you won't have to worry about salmonella.

Meat

If you are not vegetarian, you should only eat organic meat such as veal, lamb, beef, or venison once or twice a week; chicken, turkey, or duck two to three times a week; and fish two to three times a week. These must be baked or broiled, never fried, and eaten in small amounts. Remember, you need protein every day, but you do not need animal protein every day. Avoid pork sausage and bacon which are very high in saturated fat.

Butter

A little butter is okay to eat. Butter is preferable to margarine that contains hydrogenated oils. Butter is also high in vitamins A and D, which are beneficial to the eyes, immune system, and nervous system. Butter should be organic and unsalted. Use small amounts for cooking and on foods.

Ghee

Ghee is clarified butter and is easier to digest than regular butter. Look for ghee in the refrigerated section of your health food store.

Olive Oil

This is one of the few oils, in addition to grape seed and coconut oil, to be used in cooking (it is safe at high temperatures). It also can be used on salads. Olive oil helps to balance the body's pH, neutralizes acids, helps to cleanse the liver, and may dissolve gallstones and kidney stones. Combine olive oil and lemon juice to make a great salad dressing.

A Note about Acid/Alkaline Balance in Our Daily Foods

Eighty percent of our daily food intake should be alkaline and 20 percent acidic. It's easy to reach these percentages if we remember to eat six vegetables and two fruits per day to provide the 80 percent alkaline foods that we need. By eating two different fruits per day and six different vegetables per day, we will get a variety of vitamins, minerals, and phytonutrients so important to our health. The rest of the foods below are more acid forming in the body, except for almonds which are more alkaline forming. Soaked nuts of any kind become alkaline and can be included as part of the 80 percent alkaline foods per day. It doesn't work out exactly to eat just one grain and one protein, for the 20 percent, but remember that we should only eat 20 percent acid-forming foods per day. So one might have two small servings of grains (one-fourth to one-third cup each), one small serving of beans (one-fourth to one-third cup), and one to two servings of fish or chicken in a day. One should only have one to two servings of red meat per week. If you are vegetarian, use fish, eggs, cheese, beans, nuts, and seeds for proteins. Soaked, blended nuts and seeds are excellent proteins and very easy to absorb.

Tool Kit for Preparing Healthy Recipes

Many people believe that eating healthfully means eating foods that taste bad. I have taught many classes in nutrition and showed people how to prepare nutritious foods in very delicious ways. The following recipes are both healthy and tasty. Enjoy!

DRINKS

Almond Cream

> 1 cup almonds, raw
> vanilla or stevia to taste
> dates, soaked (optional)
> 1 1/2 cups purified water

Soak one cup of raw almonds in purified water for twenty-four hours. Remove the almonds, and give the water to your plants or discard it. Place the almonds in boiling water for thirty seconds to loosen the peelings. Remove the peelings. Place the almonds in a blender. Cover them with one and a half cups of purified water, and blend until thick and creamy. Add vanilla, stevia, or soaked dates with soak water (adjust with water in the recipe) to taste. This nut cream can be combined with fruit because the nuts have been soaked. Serve over berries, mango, papaya, or peaches. Enjoy! Yields three cups.

Almond Milk

> 1 cup almonds, raw
> 3 cups purified water

Make almond milk the same way almond cream is made, only with more water to make it thinner. If you are making this drink for young children, strain it well through cheesecloth. It's very high in calcium, magnesium, and other minerals, which is great for building bones and teeth. Yields one quart.

Flaxseed Tea

> 4 teaspoons flaxseeds

Bring one quart of water to a rolling boil. Add four teaspoons of flaxseeds. Turn the burner off, and let the mixture sit overnight. Strain the tea before using it. Yields four cups of brewed tea.

Good Morning Health Shake

  1 cup rice or almond milk
  1 teaspoon black cherry concentrate
  1 to 2 egg yolks
  1 to 2 bananas, chopped

Blend all the ingredients together. Yields about ten ounces.

This shake is high in potassium, natural iron, and manganese, making it great for people with hair loss, brain and nervous system disorders, attention disorders, memory loss, and anemia. The black cherry juice in this drink is especially good for relieving the pain of arthritis and gout.

Holiday Almond Nog

  1 cup almonds, raw
  8 dates, soaked, and date water
  cinnamon (to taste)
  vanilla (to taste)
  nutmeg (to taste)

Instead of eggnog, try almond nog! Prepare as almond milk, with soaked dates and date water, then add cinnamon, vanilla, and nutmeg. Delicious! Yields about one quart.

Mineral Whey Drink

  1 teaspoon mineral whey (goat milk whey)
  1 teaspoon lecithin granules
  1 teaspoon vegetable seasoning

Place all the ingredients in a large cup, and add one cup of hot but not boiling water. Let the mixture steep for five minutes and then drink. Yields one cup.

Mineral or goat milk whey is high in minerals and natural sodium, which help hold calcium in the bones and dissolve spurs and stones. The whey is the liquid part of the milk that separates from the solids when making goat cheese. It is very similar in consistency to our own clear lymph fluid that lines our eyes, sinuses, lungs, stomach, and joints. Lecithin helps keep arteries clean and lowers cholesterol. Lecithin also feeds the brain and nervous system. Vegetable seasonings may contain a variety of nourishing dried vegetables, including alfalfa, carrots, celery, parsley, pimento, spinach, or watercress; Bernard Jensen's Vegetable Seasoning (see resources) has a wonderful consistency and flavor.

Avocado Pudding

 1 cup almond milk
 $^1/_2$ cucumber
 $^1/_2$ avocado
 2 tablespoons soaked, peeled almonds
 1 teaspoon vanilla or juice of $^1/_2$ fresh lemon or 1 tablespoon
    shredded unsweetened coconut flakes
 4 to 6 drops stevia

Blend all ingredients together. Yields about twelve ounces.

This shake is delicious and completely sugar free. I recommend it for diabetics, hypoglycemics, or people with candida. It's great for everyone!

GRAINS

Millet Breakfast Cereal

 $^1/_2$ cup organic millet, uncooked
 1 cup distilled water
 1 additional cup distilled water to soak millet

Soak the millet in one cup of distilled water overnight to soften the grains. Place the soaked millet in a saucepan with the water from soaking and one additional cup of distilled water. Bring the cereal to a boil, reduce the heat, and simmer for twenty to thirty minutes, stirring occasionally, until the cereal has thickened. If using for the ten-day cleanse in chapter 6, use a food processor fitted with the S blade, and puree the cooked millet until smooth. Serve the hot cereal with almond cream if desired. Makes two six-ounce portions of cooked cereal.

SOUPS

Soups provide a delicious soothing meal that's easy to digest and warming during cold months. Soups can be made ahead of time and frozen in strong rigid plastic containers or special jars made for freezing and canning. When ready to prepare, let soup thaw for about four hours, warm it up on the stove, and your meal is ready. Enjoy soups!

Vegetable Cleansing Solution

2 tablespoons raw apple cider vinegar
1 quart of water

To prepare vegetables for any recipe, combine them with the vinegar and water and soak for five minutes. This recipe can be multiplied as necessary for larger quantities of vegetables. This solution helps wash any harmful bacteria and chemical sprays from the vegetables without changing their flavor.

Dr. Bieler's Potassium Soup

$^1/_3$ cup chopped string beans
$^1/_2$ cup chopped celery
$^1/_3$ cup chopped zucchini
1 to 2 teaspoons chopped parsley
1 teaspoon vegetable seasoning (optional)
1 teaspoon liquid aminos (optional)
basil (optional)
garlic (optional)
onion (optional)
thyme (optional)
virgin olive oil (optional)
organic butter or ghee (optional)

In a steamer, steam the string beans for five minutes. Add the celery and steam for five more minutes. Then add the zucchini. Put the mixture in a blender with two cups of the water that the vegetables steamed over, and add the parsley. You may also add one teaspoon of broth powder or one teaspoon of liquid aminos and/or basil, garlic, onion, and thyme, to taste. Blend everything together, and serve the soup warm. Some natural virgin olive oil, organic butter, or ghee may be added after blending. Yields three cups.

Raw Vegetable Juice Soup

2 large carrots, cleaned and sliced
1 small beet, cleaned and sliced
3 stalks celery, cleaned and sliced
1 bunch parsley
1 small cucumber, sliced

1 tomato, quartered
1 tablespoon pumpkin seeds, soaked
1 tablespoon sunflower seeds, soaked

Juice all the vegetables, and pour them into a bowl. Sprinkle soaked pumpkin and sunflower seeds on top. Eat the soup slowly, and chew the seeds well; even though they've been soaked, they are still crunchy and should be chewed well for optimum digestion and absorption.

Other great toppings for raw vegetable juice soup are sesame and sunflower seed sauce (see the recipe under "Dressings and Sauces"). Put a dollop of each on top. So delicious and good for you too!

Raw vegetable juice soup is great for anyone, but it is particularly good for people with chronic illness or digestive disorders. The juice is loaded with nutrients, and the seed sauce is high in minerals and protein. Both are high in enzymes. The juice and seed sauces are easy to digest and absorb. Enjoy! Yields about one cup.

Lentil Soup

2 teaspoons olive oil
1 leek, chopped
2 cloves garlic, minced
7 cups water
3 tablespoons vegetable seasoning
2 large stalks celery, thinly sliced
1 cup sweet potato, cubed
1 cup carrots, diced
1 cup green lentils, rinsed
1 teaspoon dried thyme
1 teaspoon dried basil
1 large bay leaf

Warm the oil in a large saucepan or Dutch oven over medium heat. Add the leek, garlic, and three tablespoons of the water. Cook, stirring over medium heat for five minutes or until the leek and garlic are tender. (If necessary, add more water.)

Add the vegetable seasoning. Add the vegetables, lentils, thyme, basil, bay leaf, and remaining water. Bring everything to a boil, then reduce the heat. Cover and simmer for twenty minutes or until the lentils are tender. This is a delicious soup for lunch or dinner. Serve it with cornbread or rice crackers. Makes six servings.

Split Pea Soup (Vegetarian)

2 quarts water
2 cups green split peas
2 large carrots, scrubbed and chopped
6 stalks celery, chopped
1 large yellow onion, chopped
3 large potatoes, chopped
4 tablespoons vegetable seasoning
1 tablespoon olive oil
fresh parsley, chopped, for garnish

Place the water in a large pot, add the peas, and bring it to a boil. Reduce the heat, cover, and simmer for one-half hour. Add the carrots, celery, onion, potatoes, and vegetable seasoning. Simmer for an hour. Stir in the olive oil. Garnish with parsley. Yields about two and a half quarts.

Split Pea Soup

2 quarts water
4 small soup bones with a bit of lean beef on them
2 cups green split peas
2 large carrots, scrubbed and chopped
6 stalks celery, chopped
1 large onion, chopped (optional)
3 large potatoes, chopped
$^1/_2$ to 1 teaspoon unrefined sea salt

Place the water in a large pot and add the soup bones. Bring the contents to a boil. Reduce the heat and simmer for forty minutes. Add the peas and simmer for one-half hour. Add the vegetables and simmer for one hour. Add sea salt to taste and serve. Yields about two and a half quarts.

Potato Peeling Broth

2 cups scrubbed raw potato peelings, chopped (inner potato discarded)
2 cups celery and tops, chopped
2 cups carrots and tops, chopped

1 yellow onion, chopped

2 quarts water

Place the chopped vegetables and the water in a large stainless steel pot. Bring the contents to a boil. As soon as the water boils, reduce the heat, and simmer the contents for one hour. Strain the mixture, and drink one to two cups per day. Yields about three quarts.

This broth is high in potassium, which helps relieve muscle cramps and restore calcium balance in the bones. This broth is wonderful for anyone with arthritis, muscular pain, or stress.

Hearty Vegetable Soup

2 quarts tomato juice

$^1/_2$ cup baby butter beans

$^1/_2$ cup yellow corn

$^1/_2$ cup string beans, broken

$^1/_2$ cup okra, chopped

1 cup broccoli, chopped

$^1/_4$ cup yellow onion, chopped

$^1/_2$ cup ground lean beef or turkey (optional)

2 teaspoons dried basil

1 teaspoon dried thyme

$^1/_2$ cup kidney beans, cooked

$^1/_2$ cup barley, cooked

1 teaspoon sea salt

1 tablespoon olive oil

Put all the ingredients in a large pot except the cooked kidney beans, cooked barley, sea salt, and olive oil. Bring the mixture to a boil. Reduce the heat to simmer. Simmer the mixture for one hour, then add the cooked kidney beans and barley. Simmer for twenty minutes. Add the sea salt and olive oil. Stir and serve. Yields about three quarts.

Okra is mucilaginous and very soothing to the entire digestive tract. It's a wonderful food for people with colitis or ulcers. If you have ulcers or colitis, do not add meat to the soup.

Butternut Squash Soup

1 cup onion, finely chopped
1 tablespoon garlic, minced
1 tablespoon coconut, olive, or grape seed oil
4 cups butternut squash, cubed
4 cups vegetable broth
2 cups small white beans, cooked
5 tablespoons red bell pepper, chopped
unrefined sea salt, to taste (optional)
cayenne pepper, to taste (optional)

Sauté the onion and garlic in one tablespoon of oil. Add the squash and chicken or vegetable broth. Bring the mixture to a boil. Reduce the heat. Simmer the squash and onion mixture for one hour. Place the mixture in a blender; blend to a thick puree. Place the pureed mixture back in the pan. Add the small white beans and red pepper. Cook everything over low heat for another twenty to thirty minutes. When it is done, add a pinch of sea salt and a little cayenne pepper if desired. Yields about two and a half quarts.

VEGGIES

Baked Fries

2 baking potatoes, sliced very thin or cut in oblong shapes
olive oil or butter
seasoning mix

Slice two baking potatoes very thin or cut them into oblong shapes to look like french fries. Lay the pieces on a cookie sheet that has been greased with olive oil, ghee, or butter. Bake the "fries" at 450°F for one-half hour. Sprinkle them with seasoning mix. Bake them for fifteen more minutes or until crisp. Yields about two and a half cups.

Baked Fries Seasoning Mix

$^1/_3$ stick of butter or 2 tablespoons ghee
$^1/_8$ teaspoon sea salt
$^1/_3$ teaspoon thyme
1 teaspoon basil

Place the butter or ghee in a saucepan and melt it. Add the sea salt, thyme, and basil. Stir the mixture. Spread the seasoning mix over baked fries.

*Borscht**

4 large golden beets, quartered
1 tablespoon olive oil
1 cup leeks, diced
$^1/_4$ teaspoon caraway seed
$^1/_4$ cup
celery, chopped
$^1/_2$ cup carrot, chopped
$^1/_2$ cup tomato, chopped
2 cups green cabbage, chopped
4 cups vegetable stock
1 cup russet potato, mashed
$^1/_2$ teaspoon dried dill weed
2 teaspoons lemon juice
$^1/_8$ teaspoon cayenne pepper
2 tablespoons fresh parsley, chopped
sea salt, to taste

Heat the oven to 400°F. Place all the ingredients in an oiled, covered casserole dish. Bake for one hour. You may add unrefined sea salt to taste when the borscht is done. Makes six cups.

*Onion Gravy**

$^1/_2$ cup onion, chopped
2 teaspoons ghee
$^1/_8$ teaspoon dried thyme
1 teaspoon fresh garlic, minced
2 tablespoons liquid aminos
1 cup flaxseed tea, vegetable broth, or water
1 teaspoon arrowroot powder

Sauté the onion in the ghee until translucent, about five minutes. Add the thyme and garlic, and let cook for another minute to release the flavors. Add the liquid aminos and flaxseed tea (or stock or water), and bring to a simmer. Make a slurry with the arrowroot powder and one tablespoon of cold water. Add the slurry to the onions in the pan. Cook the mixture until the arrowroot clears, adding additional tea, stock, or water as necessary to achieve the desired consistency. Serve with mashed potatoes. Makes one cup. Gravy should be creamy.

Tabouleh Salad

2 cups millet or quinoa, cooked
2 ripe tomatoes, chopped
1 large cucumber, chopped
1 small leek, chopped
1 red bell pepper, chopped
3 tablespoons lemon juice
1 tablespoon olive oil
1 clove garlic, minced
$1/3$ teaspoon sea salt
$1/4$ cup fresh mint, chopped
$1/3$ cup fresh parsley, chopped
8 leaves of romaine or butter lettuce
sprig of mint

Place the millet in a large bowl. Add the tomatoes, cucumbers, leeks, and bell pepper. Toss them together. In a small bowl, whisk together the lemon juice, olive oil, garlic, and sea salt. Stir in the mint and parsley. Pour over the millet mixture. With a fork, gently stir all the ingredients together. Cover the salad, and let it stand at room temperature for half an hour to bring out the flavors. Serve on a bed of fresh romaine or butter lettuce with a sprig of mint on top. Yields about three cups.

Tabouleh is a Middle Eastern grain salad that can be made with bulghur (cracked wheat), millet, or quinoa. If you are allergic to gluten try tabouleh made with millet or quinoa. These are delicious grains, high in protein. Tabouleh is a great salad for lunch and wonderful to take on a picnic. Enjoy!

Hummus

2 cups chickpeas (garbanzo beans)
5 cups water, distilled
2 cups raw sesame butter
2 tablespoons liquid aminos
3 cloves garlic, pressed

juice of 2 large lemons
$^1/_2$ cup fresh parsley, finely chopped
Pinch of cayenne or paprika
sprig of parsley

Soak the chickpeas in five cups of distilled water for two hours. Place the chickpeas and water into a stainless steel pot, and bring them to a boil. Reduce the heat, and simmer for two hours. Strain the mixture, and keep one cup of the broth. Place a half cup of the broth, the sesame butter, liquid aminos, garlic, and lemon juice in a blender. Blend the mixture until creamy. Pour it into a bowl and set it aside. Pour the chickpeas and another half cup of the broth into the blender, and blend until smooth. Pour this mixture into the bowl with the sesame mixture. Stir. Add the parsley and a pinch of cayenne or paprika. Stir well, and serve with a sprig of parsley on top. Yields about five cups.

Hummus can be used as a delicious dip for vegetables, a topping for baked potatoes, or a spread for a sandwich. It is easy to digest and high in protein and minerals.

DRESSINGS AND SAUCES

Sesame Seed or Sunflower Seed Sauce, Dip, or Salad Dressing

$^1/_2$ cup sesame or sunflower seeds
1 cup purified water
basil, to taste (optional)
thyme, to taste (optional)
dill, to taste (optional)
garlic, to taste (optional)
onion, to taste (optional)

Soak the seeds for twenty-four hours in one cup purified water. Discard the water. Rinse the seeds and strain them. Place them in a blender with the second cup of water and blend them. This sauce is great over salads and steamed vegetables. You may add basil, thyme, dill, garlic, or onion and serve it as a dressing or dip. Yields one and a half cups.

This topping is an excellent source of protein, calcium, and magnesium.

SANDWICHES

Sandwiches are easy, convenient, and great for picnics. They can be made with all sorts of delicious, healthy ingredients. It is best to use whole-grain bread. If you have allergies to gluten, choose bread made from rice flour or use seven-grain sprouted bread. Sprouted wheat is less "gluey," and easier for the body to tolerate than bread made from wheat flour.

Veggie Sandwiches

    2 slices whole-grain or sprouted whole-grain bread
    mayonnaise made with cold-pressed oils
    butter lettuce, green leaf lettuce, red leaf lettuce, or romaine
    buckwheat sprouts
    avocado slices
    feta cheese, goat cheese, raw cheese, or seed cheese
    fresh turkey or chicken slices, optional

Be creative with a variety of fixings to suit your taste. Have fun!

FISH AND POULTRY

*Baked Halibut with Basil**

    2 halibut or salmon filets
    1 tablespoon lemon juice
    1 teaspoon dried ground basil
    $1/8$ teaspoon cayenne pepper
    $1/3$ teaspoon unrefined sea salt

Heat the oven to 350°F. Place the halibut filets in a small baking dish. Pour the lemon juice over the fish. Sprinkle it with basil and cayenne pepper. Bake for about twenty minutes, until the fish is opaque throughout the thickest part. Sprinkle it with sea salt. Makes two servings.

Pan-Fried Fish

    4 red snapper or flounder filets
    1 cup cornmeal, stone ground

$^1/_2$ teaspoon basil
$^1/_4$ teaspoon thyme
$^1/_3$ teaspoon dill
$^1/_3$ teaspoon unrefined sea salt
3 tablespoons olive, grape seed, or coconut oil

Place one cup of stone-ground cornmeal in a plate, and mix in the basil, thyme, dill, and a little sea salt. Roll the fish into the mixture. Put three tablespoons of olive, grape seed, or coconut oil in a stainless steel pan, and heat it on medium high. Add the fish when the oil starts to bubble. Watch the fish carefully and turn it regularly until golden brown. Serve with coleslaw, steamed broccoli, and yellow squash. Serves four.

Baked "Fried" Chicken

1 cup cornmeal, stone ground
$^1/_3$ teaspoon basil
$^1/_4$ teaspoon rosemary
$^1/_2$ teaspoon sage
$^1/_4$ teaspoon cayenne pepper
pinch of sea salt or vegetable seasoning
4 chicken breasts, thighs, or legs, skinless
1 tablespoon olive oil

Place one cup of stone-ground cornmeal on a plate, and mix in the basil, rosemary, sage, cayenne pepper, and sea salt or Jensen's vegetable seasoning. Roll the chicken into the mixture. Place the coated chicken in a stainless steel or glass dish that has been oiled well with olive oil and bake at 375°F for forty-five minutes or until done. The chicken should be crispy and golden brown.

If you use animal products, make sure they are organic (so they're not full of steroids or hormones). Salmon should be wild and not farm raised.

DESSERTS

Banana Ice Cream

4 ripe bananas, chopped
1 cup rice milk or almond milk
1 teaspoon vanilla

Freeze the chopped bananas in a plastic bag. Place the bananas in a blender, cover with rice or almond milk, and add the vanilla. Blend the mixture until it is thick and creamy. Makes two and a half cups.

Carob Walnut Syrup

4 to 5 tablespoons water
4 tablespoons maple syrup
$1/2$ cup carob powder
$1/3$ cup walnuts, chopped

Place the water and maple syrup in a pan. Warm them on low. Add the carob powder. Stir the mixture until it's free from lumps and creamy, adding water if needed. Simmer the mixture for three to five minutes. Add the chopped walnuts, and pour the syrup over banana ice cream. Makes one cup.

Almond Cream Pie

1 $1/2$ cups pecans and almonds, finely chopped
1 teaspoon cinnamon
2 cups almond cream
1 cup kiwis, mangoes, papayas, peaches, raspberries, or strawberries, sliced (noncitrus fruit in season)
$1/3$ cup dried coconut (optional)

Combine the chopped nuts and cinnamon. Spread them in a glass dish. Pour in half of the almond cream. Cover the mixture with sliced fruit. Top with another layer of almond cream. Decorate the pie with fruit on top. You may sprinkle it with dried coconut too. Enjoy! Serves six to eight.

Sesame Cookies

1 cup butter, soft, or $1/3$ cup olive oil
1 cup oat flour
1 cup rye or spelt flour
1 cup sesame seeds
2 cups dates, chopped
2 cups unsweetened coconut, shredded
(may use 1 cup oatmeal instead)
1 cup pecans, chopped

2 cups almonds, chopped
1 egg, beaten, or 2 tablespoons flaxseed tea
$^3/_4$ cup vanilla rice milk
1 tablespoon vanilla
4 tablespoons maple syrup

Mix together the butter, flour, and sesame seeds. Add the remaining ingredients, and mix to form a stiff dough. Shape the dough into flat circles, and place them onto a greased cookie sheet. Bake at 350°F for twenty to thirty minutes. Makes fifty cookies.

* Denotes recipes by Kelly Worrall.

OTHER SUGGESTIONS FOR HEALTHY DESSERTS

Carob brownies
Pumpkin pie made with maple syrup
Apple pie made with spelt flour and sweetened with fruit juice
Pecan pie sweetened with maple syrup
Ice cream made with rice milk
Rice pudding
Cookies made with rice flour and sweetened with fruit juice
Cookies made with oats and rice flour and sweetened with maple syrup
Tapioca pudding made with rice milk
Dates stuffed with almonds or walnuts
Baked apples stuffed with cinnamon, maple syrup or stevia, almonds,
    walnuts, and pecans

RECIPE BOOKS

Here are several recipe books that offer great ideas for creating healthy meals.

A Cookbook for All Seasons, Elson Haas, MD
The Best Vegetarian Recipes, Martha Rose Shulman
Blending Magic, Dr. Bernard Jensen
The Cleanse Cookbook, Christiane Dreher, CCN, CCH
Back to the House of Health, Shelly Redford Young, LMT, and
    Robert O. Young, PhD
Fresh Vegetable and Fruit Juices, Norman Walker
Gaia's Kitchen, Julia Ponsonby

Gourmet Uncook Book, Elizabeth and Dr. Elton Baker
Intuitive Eating, Humbert "Smokey" Santillo, ND
The Quintessential Recipes for Vibrant Health, F. Naragali
Cooking for Health, Cheryl A. Matschek, PhD
Recipes for Better Health, Nenita Sarmiento and Leonard Mehlmauer
Ten Talents, Frank J. Hurd, DC, MD, and Rosalie Hurd, BS
Vibrant Health from Your Kitchen, Dr. Bernard Jensen
The Good Herb, Judith Benn Hurley
Organic Annie's Green Gourmet Cookbook, Ann Miller-Cohen
Nourishing Traditions, Sally Fallon
Living in the Raw, Rose Lee Calabro
The Raw Gourmet, Nomi Shannon

Summary of Practical Tools to Help You Eat Healthy Foods

You now have practical tools for making healthy food choices, creating healthy meal plans, choosing healthy snacks, and preparing healthy recipes. The following is a summary of these healthy food tools. A good way to use this list is to type it on a separate piece of paper and hang it somewhere in your kitchen. Slowly work toward following each item on the list. When you have accomplished one of the items and are practicing it on a regular basis, check it off or put a gold star beside it. With each check or gold star you will be closer to practicing good food habits that will keep you nourished, healthy, happy, and wise. Take your time and move at your own pace, but be determined. Building good eating habits is a very important foundation for good health.

- Eat foods that are pure, whole, fresh, and natural.
- Avoid denatured, preserved, and processed foods. Replace them with natural whole foods.
- Cook foods with a minimum of water. Steam your foods or use a Crock-Pot or waterless cookware.
- Never deep-fry foods.
- Bake or broil foods rather than frying them.
- Practice combining foods.

· Choose from a variety of foods each day. Variety is the spice of life and our bodies need a variety of foods to get all the vitamins and minerals they need.
· Add fiber to your nutritional program each day.
· Eat some raw vegetables with your meals.
· Get 80 percent of your food intake from alkaline-forming foods and 20 percent from acid-forming foods.
· Add essential fatty acids to your nutritional program. Avoid hydro-genated oils.
· Avoid sugar, corn syrup, and artificial sweeteners and replace with stevia, agave, pure maple syrup, or honey.
· Avoid salt and replace with vegetable seasoning or unrefined sea salt.
· Eat only when you are truly hungry, and stop eating when you are full. Learn to recognize when you are full. This may take practice at first if you are used to overeating. The more you eat nutritious foods, the less you will feel the need to overeat.
· Eat in peace.
· Chew your food well.
· Never consume beverages that are too hot or too cold.
· Eat your evening meal before 7:00 P.M. so you will have a restful sleep.

chapter 2 ❧

Healthy Drinks

Let us drink for good health!
–Dr. Bernard Jensen

THERE ARE MANY DRINKS AVAILABLE on the market today. Many of them are loaded with refined white sugar, caffeine, aspartame, artificial color, preservatives, and chemicals. All of these additives are detrimental to the body. In order to build pure blood, vital organs, healthy muscles, and strong bones, we should enjoy delicious, refreshing drinks that are natural.

Tool Kit for Choosing Healthy Popular Beverages

Sodas, slushies, milkshakes, frappuccinos, cappuccinos, coffee, tea, beer, wine, lemonade, water—beverages are available everywhere, so which ones should we choose? In order to be healthy, we should make wise choices about the liquids we consume. Remember, we are organic creatures made from the natural elements of the earth. When we consume unnatural, synthetic substances in either our foods or our beverages, our bodies will rebel—sometimes immediately with an allergic reaction or sometimes slowly over time. Unnatural substances can weaken our immune systems, cause our adrenal glands, heart, and pancreas to overwork, and congest our arteries. Some good questions to ask when choosing what to drink are the following:

- Are the ingredients in this drink completely natural and without artificial colorings and preservatives? If so, this is a good drink to choose.
- Is this drink sweetened with natural sweeteners including stevia, xylitol, or agave? If so, this is a good drink to choose.
- Is this drink sweetened with natural sweeteners including raw organic honey, real maple syrup, or whole cane sugar? This drink is good for most

people, but diabetics, hypoglycemics, people trying to lose weight, and people with candida (yeast infections) should avoid these drinks.
· Is this drink sweetened with refined white sugar, aspartame, or Splenda? If so, this drink should be avoided by all for reasons previously mentioned.
· Does this drink contain refined white sugar, caffeine, or alcohol? If so, people with diabetes, hypoglycemia, and chronic fatigue should avoid these drinks. Even healthy people should proceed with caution.

In this section, we will review various different drinks and popular beverages in order to help you make wise choices based on your current health conditions.

WATER

The body is composed of approximately 60 to 70 percent water. Our digestive juices are 98 percent water. The human body excretes about one gallon of water every twenty-four hours. All of the body's cells need water to function. Clearly, water is an essential ingredient to good health.

F. Batmanghelidgj, MD, has written a fascinating book based on years of research called, *Your Body's Many Cries for Water*. In it he writes about water: "It is the solvent—the water content—that regulates all functions of the body . . . every function of the body is monitored and pegged to the efficient flow of water." He goes on to explain that a dry mouth is not the only indicator of thirst. He says: "When the neurotransmitter histamine generation and its subordinate water regulators become excessively active, to the point of causing allergies, asthma, and chronic pains in different parts of the body, these pains should be translated as a thirst signal—one variety of the crisis signals of water shortage in the body." So we can see, based on this important research study, the vital importance of drinking water!

The healthiest water can be found in pristine regions of the world, where it is clean, pure, and vibrant. Its molecules, if viewed under a microscope, look a lot like snowflake crystals. All the water on our planet used to be this way until it became tainted and polluted with pesticides and chemicals. Tap water contains chlorine and often fluorine, both of which are toxic and place a burden on the liver. Chlorine not only kills harmful bacteria, it also kills good bacteria in the digestive tract, an important part of our immune system. Some water contains heavy inorganic minerals, the same ones that you see clogging up your iron, creating a ring in your teapot, and even staining your bathtub! It is impossible for the body to break down and digest inorganic minerals, and they can accumulate in the body's vessels and joints.

Steam-distilled water has had the heavy minerals, bacteria, and harmful chemicals removed. Steam-distilled water and water purified by reverse osmosis are two of the best water choices we can make. Distilled water is "empty" water because it does not contain minerals. Distilled water helps to cleanse the vessels and joints of mineral deposits. Herbal tea should be made with distilled water.

A small amount of minute minerals in our water is actually good for us. Thus, it's a good idea to add liquid ionic trace minerals to your distilled water. Ionic minerals are the smallest minerals and therefore more bioavailable and absorbable by the cells than the large inorganic minerals found in most water. Ionic trace minerals provide electrolytes that give us energy and neutralize the body's pH. Trace minerals nourish and strengthen the cells, giving them the life force necessary to throw off toxins and perform their jobs. Drink eight glasses of purified water daily; use about three drops of ionic trace minerals in each eight-ounce glass of water. It will help cleanse and build every organ of your body!

SOFT DRINKS

Soft drinks are addictive and very harmful to the body. One canned soft drink contains thirteen teaspoons of sugar. Some diet drinks are even more toxic because they contain aspartame—a serious poison! Beware of those sweetened with Splenda as well. Most soft drinks are high in caffeine and can cause heart palpitations. Many of our youth in high school and on college campuses are seriously addicted to soft drinks, and they are beginning to rot their teeth and destroy their pancreases at a young age!

If you are drinking soft drinks, you can replace them with delightful fruit juice drinks. Mix pure fruit juice with sparkling mineral water, half and half. Or mix sparkling mineral water with a dash of lemon or lime juice. Add some liquid stevia, agave, or xylitol as a sweetener. Drinks made with water and lemon or lime sweetened with stevia, agave, or xylitol actually nourish your body, balance the pancreas, add few or no calories, and place no burden on the liver. They don't cause blood sugar highs or lows. When people consume drinks sweetened with refined white sugar or high fructose corn syrup, the pancreas must produce lots of insulin to manage the influx of concentrated sugar. They may feel energized for an hour, then weak when the sugar passes out of their systems. Stevia nourishes the body without making the pancreas have to work so hard. Blue agave nectar and xylitol also cause very little burden to the pancreas. If you are diabetic or hypoglycemic, use stevia, blue agave nectar, or xylitol for sweetening your drinks; or make drinks by mixing three-quarters sparkling mineral water and one-quarter fruit juice. Black cherry and apple juice are especially good with mineral water. Natural soft drinks, such as ginger ale are also available. These natural soft drinks contain good ingredients such as water, fruit juice, stevia, agave, xylitol, ginger, vanilla, or other natural flavorings. If you are diabetic or hypoglycemic consume drinks sweetened with fruit juice sparingly. Read labels when purchasing natural soft drinks. Some will say they are natural although they contain Splenda, artificial colorings, and preservatives.

COFFEE

Most coffee on the market is highly processed and loaded with chemicals because crops are heavily sprayed. Organic coffees are better and even contain some antioxidants but still contain caffeine. Some decaffeinated coffees are also toxic because of the decaffeinating process, which uses chemicals such as methylene chloride to extract the caffeine. Methylene chloride is used by many industries for things such as metal cleaning and paint stripping. Methylene chloride is considered a potential carcinogen by Occupational and Safety Health Administration (OSHA). Water-decaffeinated coffees are better for you. Organic water-decaffeinated coffee is the best option, but remember that a bit of caffeine remains in it. A healthy person's liver can process caffeine better than an unhealthy person's. A new study has revealed that decaffeinated coffee is higher in fats and oils than regular coffee and more than two or three cups per day is not good for a person with high cholesterol. If you are a coffee drinker, and especially if you are ill, replace coffee with delicious substitutes such as Pero, Inka, Postum, and Caffix. These "coffees," made from chicory, are instant, so you only have to add water. If you like to drip or perk your coffee, try Teeccino. Delightful with a rich, full-bodied flavor, Teeccino is made from carob, barley, chicory, figs, almonds, and dates. It is high in potassium and gives you a boost of energy. It also contains inulin, a soluble fiber that enhances digestion and promotes regularity. Add a little rice milk and stevia if you are accustomed to cream and sugar. Delicious! All of these coffee drinks may be purchased in health food stores.

The caffeine in coffee "kicks" the adrenals to produce an overabundance of adrenaline, which causes the heart to race and the pancreas to produce too much insulin. The insulin then drops the blood sugar and causes you to feel hungry or crave sweets an hour or two after drinking the coffee. Because of this, we often eat more and gain weight.

Some people think coffee keeps their bowels moving, because the caffeine kicks them into action. In reality caffeine increases acid production and may cause constipation.

If you are addicted to caffeine, wean yourself from it slowly. Start drinking half regular and half decaf coffee the first week, then change to one-third regular and two-thirds decaf coffee the second week. By the end of a month, you can be completely free from a caffeine addiction and able to switch to herbal teas or coffee substitutes.

BLACK TEAS

Like coffee, black teas are high in caffeine and can be addictive. Replace black tea with any of the hundreds of herbal teas on the market. Try apple cinnamon, black cherry, peppermint, or whatever you prefer. Many herbal teas are already prepared for you in tea bags. Study the wide variety of herbal teas listed for you in this book. By learning what they do for you, you will be able to make wise choices about what your body needs at the moment. Green tea can be a great substitute for black tea, and it is a wonderful antioxidant.

BEER AND WINE

In addition to containing alcohol, which can be harsh on the liver, beer is high in sugar and calories, which is why drinking lots of it over a long period of time can create a beer gut. Beer also contains yeast, which can promote the growth of *Candida albicans* and cause yeast infections. There are organic beers and alcohol-free beers, but they also contain sugar and yeast.

Red wine has been reported to be beneficial in cleaning the arteries and lowering cholesterol. Look for organic wines made from grapes that were not sprayed with pesticides. There are alcohol-free wines as well. Drinkers who are hypoglycemic often become alcoholics because their overproduction of insulin causes them to crave the sugar and alcohol in alcoholic beverages.

Hard liquor used daily can be extremely damaging to the liver, brain, and nervous system. It is best for those who are ill to avoid all alcoholic beverages.

Tool Kit for Choosing Healthy Juices

Raw vegetable and fruit juice is one of the finest foods we can take into our bodies. Because of its nourishing contents, raw juice can help heal all sorts of ailments, mend bones, reverse osteoporosis, cleanse and repair the cells, improve immune function, fight viruses and bacteria, oxygenate the cells, fight free radicals, energize, and invigorate. Raw juice can save the life of a person who cannot digest food, because it is so easily absorbed.

Raw juices build healthy red blood cells. For this reason you should take out your juicer, dust it off, and start juicing for your health! If you don't have a juicer, use your blender. A blender will not extract the fiber from the vegetables, so your drink will have more fiber and be more filling.

ENZYMES

Enzymes are molecules that catalyze or initiate chemical reactions. Most enzymes are proteins that have special catalytic activity, but there are some RNA molecules that also have this property. Enzymes are responsible for the life force in our bodies with high levels of specificity. For example, the enzyme lactase catalyzes the breakdown or digestion of lactose. Raw juice is high in enzymes. These vital nutritional elements constitute the life principle in every atom and molecule of all living organisms. Enzymes are involved in all the body's activities and functions and are vital to healthy cellular activity. Thus, enzymes help our immune system function well by breaking down toxins that could cause illness. They help keep the arteries clean and are essential to our organs and metabolic pro-cesses. We would not be able to see, move our limbs, smell, taste, breathe, or think without enzymes!

Without enzymes, we become lethargic and exhausted. Edward Howell conducted extensive research on the effect that food enzymes have on our health. In *Enzyme Nutrition*, he says, "Enzymes offer an important means of calculating the vital energy of an organism. That which we call energy, vital force, nerve energy and strength, may be synonymous with enzyme activity."

Enzymes are destroyed at temperatures of 130°F or higher. People who live only on cooked foods deplete all their stores of enzymes and age more rapidly or become ill more often than people who eat plenty of raw foods. Undigested food ferments in the intestinal tract and becomes food for parasites and candida. Eat raw vegetables with meals to provide enzymes for good digestion.

Raw juices are delicious and nutritional as well as medicinal. If you are healthy, drink twelve to sixteen ounces of vegetable juices daily to stay strong and well and prevent illness. Max Gerson, MD, helped hundreds of patients recover from otherwise "incurable" diseases. In *A Cancer Therapy*, he writes:

1. Juices consist of living matter with active ferments, fast-neutralizing oxidizing enzymes, which are most necessary for the sick body.
2. The body needs an equilibrium of active oxidizing enzymes supplied throughout the day. These cannot maintain active states except in freshly pressed juices, given at hourly intervals.

If you are ill, try to drink several eight-ounce glasses of raw vegetable juice each day.

TYPES OF JUICERS

The best juices are those that have been freshly extracted by a juicer. A juicer is one of the most important health-building appliances you can have in your kitchen. There are several types of juicers on the market. One is the centrifugal juicer, which works by grinding the fruits or vegetables and throwing the pulp against a round spinning screen. Another type of juicer has a round blade that grinds the fruit or vegetable, separates the juice through a screen, and expels the pulp into a bucket fitted in back. Then there is the heavy-screen juicer that presses the pulp through a stainless steel screen and tosses it out the front while the juice falls through the screen into a bowl below. The wheatgrass juicer grinds very slowly and extracts juice from delicate wheatgrass or spinach leaves.

The latest juicer has twin gears and can be used to extract juice from both fruits and vegetables and from wheatgrass. This machine's gears run slowly, which eliminates oxidation caused by faster machines.

PREPARING FRUITS AND VEGETABLES FOR JUICING

Use fruits and vegetables that are organic and free from pesticides. Wash your produce thoroughly, since it can contain certain parasites or their eggs. Prepare a solution with one tablespoon of raw apple cider vinegar to each quart of water. Soak your fruits and vegetables in this solution for five minutes. Then scrub them well with a natural-bristle vegetable brush. Make sure the vinegar you use is raw. Most vinegar is made from apple peelings that have been sprayed with pesticides and cooked at high temperatures, killing all living enzymes. Raw apple cider vinegar is high in enzymes and can kill parasites and streptococci germs.

RAW FRUIT JUICES

Fresh-squeezed fruit juices from organic fruits are best. A glass of freshly juiced fruit juice of any kind is delicious and much better for you than soft drinks. However, fruit juice is still high in sugar content and should be used sparingly. Sugar in fruit juice feeds candida and parasites. You can dilute fruit juice with water and reduce the sugar content.

Black Cherry Juice

Black cherry juice is a very healthy juice and is high in organic iron. Organic black cherry concentrates are available. If you are tired or anemic, this is a great juice for you. It helps dissolve uric acid crystals in the body and may relieve the pain of gout and arthritis. Freshly juiced black cherry juice is even better for you when the cherries are in season. Black cherry juice diluted with distilled water is a good juice to give your baby when the baby is about four months old. By this time, the supply of iron in mother's milk becomes depleted, and the juice helps to supply iron.

Citrus Fruit Juices

Citrus fruits should be ripened on the vine before they are picked or they will be very acidic in the body. Fresh-squeezed lemon, lime, and grapefruit juices cleanse the liver. Lemon, lime, grapefruit, and orange juice are high in vitamin C.

Cranberry Juice

Cranberry juice can help heal a kidney or bladder infection. Cranberry juice has also been used in the treatment of asthma and kidney stones. It is very cleansing to the lymph system. Some of the key nutrients in cranberry juice are vitamin C, B vitamins, potassium, and beta-carotene. It also contains quercitin and ellagic acid, which are powerful antioxidants. The nutrients in cranberry juice keep bacteria from adhering to the cells of the bladder and thus flush it out of the body.

Grape Juice

Use only organic grapes with the seeds in them. Never use seedless grapes. Juice the grapes, seeds and all. Grape seeds are a source of oligomeric proanthocyanidins, or OPCs, which combat free radicals and improve immune function. They help to strengthen the capillaries in the eye and improve vision, including night blindness. OPCs also help repair connective tissue and thus heal varicose veins and hemorrhoids. Grape juice from the whole grape and seed can cleanse the veins and arteries, eliminate plaque, and promote cardiovascular health.

Dark purple grapes are high in iron. They help relieve gout and cleanse the liver. Grapes also fight some types of viruses, and bacteria. Johanna Brandt wrote a book titled *The Grape Cure*, in which she used grapes and their seeds to help heal cancer.

If you are hypoglycemic or diabetic, drink grape juice in small quantities or diluted.

Lemon and Lime Juice

The juice from fresh lemons and limes helps dissolve kidney stones and gallstones. Lemon pulp is high in bioflavanoids, which help strengthen the weakened tissue in those areas. Stanley Burroughs wrote about a "Master Cleanser" drink that was made of lemon juice, organic maple syrup, and cayenne pepper. Here is a great way to prepare this drink:

Peel two lemons or three limes, cut them into quarters, and remove seeds. Place the chunks in a blender with twenty ounces of water, and add a half cup of pure organic maple syrup and one-eighth to one-fourth teaspoon of cayenne pepper or ginger powder. Blend for two to three minutes. Makes two servings.

Cayenne and ginger help to promote circulation and strengthen the heart. Cayenne also helps stop internal or external bleeding.

Orange Juice

It's a good idea for nursing mothers to supplement breast milk with fresh-squeezed, strained orange juice. Breast milk is not high in vitamin C. Orange juice can be given to the baby by the third or fourth month. Oranges should be fresh, organic, and ripened on the vine. Dilute the juice to half-potency with distilled water. Fresh squeezed OJ is good for people of all ages since it's high in vitamin C and calcium and also contains bioflavanoids including rutin and hesperidin, which helps strengthen connective tissue in the body.

Papaya Juice

Papaya juice is available in health food stores in concentrated form and helps facilitate digestion because it is high in enzymes. Papain is an enzyme that aids in protein digestion. Papain has proven valuable in the reduction of inflammation. Some important nutrients in papayas are vitamins C and A, pantothenic acid, and beta-carotene. These nutrients in combination with its soothing alkaline properties make papaya juice healing for ulcers and colitis. Papayas can be juiced or blended at home as well.

Pineapple Juice

Fresh-squeezed pineapple juice is high in bromelain, an enzyme that helps digestion and reduces inflammation. Studies have shown that bromelain prevents the aggregation of blood platelets and may be beneficial in the prevention of heart attacks and stroke. It also contains vitamin C, calcium, and potassium.

Pomegranate Juice

Pomegranate juice is packed with wonderful nutrients that help clear up kidney infection, tighten the gums around the teeth, strengthen varicose veins and hemorrhoids, stop diarrhea, and improve bad breath. It contains vitamin C, riboflavin, and niacin. Its mineral content includes iron, potassium, calcium, and magnesium. The phytonutrients in pomegranate juice provide antioxidants and astringent properties; these include ellagic acid, beta-carotene, tannin, and pectin.

Watermelon Rind Juice

When you juice watermelon, add the rind! Watermelon juice is delicious and great for the kidneys and bladder. It acts as a natural diuretic. The juice of the rind is high in sodium, which nourishes the lymph fluids and stomach lining. You will also receive chlorophyll from the rind, which builds the blood.

RAW VEGETABLE JUICES

Raw vegetable juices are powerful antioxidants and slow the aging process. They provide highly absorbable vitamins and minerals of the finest quality. They both build and cleanse the body. Vegetable juices provide minerals including sodium and calcium in a balanced ratio that can assist the body in proper absorption so that calcium can be restored to the bones in cases of osteoporosis and arthritis. Bottled or canned juices have been heated or cooked, and all the living enzymes have been destroyed. Raw juices contain minerals that the body can absorb. On the other hand, the minerals in most water, such as lime, iron, and chalk, are hardened and not easily absorbed or utilized and can actually cause stones to form.

Blended salads and blended raw soups are very good for you, but not the same as juice because they still contain fiber. Fiber has its place and helps promote good peristalsis in the bowel and acts as little brooms to sweep the intestine clean. Juices contain more concentrated vitamins and minerals than blended salads and soups because the fiber is missing. Nutrients from the juice are more easily absorbed than when the fiber is included. I'm not suggesting you omit blended soups or blended salads. To use both in the diet is very beneficial. The only time juice alone is appropriate is during some types of cleanses or when a person is very ill and having trouble digesting fiber. Hypoglycemics and diabetics should stick with green vegetable juices in order to avoid the sugar content that is in carrot, beet, and fruit juices. To make raw vegetable juice in your blender, put the vegetables in the blender with water. Blend well, strain off the juice, and drink it. You will absorb more nutrients from the juice.

Alfalfa Juice

Alfalfa juice is rich in nutrients including protein, vitamins E and K, beta-carotene, chlorophyll, calcium, magnesium, and potassium because the alfalfa plant's roots reach as far as 120 feet into the earth, absorbing vitamins and minerals from many different levels of soil. Alfalfa juice builds bones and blood, helps reverse arthritis, and promotes good bowel function.

Asparagus Juice

A wonderful diuretic, asparagus juice cleanses oxalic crystals from the kidneys and muscles and is a great blood builder. It's high in potassium, folic acid, thiamine, and vitamins C and A. It works best when combined with carrot and cucumber juice.

Beet Juice

Beet juice is high in iron and helps build red corpuscles. It contains vitamin C, B vitamins, calcium, magnesium, and phosphorus. All of these nutrients along with beta-carotene and lutein work together synergistically to cleanse the liver and gallbladder, prevent jaundice, cleanse and soften hardened arteries, and strengthen varicose veins. It is high in organic sodium, which restores calcium to the bone, helps dissolve crystals in the joints, and may prevent or dissolve kidney and gallstones. It is also high in potassium, which strengthens the muscles, including the heart.

Do not drink more than one to three ounces of beet juice if you are not used to it. It is so cleansing to the liver and gallbladder, it can cause nausea. Combine beet juice with carrot and celery juice or carrot and cucumber juice to dilute its cleansing effects.

Beet Greens Juice

High in chlorophyll, potassium, calcium, magnesium, iodine, and iron, beet greens juice cleanses and builds the blood. It also strengthens the heart and thyroid gland, builds bones, and relaxes muscles.

Broccoli Juice

Broccoli has tremendous cancer preventive properties. High in vitamin C, calcium, and phosphorus, it strengthens the immune system and builds bones. The American Cancer Society recommends eating broccoli several times a week to help prevent cancer. The best way to get the most benefit from broccoli is to juice it! A pound of broccoli makes three ounces of juice. NOTE: While broccoli juice can be very beneficial to those with hyperthyroidism, people with hypothyroidism should use in moderation. (See "Thyroid Disorders" in chapter 4.)

Cabbage Juice

More of a cabbage's beneficial nutrients are in its outer leaves, which most people discard. Why not juice them? A very important nutrient in cabbage juice is vitamin U or ascorbigen, which is one of the most effective cures for ulcers. The chlorophyll in cabbage juice provides iron and stimulates the flow of bile and cleanses the intestinal tract. Cabbage juice is high in vitamin C, which also boosts the immune system and helps protect the body from cancer. Cabbage is high in sulfur so it helps improve circulation and relieves arthritic pain as well as allergies. Other wonderful nutrients in cabbage are vitamin K, which helps the blood clot properly, and calcium, which strengthens the bones.

Carrot Juice

High in beta-carotene, carrot juice has tremendous cancer-preventing properties. Beta-carotene is a powerful antioxidant and protects the body against free radicals. Carrots and carrot juice boost the immune function by enhancing the performance of white blood cells. Carrots are also high in calcium and strengthen the bones. People with osteoporosis or arthritis should drink lots of carrot juice! Carrot juice also cleanses the body and helps fight infection. The fiber in carrots can help lower serum cholesterol. And everyone knows carrots help improve sight. Our bodies convert beta-carotene to vitamin A, which helps keep the retina healthy. NOTE: Diabetics, hypoglycemics, and those with yeast or fungal infections should use sparingly becaue of the sugar content in carrot juice.

Celery Juice

Celery juice is high in chlorophyll, which cleanses the blood. It is also high in organic sodium, which nourishes the lymph fluid and helps hold calcium in solution. Celery juice thereby helps prevent, as well as to dissolve, the crystals that occur with arthritis, gout, kidney stones, and gallstones. The stomach is lined with natural sodium, and fluid in the eyes is high in sodium. Celery juice can be helpful in cases of dry eyes or stomach disorders, acting to neutralize acids in the stomach as well as throughout the body. It contains coumarin which enhances blood flow and has antifungal and anti-tumor properties. It also contains pthalides, a phytochemical which can assist with lowering high blood pressure. Celery juice can calm the nerves, improve bowel function, help to lower cholesterol, and release excess fluids that cause swelling. It is high in potassium and can relieve muscle cramps. It is delicious mixed with carrot juice! NOTE: People taking blood thinners should use sparingly.

Cucumber Juice

Cucumber juice is a delicious juice that is high in water content. It helps hydrate cells when you have a fever or are just "dry" and thirsty. A cucumber's precious naturally distilled water helps cool the body and calm the nerves. It acts as a natural diuretic and flushes the kidneys, and it assists in lowering high blood pressure. Please use only organic cucumbers, and juice the entire vegetable, including the skin. The peel is high in chlorophyll, which cleanses the blood, as well as silicon, a mineral that nourishes the nerves and connective tissue, helping prevent wrinkles, varicose veins, and hemorrhoids.

Garlic Juice

Garlic juice may sound terrible, but it can get rid of a cold or flu in a short period of time. Juice one clove of garlic with one apple. Drink two to three of these cocktails per day when ill, and you will heal rapidly. Garlic is high in a very potent antioxidant called allicin which helps fight many different types of bacteria and viruses. Garlic can also be juiced with carrots and celery or any other vegetables you prefer. If you are ill with salmonella, *Candida albicans*, or any bacterial infection, garlic is a must. According to research done by Steve Meyerowitz for his book, *Power Juices, Super Drinks*, "Garlic can even help in the war against AIDS." He found that ". . . garlic is also a powerful agent in the war against cancer." In addition to garlic's antibacterial properties, it is also high in sulfur, which can help with hardening of the arteries (atherosclerosis), high blood pressure, and cholesterol. NOTE: If you are taking any medications to dissolve blood clots or thin the blood, be careful with garlic, because it also acts as an anticoagulant in the blood.

Ginger Juice

When combined with other juices, ginger juice is both delicious and good for us. I like to drink a combination of carrot, beet, celery, and ginger juice; or carrot, cucumber, apple, and ginger juice. Ginger warms the body and promotes circulation. It helps relieve nausea. Ginger juice can be added to hot water and honey for tea when you feel queasy or nauseous. Ginger helps people who are undergoing chemotherapy avoid nausea and pregnant women alleviate morning sickness. It can also help with motion sickness and vertigo. Ginger juice relieves inflammation associated with rheumatic pains, improves circulation, and loosens phlegm from the sinuses and lungs. The medicinal properties of ginger are in its volatile oils and pungent phenol compounds such as gingerols, shogaols, and zingibain. Important vitamins in ginger are vitamin C, vitamins B-1, B-2, niacin, and B-6. Its minerals include zinc, calcium, phosphorus, and postassium. Key phytonutrients are curcumin which is anti-inflammatory and quercitin, a powerful antioxidant. NOTE: Ginger also helps thin the blood so use with caution if taking anticoagulant drugs.

Green Leafy Vegetable Juice
Juice made from beet tops, turnip greens, celery tops, kale, broccoli, collards, chard, Chinese cabbage, or spinach will make you as strong as the cartoon character Popeye! These vegetables are loaded with minerals and chlorophyll that help improve red blood cell counts. All are high in iron, and spinach is twice as high in iron as the rest, making them wonderful remedies for anemia. These juices are also very high in absorbable calcium and can help reverse osteoporosis! One cup of green juice from these vegetables contains more calcium than a glass of milk and is much easier for the body to absorb and utilize. Green leafy vegetable juices have phytochemicals, which can help prevent cancer and strengthen the eyes. If you don't like to drink these juices straight, combine them with carrot juice.

Parsley Juice
Parsley juice is high in chlorophyll and helps oxygenate the blood and build red blood cells. Parsley juice is a natural digestive aid. It is also a natural diuretic and flushes the kidneys. It assists with healing kidney and bladder infections and with preventing kidney stones. It is also high in calcium, so it can help with tissue and bone repair. It is high in potassium and can prevent cramping. Carrot and parsley juice combined is delicious and great for you! Both contain beta-carotene, which is super for the eyes and immune system.

Radish Juice
Radish juice is a bit hot because it contains a potent oil, much like mustard oil, that's great for clearing the sinuses and lungs of excess mucus, relieving

sore throat, and improving circulation. Radish juice contains salicylates (also in aspirin) that have been known to help relieve arthritis pain. Other important nutrients in radish juice are vitamin C, iodine, iron, calcium, and sulfur. Mix it with carrot and parsley juice, and you'll have a delicious drink!

Red Bell Pepper Juice

Red bell pepper juice is sweeter and better for you than green bell pepper juice. Red bell peppers are ripe, while green ones are not ripe and contain fewer nutrients. Red bell peppers are high in vitamin C and are great for the immune system. They are also high in silicon, which helps strengthen and repair connective tissue and prevent bruising.

Tomato Juice

Tomato juice should be made only from organic, vine-ripened tomatoes. Some of the tomatoes available in grocery stores in the winter are void of nutrients and hardly taste like tomatoes at all! Tomato juice is high in beta-carotene and vitamin C, which boost the immune system. They contain lycopene, a powerful antioxidant that helps prevent cancer and heart disease. Tomato juice is also rich in the amino acid lysine, which helps heal cold sores, and potassium, which is a great mineral for the muscles and heart. Some people worry that tomato juice contains too much sodium. This is because most people are drinking canned or bottled tomato juice that has added salt for flavor. Freshly juiced tomato juice contains some organic sodium, but this natural sodium is very helpful in dissolving crystals in the joints and holding calcium in the bone. Some tomatoes are a bit too acidic for some people and may cause indigestion. If this is the case, I suggest trying the more alkaline Roma tomatoes. Enjoy tomato juice! NOTE: If you have arthritis and are concerned that the foods from the nightshades including tomatoes, peppers, potatoes, and eggplants could be bothering you, leave out all nightshades for a week and introduce one at the time into your diet. If pain is worsened due to the nightshades, omit them from the foods you eat. It may be that after following a healthy nutritional plan for a year, your body will grow strong enough to tolerate the nightshades. If not, continue to avoid them completely.

Watercress Juice

Watercress juice has a bittersweet taste and is great juiced with carrot and cucumbers. It is a natural diuretic and helps prevent fluid retention. Drink watercress juice to strengthen your hair—it contains a lot of amino acids. It is also a good source of minerals, including sulfur, which helps arthritis and prevents cancer growth, and iodine, which is great for the thyroid gland. Watercress is also great for the immune system because its high in vitamins A and C.

Wheatgrass Juice

Wheatgrass juice cleanses the blood and acts just like a drain cleaner, killing bacteria and parasites as it goes through the system. If you don't have a wheatgrass juicer, the juice is often available in health food stores. It is also available in powder form. Barley grass and green kamut are similar because they are both good blood cleansers and detoxifiers and also come in powdered form. Ann Wigmore, who founded the Hippocrates Health Institute in Boston, is credited with discovering the benefits of wheatgrass juice. She had gangrene in her legs, and the doctors wanted to amputate. She started drinking wheatgrass juice and using poultices on her legs. Not only did her legs heal, but she went on to run the Boston marathon! Since then, many people with "incurable" diseases have gotten well using wheatgrass juice. I drink two ounces of wheatgrass juice often and feel energized! People with allergies to wheat will have no problem using wheatgrass juice, as wheat is a grain, while wheatgrass is a grass (not a grain). Wheatgrass juice is about 70 percent chlorophyll, which closely resembles hemoglobin in chemical composition. Chlorophyll has antiseptic cleansing properties. Wheatgrass juice is a wonderful source of protein, beta-carotene, B vitamins, and vitamins C, E, H, and K. It is said to contain a wide variety of minerals with more iron than spinach. Its nutrients nourish the body and give it a real boost.

Tool Kit for Choosing
Therapeutic Herbal Teas

Herbal teas have been used for centuries both for healing and enjoyment. There is something wonderful about sitting with a cup of soothing tea in the midmorning, afternoon, or evening. You can curl up on a rainy afternoon on the couch with a blanket, a good book, and a delicious cup of warm tea or enjoy tea with a friend. When choosing a tea, make sure it is right for you. There are such a variety of teas with various benefits. For example, cramp bark tea is very useful to a woman with menstrual pains and may be helpful during pregnancy. When pregnant however, it would be wise to consult a knowledgeable herbalist or your physician before taking. Herbs are our friends and can comfort and delight. Some are medicinal and should be used with respect. To prepare a tea, it is best to use distilled or purified water. Never use tap water because in most places it is full of chlorine and other harmful chemicals.

MAKING PERFECT TEA

Follow these rules when preparing your tea, and you will have wonderful tea each time.

- If the tea is leaves or blossoms, bring water to a boil, add the tea, turn off the burner, cover, and let it steep for about twenty minutes. Covering tea while it's steeping is most important in order to hold in the volatile healing properties.
- If the tea is seeds, bring the water to a boil, add the seeds, and reduce the heat to simmer. Simmer the tea for ten minutes, covered. Then turn off the heat, cover, and let it steep for twenty to thirty minutes.
- If the tea is roots, straw, or bark, bring the water to a boil, add the tea, cover it, then reduce the heat to simmer. Simmer the tea for twenty minutes. Then turn off the heat, and let it steep for thirty minutes.
- If the tea is a powder, pour boiling water over the powder, cover it, and let it steep for ten minutes.
- Use a teaspoon of each type of tea per cup unless directed otherwise.

HERBAL TEAS

Tea can make us more alert at work, help heal a sore throat, or help us to sleep at night. If you know the healing values in herbal teas, you can choose the best ones for your current needs. Herbs are rich in vitamins, minerals, and healing oils, and I have listed the most important of these for each tea. It is good to understand, however, that an herb's healing power lies within the synergistic interaction between all of the nutrients within it and not in one single element. Following is a list of various herbal teas and their medicinal benefits. These teas can be drunk with or without sweeteners. If you like your tea a bit sweet, add stevia, agave nectar, xylitol, pure maple syrup, or raw honey. Learn about the different teas and use them appropriately for yourself, your friends, and your family. Enjoy!

NOTE: If you do not want to drink these herbs as teas, but feel they would be beneficial to you, you may take them in capsule or tincture form. Check with a knowledgeable herbalist or physician to make sure they are right for you.

Alfalfa Leaf Tea

Alfalfa leaf tea is rich in minerals, including calcium, magnesium, iron, and potassium. It is also high in chlorophyll and vitamins A, B, C, D, K, and P. It contains all eight of the essential amino acids. Alfalfa leaf tea aids digestion, builds blood, and relieves inflammation. It can also be helpful with ulcers, urinary tract infections, and arthritis.

Anise Seed Tea

Anise seed tea is a wonderful digestive aid. It relieves nausea, flatulence, and cramping. It can also be given to babies to relieve colic. Anethole, often referred to as the oil of anise seed, is aromatic and gives anise its licorice flavor. Anethole has carmitive properties, which help get rid of gas and settle the digestive system, and antispasmodic qualities, which soothe cramps. The anethole in anise is also an expectorant with antimicrobial abilities, which makes it excellent for releasing mucus and healing sore throats. Anise contains several phytonutrients including rutin, which helps tighten connective tissue in the gums. Key nutrients are vitamins A, B vitamins, C, and E. Its minerals include magnesium, calcium, iron, zinc, and potassium.

Burdock Root Tea

Burdock root tea purifies the blood, cleanses the liver, aids digestion, and balances blood sugar because it contains inulin, a plant starch that has been shown to have a favorable effect on the pancreas. Burdock root has been used as a diuretic and to help release uric acid from the kidneys and blood, thus relieving gout. It contains nutrients called polyacetylenes that have antibacterial and anti-inflammatory properties. Inulin, which helps to manage blood sugar in hypoglycemics and diabetics, makes up a large percentage of burdock root. Burdock is a fine blood purifier and has been used to heal arthritis and skin disorders. Burdock root is rich in vitamins A, B, C, E, P, as well as minerals chromium, phosphorus, selenium, iron, potassium, sulfur, iodine, silicon, zinc, magnesium, and calcium. Active compounds in burdock root are called sesquiterpene lactones (antimicrobial), volatile oils, and phytochemicals.

Cardamom Seed Tea

Cardamom seed tea relieves the gripping pain of stomach and intestinal cramps. It is both delicious and soothing. There are monoterpenes in the cardamom seeds that have antispasmotic, antiviral, antibacterial, and antifungal properties. The oil in cardamom contains limonene, terpineol, and terpenene, which have been found to relieve inflammation and pain. Cardamom seed oil also helps release mucus from the respiratory tract as well as improve digestion. Add some rice milk and have a cup in the evening.

Cascara Sagrada Bark Tea

Cascara sagrada bark tea is a safe, natural laxative that stimulates the liver to produce bile and the stomach and pancreas to produce enzymes. It contains anthraquinones, or natural phytochemicals, that help promote peristalsis in the bowel. A liver cleanser, it is useful in cases of jaundice. Take cascara sagrada together with cardamom and cinnamon to improve the flavor and prevent possible cramping.

Use cascara sagrada bark tea only when necessary. Though it is not harmful, our bowels should function without the aid of laxatives. Constipation is often related to a magnesium deficiency. Enhance your diet with foods containing magnesium. See more about constipation under "Remedies" in chapter 4.

Catnip Leaf Tea

Catnip leaf tea calms the nervous system and helps induce sleep. It also lowers fevers, eases symptoms of flatulence, stomach acids, intestinal spasms, and colic. This a wonderful tea to relieve colic in infants and promote rest. Catnip tea contains several minerals including calcium and magnesium that help calm the nerves and relax the body. It is rich in iron. Key vitamins are A, B-1, B-2, niacin, and B-6. B vitamins are very soothing to the nerves. It also contains a compound called valeric acid, a natural seditive also found in valerian root.

Chamomile Blossom Tea

Chamomile blossom tea soothes and relaxes the nervous system. It has a mild sedative effect, which can induce sleep. It also relieves digestive disorders, such as diarrhea, flatulence, and cramps. This tea can help relieve flu-like symptoms such as aching muscles, inflammation, and coughing. Add four cups of chamomile blossom tea to the bath water to relieve muscular pain or sunburn. Chamomile contains the phytochemicals azulene (an anti-inflammatory), borneol (a digestive aide), salicylic acid (relieves pain), rutin (tightens tissues), and quercitin (an antioxidant). It's vitamins are B and C. Blondes can use this tea as a hair rinse to lighten their hair. NOTE: Those with an allergy to ragweed should drink chamomile tea with caution because it is very similar in nature to ragweed. Don't mix chamomile tea with alcohol or sleeping medications.

Chickweed Leaf and Stem Tea

Chickweed makes a nice herbal tea with natural fatty acids that help with weight loss. It is also high in vitamin C, iron, and potassium and helps to cleanse the blood and reduce fevers. Add a little raw organic honey to the tea and it will soothe a sore throat.

Cinnamon Bark Tea

Cinnamon bark tea relieves symptoms of indigestion and helps stop diarrhea, stomach cramps, and nausea. The oils in cinnamon improve circulation and can encourage menstrual bleeding if a menstrual period is late. This tea has antifungal, antibacterial, and antiviral properties. Cinnamon contains beta-carotene—a form of vitamin A that boosts immunity and chromium that helps balance blood sugar in diabetics and hypoglycemics. NOTE: May take only small amounts during pregnancy, no more than one cup every few weeks.

Collinsonia Root Tea

Collinsonia root tea is wonderful for healing hemorrhoids and varicose veins because it strengthens the walls of the veins. The resin in it strengthens tissue and helps wounds to heal. The tannins in it are astringent and are beneficial in helping stop diarrhea. Tannins help fight bacteria and fungi. It also contains saponins which have cholesterol lowering abilities.

Cramp Bark Tea

Cramp bark is a wonderful tea for cramps of any kind, especially menstrual because it contains valerianic acid, the phytonutrient also found in valerian root that has relaxing properties. It can help regulate menstrual cycles and may be beneficial when there is potential for miscarriage. Cramp bark can also help ease heart palpitations because of its relaxing nervine properties. It contains the minerals calcium, magnesium, and potassium—also great muscle relaxants. It works wonderfully to relieve cramps when blended with false unicorn. NOTE: Consult an herbalist or knowledgeable physician before taking if you are pregnant.

Dandelion Leaf and Root Tea

Dandelions are high in vitamins A, B, C, and D and the minerals calcium, iron, potassium, and sulfur. The tea is a wonderful spring tonic and blood and liver purifier. Dandelions are also high in inulin, which helps regulate the blood sugar and is a gentle laxative and natural diuretic. Dandelion leaf and root tea can alleviate anemia, jaundice, diabetes, gout, hepatitis, and constipation. It can also help reduce levels of uric acid and serum cholesterol. NOTE: Dandelion is a natural diuretic so do not drink this tea if you are taking medicinal diuretics. Also avoid this tea if you have gallstones.

Echinacea Root Tea

Echinacea root tea purifies the lymph and blood, thus helping fight off colds, bronchitis, sore throat, urinary tract infections, and flu. It contains the phytochemicals alpha-pinene, an antibacterial, and beta-carotene, a plant form of vitamin A that strengthens the eyes. It also contains the phytochemicals apgenin, a natural anti-inflammatory, and arabinogalactan, which boosts the immune system and protects against allergies. The tea stimulates white blood cells, which help attack germs, as well as interferon, which is a front-line component known to fight the development of cancer cells. It is antiviral and antibacterial. It is high in vitamin C, phosphorus, iron, and zinc. NOTE: This tea should not be taken for more than four to six weeks or it loses its potency in the body. Since this tea stimulates the immune system, it should be used with caution by those with auto-immune disorders. It should also be used with caution if you have an allergy to ragweed, daisies, chrysanthemums, or marigolds because echinacea has similar properties to these plants.

Eyebright Leaf Tea
Eyebright is high in beta-carotene and vitamin C. The tea is extremely beneficial in strengthening the eyes and maintaining good vision.

False Unicorn Root Tea
This wonderful tea helps regulate irregular menses and relieve cramping. False unicorn root tea relieves nausea that may come with menstruation or pregnancy. It has also been used successfully to help women become pregnant. Men who want to increase sperm count should drink false unicorn root tea. This tea helps rid the bowel of parasites as well. It contains the phytonutrients helonin, known to tone the female glands, and chamaelirin, known to strengthen both male and female systems, help impotence, and also act as a vermifuge.

Fennel Seed, Leaf, and Flower Tea
Fennel tea can be made from the seed, leaf, or flower. It is an excellent sore throat remedy. It also helps relieve coughs and colds and helps expel mucus. Fennel tea relieves colic, intestinal cramping, and flatulence. Fennel is very alkaline in nature so it's a great tea for an acid stomach or for those who have undergone chemotherapy. Its active constituents include terpenoid anethole, which has an estrogen-like activity that inhibits spasms in the smooth muscles due to coughing or abdominal cramping. It contains alphapinene, a phytonutrient which is antibacterial. Other key nutrients are beta-carotene, qurecitin, vitamin C, iron, and selenium.

Fenugreek Seed Tea
Fenugreek seed tea strengthens the liver. The seeds contain steroidal saponins, which have cholesterol lowering properties. These saponins also reduce the formation of secondary bile acids which are known to lead to colon cancer. Fenugreek contains the phytonutrient coumarin, which is antifungal, and kaempferol and quercetin, which are strong antioxidants and together have been known to reduce the proliferation of cancer cells. Oil of fenugreek helps soothe the throat and lungs and lubricate the intestines, and acts as a mild laxative. The oil may also reduce fevers and help asthma and sinus problems by clearing away mucus. Fenugreek contains amino acids, essential fatty acids, calcium, magnesium iron, phosphorus, zinc, potassium, B vitamins, and vitamin C. Because it is so nutritious, it

strengthens the endocrine system and can help increase the flow of breast milk in nursing mothers.

Feverfew Bark, Leaves, and Flowers Tea

A wonderful anti-inflammatory, feverfew tea can relieve headaches, migraine headaches, and arthritic aches when used faithfully over a period of several months. It contains the phytonutrient parthenolide, which has been shown to be effective in relieving migraines and fighting leukemia. Parthenolide is anti-inflammatory. Key nutrients in feverfew are calcium, magnesium, potassium, selenium, zinc, iron, B vitamins, and vitamin C. Synergistically, its constituents help fight bacteria, yeasts, and fungi as well as inhibit the release of histamine in allergic reactions. NOTE: People who take pain killers or medicines that thin the blood should not take feverfew without consulting a physician. Feverfew should not be taken during pregnancy.

Flaxseed Tea

Flaxseed tea is mucilaginous and soothes the digestive tract, thereby helping relieve constipation. It is excellent for soothing and cleansing the urinary system as well. It contains the phytochemicals beta-sitosterol and campesterol, which are known to help in lowering cholesterol. Another phytochemical in flaxseed is apigenin, which is a natural anti-inflammatory and helps reduce cramping. Flaxseed are high in iron, potassium, sulfur, magnesium, zinc, B vitamins, and vitamin E.

Ginger Root Tea

Ginger root makes one of the finest teas to help relieve vertigo, nausea, and vomiting. It helps stop morning sickness in pregnant mothers and relieves menstrual cramps. It is also very helpful with colitis, stomach cramps, and flatulence. Ginger root tea increases circulation and warms the body, and it is wonderful for colds and flu. Please see the medicinal and nutritive benefits of ginger on page 84.

NOTE: It's best to avoid ginger if you have gallstones or are taking a blood thinner. Pregnant women should take small amounts or consult their midwife or herbalist.

Ginkgo Biloba Leaf Tea

Gingko biloba leaf tea increases blood and oxygen circulation to all parts of the body, including the brain, thereby improving memory and easing the symptoms of Alzheimer's disease, headaches, and depression. It helps improve the transmission of information at a nerve cell level, thus improving mental performance. Ginkgo has been shown to improve the mental clarity of geriatric subjects and of people with attention deficit disorder. Ginkgo contains the flavonoids, ginkgolide, quercitin, and kaempferol. Flavonoids are compounds found in fruits, vegetables, and herbs that have powerful antioxidant, anti-inflammatory, antiviral, antifungal, and anti-tumor activities. Three important flavonoids in ginkgo are ginkgolide, quercetin, and kaempferol. Ginkgo has wonderful nutrients that are excellent for the brain, including manganese, phosphorus, potassium, and zinc. It contains vitamins A, B-1, B-2, niacin (helps circulation), and C.

NOTE: Children twelve years old and younger should not take gingko; nor should those using pain killers or blood thinning medicines.

Panax Ginseng Root Tea

Panax ginseng root tea is a wonderful tonic for the immune system. It has been used in Asia since ancient times as a tonic, stimulant, and digestive aid. Panax ginseng is the only true ginseng and there are American, Chinese, and Korean panax ginsengs. Siberian ginseng, which is much less expensive, has similar properties, but it is important to note that it's not a true ginseng. There are two types of Panax ginseng, white and red. Red ginseng is made from the carmel-colored steamed root and is resistant to the invasion of worms and fungi. White ginseng has had the skin peeled off and is made from the dried underlying white part of the root. It is the red ginseng that is more commonly used in Oriental medicine. Panax ginseng contains phytochemicals called ginsenosides, saponins, panaxans, flavonoids, and volatol oils that work together as antioxidants, anti-inflammatories, and immunity builders. They help to strengthen both male and female reproductive organs as well as the adrenal glands. Ginseng has been used to enhance physical endurance, increase energy levels, elevate mood, and improve memory. Ginseng root tea stimulates blood circulation and improves energy levels. Start slowly with ginseng; use small amounts at first. Studies have shown an absence of harmful effects, but some people may experience a feeling of hypertension. NOTE: Ginseng should not be used by anxious, nervous, or hyperactive people. People should avoid caffeine while using ginseng. Ginseng should not be taken if using aspirin or blood-thinning medications. Ginseng may exaggerate the effects of antipsychotic medication so they should not be taken together. It should not be taken if one is using an antidepressant. Ginseng may block the pain-reducing effects of morphine. It should not be used by children twelve years old and under. It should not be used by anyone with a heart problem, high blood pressure, insomnia, or asthma. Pregnant women and nursing mothers should avoid ginseng.

Goldenseal Root Tea

Goldenseal boosts the immune system. It contains an alkaloid constituent called berberine that has been widely studied. According to research, berberine has powerful antibiotic, anti-inflammatory, and antibacterial properties. Goldenseal root tea soothes irritated mucous membranes and is helpful in healing gum diseases, yeast infections, colitis, colds, and flu. NOTE: Goldenseal also has been known to raise blood pressure. Do not use goldenseal for more than two to three weeks at a time, and do not use it at all in cases of high blood pressure. It should not be used in cases of insomnia or by pregnant women or nursing mothers. Since goldenseal is endangered, Oregon grape root is a good alternative.

Gota Kola Nut, Leaf, and Root Tea

Gota Kola is native to India and has been used in Ayurvedic medicine for thousands of years. In China, it has been called a miracle elixir of life. Gota Kola is a great blood purifier and helps relieve high blood pressure. It decreases fatigue, increases sex drive, and helps with combating depression. Gota Kola contains several important sterols, including beta-sitosterol, campesterol, and stigmasterol. These natural lipids help lower cholesterol and nourish the brain and nervous system, enhancing memory. Important antibiotic properties are found in Gota Kola that support the immune system and promote wound healing. It is very alkaline in nature and may help reduce acidity in the body. Gota Kola contains beta-carotene, amino acids, vitamins B, C, and K as well as the minerals iron, calcium, magnesium, phosphorus, potassium, selenium, and zinc.

Gravel Root Tea

Gravel root tea is used to strengthen the urinary tract and dissolve stones. It can be very beneficial in slowing the frequency of excessive nighttime urination, as well as with enuresis (the involuntary discharge of urine). Gravel root contains the phytonutrients eupatorin and euparin, which work together as a urinary tract tonic. Gravel root helps strengthen the prostate and dissolve kidney stones.

Green Leaf Tea

Research shows that green tea is high in polyphenols, which are powerful antioxidants that help fight free radicals. Free radicals can cause disease and premature aging. Green tea has been shown to prevent the growth of tumors, lower blood pressure, and prevent blood clots. Green tea also assists in fighting bacteria in the mouth that can produce cavities. It is antiviral and can aid in fighting influenza as well as the common cold. It is high in vitamin C and the bioflavonoids rutin and quercitin. It also contains B vitamins, potassium, zinc, and iron. Green tea does contain some caffeine, so drink it in the morning. It might help you kick the coffee habit. Decaffeinated green tea is also available.

Hawthorne Berry Tea

Hawthorne berry tea is great for the heart. It is high in bioflavonoids, which build and repair connective tissue of arterial walls. It also helps reduce cholesterol levels and lower high blood pressure. Hawthorn contains amino acids, potassium, calcium, magnesium, and zinc as well as B vitamins and vitamin C.

Horehound Leaf and Flower Tea

Horehound is a must-have during times of coughs, respiratory infections, and colds. Horehound tea contains limonene, the same oil that is found in citrus and it helps clear the sinuses and lungs of mucus and helps the throat rid itself of thick phlegm. It soothes a sore throat and helps ease a cough. It contains tannins, which are antimicrobial and help the body to ward off infection. Horehound tea, made from leaves or flowers that also contain pectin, may help cleanse the liver, reduce indigestion, and rid the body of jaundice. Key nutrients in horehound are vitamins A, B, C, and E and potassium, and iron. NOTE: Use no more than one or two cups of horehound a day for no more than four to six weeks. Larger amounts may cause heartbeat irregularities. If you have heart concerns, consult your physician before taking.

Horsetail Plant Tea

The horsetail plant, also called shavegrass, looks like a green horse's tail. Use only the plant, not the roots, for tea. When I hiked in the Swiss Alps in the summertime, we broke open the stem of a horsetail plant and used the white creamy milk inside to relieve rashes we got from the nettles that grew all around. High in silicon, zinc, phosphorus, calcium, and fluorine, horsetail taken internally helps repair weak or broken bones and strengthen the skin, hair, teeth, and fingernails. It is high in vitamin C, has been used to help stop bleeding, and can be very beneficial in treating ulcers.

Juniper Berry Tea

Juniper berry tea is great for the bladder and helps heal bladder infections and prostate disorders. A natural diuretic, it releases fluids from the body when there is excessive swelling. It aids in relieving indigestion and gas. Its anti-inflammatory qualities help relieve arthritic and rheumatic pains. It is also useful in treating gout. Juniper berries are high in the antibacterial tannins, beta-carotene, and bioflavonoids. It contains chromium, which helps balance blood sugar, potassium, selenium, calcium, zinc, B vitamins, and vitamin C. NOTE: Large amounts of juniper berry tea—more than two cups per day over extended periods of more than four weeks—may interfere with iron absorption. Avoid juniper berry tea if you have a kidney disease until you have consulted with a knowledgeable health practitioner. Do not drink juniper berry tea during pregnancy.

Kava Kava Root Tea

Kava kava is a wonderful tea that contains the phytonutrients kavapyrones and kavalactones, which help to relax the nervous system thereby making it a natural sleep aid. Kava kava helps relax tight muscles and relieve pain. It's great for anyone with a pinched nerve, muscle spasms, muscle aches, or cramping. It could be very useful during moments of anxiety and panic. Kava kava also contains cinnamic acid, which is a natural antiseptic. NOTE: Should not be used with alcohol, sleep medications, or antidepressants. May cause drowsiness (if so, use only at night when you are ready for sleep). Not for those eighteen years old or younger. Pregnant women and nursing mothers should avoid.

Kombucha Tea

Kombucha tea is made from a mushroomlike fungus along with black or green tea, apple cider vinegar, and sugar. Some health food stores carry the brew ready-made. It has been reported to boost energy levels, strengthen immune function, normalize blood pressure, lower cholesterol, bring hair color back, ease arthritis pain, and fight AIDS and cancer. It has anti-inflammatory and antimicrobial properties. It helps fight bacteria, fungi, and viruses. NOTE: Kombucha should not be taken by those with a weak liver. It is a powerful detoxifier and will pull toxins from the body and pass them through the liver. Because the tea is made with white sugar, people with blood-sugar imbalances and diabetics should use it with care. Pregnant or nursing women should not drink it at all because it contains some caffeine and alcohol and thereby may cause a toxic effect on the liver. Children twelve years and under should not take kombucha for the same reasons. Alcoholics in recovery should avoid kombucha because the small amount of alcohol contained in it could have a negative reaction in their bodies.

Lemon Balm Leaf Tea

Lemon balm leaf tea also known as Melissa tea contains balsamic oils and tannins that have antibacterial and antiviral properties that help fight colds, cold sores, and flu. It contains phytonutrients called terpines that help relax nerves and relieve feelings of anxiety or panic, relieve headaches (possibly migraines), and if taken at night, promote restful sleep. It contains another nutrient called eugenol which calms muscle spasms and aids with digestive disorders, such as cramping, flatulence, and nausea. Lemon balm has been effective with the relief symptoms associated with hyperthyroidism. Because of its special essential oils, it can help gently break a fever in children. NOTE: No toxic effects are known, but this herb should not be taken by pregnant women or nursing mothers. It also should not be taken with barbiturates or sleeping medicines, as it can enhance their sedative effects.

Lemongrass Leaf Tea

Lemongrass leaves are high in lemongrass oil and the phytochemicals citral, geraniol, terpineol, limonene, spononin, and the bioflavonoids quercitin and rutin. The synergistic effects of these nutrients help reduce fevers, relieve headaches, soothe digestive disorders, and reduce flatulence. Its anti-spasmodic qualities may help relieve abdominal muscle cramps during menstruation. The oil also has antifungal and antibacterial properties. It is high in potassium, calcium, magnesium, and zinc.

Lemon Verbena Leaf Tea
Lemon verbena leaf tea is an astringent herb with volatile oils that relieve cramping, including that which occurs during menstruation, and nausea, and it soothes the nervous system. It contains the phytonutrients limonene, geraniol, and terpineol, great antioxidants that help clear a stuffy nose or congested bronchial tubes. These phytonutrients have anti-inflammatory properties as well.

Licorice Root Tea
Licorice is a sweet, very nutritious root that helps to balance the adrenal gland, protect the liver, and dispel depression. The root can be chewed during hikes to help maintain energy levels. It also helps smokers kick the smoking habit and not gain weight. People who crave caffeine or sweets or are hypoglycemic can chew on the root as well to eliminate cravings and regulate blood sugar. The tea is delicious and can be added to other teas to sweeten them. Licorice root tea contains camphor, is antispasmotic, and reduces muscle spasms, soothes the digestive tract, helps heal ulcers, relieves nausea and gastritis, and helps ease colitis. Licorice root can also relieve sore throats, allergies, and asthma, help expel mucus, and fight colds, inflammation, and bronchitis. Licorice root contains a nutrient called glycyrrhizin that is known to be antiviral. Another one of its constituents is manitol, which helps scavenge free radicals and may act as a natural diuretic. Licorice root contains salicylic acid, the same ingredient in aspirin that relieves pain and fights inflammation. It also contains antioxidants including beta-carotene and quercitin. Another phytonutrient in licorice is geraniol, a natural antioxidant that may help prevent the growth of tumors. It is rich in nutrients including iron, calcium, magnesium, phosphorus, potassium, selenium, silicon, and zinc, as well as B vitamins and vitamin C. NOTE: Licorice root should not be used on a daily basis as it can raise the blood pressure. It should not be used by people with high blood pressure, glaucoma, diabetes, or heart disease. It should be avoided by people that have seizures or who have had a stroke. It should not be taken by pregnant women or nursing mothers.

Linden Flower Tea

Linden flower tea helps calm tension and relax the body because of its anti-spasmodic properties. It is high in flavonoids including quercetin and kaempferol, as well as p-coumaric acid, that act as diaphoretics that promote sweating. These nutrients work together to reduce fever and congestion during a cold or flu and soothe a sore throat.

Lobelia Leaf and Flower Tea

Lobelia tea, made from the leaves and flowers of the Lobelia plant, is excellent for healing coughing, wheezing, colds, bronchitis, sore throats, asthma, and pneumonia. It helps the bronchial muscles relax and liquefies thickened mucus that needs to be expelled from the sinuses or lungs. Lobelia tea can also help people addicted to nicotine let go of the habit with few withdrawal symptoms. Lobelia contains the active ingredient lobeline, which is similar to nicotine in its effect on the central nervous system. It stimulates the adrenal glands to release the hormone epinephrine, which relaxes and dilates the bronchioles (air passages in the lungs), thereby increasing respiration.

Lobelia is an herb to be respected and should be used in small amounts. Use no more than one-third teaspoon of dried lobelia to eight ounces of hot water. Sip it slowly and drink no more than three cups per day. NOTE: Too much lobelia causes vomiting, dizziness, and nausea. Consult your health-care practitioner before taking. Children should not take lobelia unless under the care of a qualified physician. Lobelia should not be taken by pregnant women or nursing mothers.

Ma Huang Stem Tea

Ma huang stem tea has been used as a bronchial dilator and decongestant to help reduce the symptoms of asthma, allergies, bronchitis, colds, and flu. It has also been used in weight reduction programs because of its ability to suppress the appetite and stimulate the metabolism. Ma huang contains two widely used alkaloids called ephedrine and pseudo ephedrine. Ephedrine stimulates the thyroid gland and nervous system, thereby increasing the metabolic rate and suppressing the appetite. It can also alleviate feelings of fatigue and depression, and increase energy levels, alertness, and perception. Psuedo ephedrine is a nasal decongestant and bronchodilator. It is a key ingredient in several over-the-counter cold and flu remedies.

NOTE: Ma huang should not be used by people with high blood pressure, heart disease, diabetes, prostate disorders, or thyroid problems. Nor should it be used by people on medications for hypertension or depression. Ma huang can cause insomnia and anxiety, so it should be used in small amounts and with respect. Consult your health-care practitioner.

Malva Leaf Tea

Malva leaf tea is high in vitamin A, which helps to strengthen the eyes and the immune system. Malva contains flavonoids and demulcent qualities and is excellent for relieving inflammation in the mucous membranes. It is said to loosen phlegm in congested lungs. It soothes the digestive and urinary tract and acts as a mild diuretic. It has a mild laxative effect and works well as a laxative for children. When combined with eucalyptus in tea, it is an excellent remedy for coughs and other chest ailments.

Marigold Petal Tea (Calendula)

There are different varieties of marigolds (including African) which are often called American *(Tagetes erecta)* because they grow in North America, or French *(Tagetes patula)*. The marigold that is used for tea and medicinal purposes is called the pot marigold or *Calendula officinalis.* Actually the pot marigold, though called marigold, is not a true marigold. It has beautiful orange and yellow flowers similar to the marigold family. The pot marigold petal tea contains calendula oil and vitamin E, which help soothe ulcers, lower or break fevers, and regulate the menstrual cycle. It also helps alleviate skin disorders, such as boils and shingles, and soften varicose veins and hemorrhoids. It has salicylic acid, which gives it antiseptic and antifungal properties that make it useful in reducing infections and treating gingivitis (gum disease), *Candida albicans* yeast, acne, and athlete's foot. It also contains beta-carotene, which is an excellent antioxidant that fights the signs of aging and assists in healing wounds and eczema. The tea is mucilaginous and soothing to the digestive tract, especially in cases of colitis, diverticulitis, and ulcers. This soothing tea also makes a wonderful eyewash for dry burning eyes.

Marshmallow Flower, Leaf, and Root Tea

Marshmallow root tea soothes inflammation in the body. As marshmallow root is mucilagenous and slippery, it is great for relieving ulcers, diverticulitis, or colitis. It contains beta-carotene, quercitin, salicylic acid, and tannins, which make it an antioxidant and antimicrobial. It helps fight kidney and bladder infections, sore throat, and sinusitis, and helps the body release mucus from the lungs. Key nutrients in marshmallow flower are vitamin C, calcium, magnesium, potassium, selenium, and iron.

Motherwort Leaf and Flower Tea

Motherwort tea, made from leaves and flowers, is great for strengthening the heart because of its special oils and the antioxidants quercitin and vitamin C. It slows heart palpitations and a rapid heartbeat. It can also help lower blood pressure. It contains alkaloids, derivatives of amino acids, which may have a sedative effect. This tea calms muscle spasms, including leg cramps. It is great support for women's health, easing symptoms of PMS, menstrual cramping, and the hot flashes associated with menopause. It helps relax the nerves, calm anxiety, reduce stress, and ease depression. Motherwort may calm a hyperactive thyroid. The healing constituents of motherwort are rutin, which strengthens connective tissue and is especially helpful with hemorrhoids and varicosities, and alpha-pinene and tannins, which have wonderful antibacterial properties.

Mullein Leaf and Flower Tea

Mullein is an exotic-looking plant, tall with soft velvety green leaves. It contains the phytonutrients hesperidin, which strengthens veins; coumarin, which has antifungal and blood vessel strengthening properties; beta-carotene, an antioxidant; and saponins, which have antibacterial and cholesterol lowering abilities. The mullein oil in mullein tea is a valuable destroyer of germs and viruses and has even been known to help get rid of warts. It is also high in mucilage. Because of these nutrients and its slippery consistency, mullein is a great decongestant and is very helpful in ridding mucus from the lungs and sinuses. It soothes the membranes in the throat and entire intestinal tract and may act as a mild laxative. It has been used for coughs, asthma, influenza, and urinary tract infections. Mullein has sedative properties and helps relax the body and relieve abdominal cramps.

To prepare the tea, use two heaping teaspoons in eight ounces of boiling water. Cover and let it steep for five minutes, strain, then drink.

Nettle Leaf, Flower, Root Tea

If you are going out to pick nettles, be sure to wear gloves. They are full of little stingers that are high in formic acid, which can cause a skin rash and itching. If you accidentally touch nettles, there are usually some horsetail plants growing nearby. Break open the stem of the horsetail, and use the creamy juice to coat the stinging area of your skin. This will greatly reduce the rash and promote healing.

Once nettles are dried or cooked for about eight minutes, they lose their stinging quality. Nettles, also called stinging nettles, are high in vitamins C, K, pantothenic acid (B-5), and E, and minerals, including iron, calcium, magnesium, phosphorus, and potassium, and can be very beneficial in treating anemia. A cup of nettles tea may help prevent internal bleeding because the high dosage of calcium acts as a "knitter" to repair tissues (check with your physician). The tea helps purify and build the blood. Nettle tea can also be beneficial in calming allergic reactions. It can even help stop the itching and burning that often comes with allergies. Because of its rich nutritional content, which includes protein, natural lecithin, and essential fatty acids, nursing mothers will produce more milk while drinking this tea. Nettles tea has been know to stimulate hair growth. In cases of baldness, drink the tea and rub it into the hair follicles as well.

Oatstraw Tea

A horse that eats oats has a shiny coat, silky mane, and great stamina. Oatstraw contains the minerals silicon, calcium, iron, copper, zinc, and magnesium, as well as the B-complex vitamins. It strengthens and nourishes the skin, hair, fingernails, connective tissue, cartilage, and bones. It can also help people with hair loss or skin troubles such as acne, dandruff, eczema, and psoriasis. It can improve the sperm count in men. Oatstraw tea is a super nerve tonic that has a calming effect and strengthens the brain and nervous system. It has been known to decrease or stop bed-wetting. It is great for anyone who is trying to stop smoking, as it lessens withdrawal symptoms. Oatstraw tea is wonderful for athletes or anyone desiring more energy and stamina. This tea can be used as a delicious base for soups and broths.

Orange Peel Tea

The inner portion of an orange peel is high in bioflavonoids, which build connective tissue, preventing bruising and promoting the healing of wounds and tissues. Orange peel tea can relieve flatulence and improve digestion. Be sure to use organic peelings that are free from chemicals.

Oregon Grape Root Tea

Oregon grape root is a powerful natural antibiotic with many of the same qualities as goldenseal. They are both high in berberine and Oregon grape root also contains tannins, which help strengthen the immune system and fight bacteria. Oregon grape root tea is a blood purifier and is remedial in treating skin disorders, including acne, cold sores, psoriasis, and eczema. It strengthens a weak liver and gallbladder and aids in digestion. NOTE: Pregnant women and nursing mothers, people with high blood pressure, insomnia, and people with an overactive liver should not drink this tea.

Parsley Leaf, Stem, and Root Tea

Parsley leaf, stem, and root is a natural diuretic that is rich in chlorophyll. It helps cleanse the liver, kidneys, and bladder and fight urinary tract infections. It helps stop bed-wetting. The root is particularly helpful in dissolving stones. The entire parsley plant, including leaves, stems, and roots, is high in iron, phosphorus, calcium, manganese, B vitamins, and vitamins A, C, and K, making it great for building blood. The tea is also a wonderful digestive aid, helps relieve gas, and freshens the breath.

NOTE: Parsley tea can stop the flow of milk in nursing mothers. They should use the tea only after they have stopped nursing and are ready for their milk to dry up. Pregnant women should avoid using parsley tea completely because it can cause early labor.

Pau d'Arco Bark Tea

Pau d'Arco bark tea has also been called La Pacho, Ipe Roxo, Taheebo, and Tecoma. It comes from the Pau d'Arco tree that grows in the forests of Brazil. This same tree grows in Argentina and is called La Pacho. Native tribes used it to treat cancers. Two primary active compounds in pau d'arco that have antifungal, antibacterial, antiparasitic, and anticancer properties are lapchol and beta-lapachone. Beta-sitosterol, a phytochemical in pau d'arco, helps lower cholesterol and is a natural anti-inflammatory. It has been reported to be beneficial in fighting Candidiasis in the intestines and vaginal tract. It has proved very helpful in treating diabetes, liver disorders, lung congestion, skin diseases, ulcers, immune dysfunction, infections, warts, smoker's cough, and allergies.

Peppermint and Spearmint Leaf Tea

The menthol oil (called carvone) in these delightful teas helps them to soothe the digestive system, relieve heartburn, cramping, nausea, and flatulence. Peppermint and spearmint leaf teas are also great for relieving menstrual discomfort and morning sickness. They contain niacin, which is known to stimulate circulation and ease headaches. The oils and tannins in these teas give them antifungal, antiviral, antibacterial, and antiparasitic properties. Tannins are useful in soothing the digestive tract in cases of diarrhea, constipation, ulcers, and colitis. They can help heal colds, flu, and upper respiratory tract infections. Children tend to like spearmint tea because it's milder in taste. It can help them with the relief of stomachaches, coughing, and sinus congestion.

Red Clover Tea

Red clover is a natural blood purifier and tonic and contains salicylic acid, which has anti-inflammatory and antiseptic properties. It helps fight infection, cancers, and tumors. Red clover tea is great for helping heal skin conditions such as acne, eczema, and psoriasis. It is also wonderful for strengthening the immune system in both adults and children. Red clover has been used to treat asthma, bronchitis, pneumonia, arthritis, and gout. Its antispasmodic properties make it useful in treating coughs. Red clover tea can be beneficial to those who are trying to lose weight because it is a natural appetite suppressant. It is a good source of beta-carotene, calcium, chromium, magnesium, potassium, phosphorus, niacin, and vitamin C.

Red Raspberry Leaf Tea

Red raspberry leaf has often been called the herb for women because it helps stop frequent and excessive menstrual bleeding and relieves menstrual cramps. It can also relieve hot flashes. Red raspberry leaf strengthens and tones the uterus wall, helping to ease labor pains and facilitate childbirth. Pregnant women should not drink red raspberry leaf tea before their eighth month of pregnancy unless advised differently by their doctor or midwife. After pregnancy, because of its rich content of calcium, iron, phosphorus, the B vitamins, vitamin D, and vitamin E, red raspberry leaf enriches breast milk and helps the uterus return to its normal size and tone. Red raspberry leaf strengthens bones, skin, fingernails, and teeth, making it especially beneficial for children and elderly people. It is helpful in soothing urinary tract inflammations, treating colds, cold sores, flu, diarrhea, ulcers, bleeding gums, and colitis. NOTE: Herbalists may advise small amounts of raspberry leaf tea after the first trimester and increase the dosage during the last trimester depending on each individual, her history, and her needs.

Rosehips Tea

Rosehips tea is higher in vitamin C and bioflavonoids than oranges. Bioflavonoids help build connective tissue. Rosehips tea is useful in preventing bruising, treating sore throats, colds, flu, and sinus infections.

Sage Leaf Tea

The term sage describes someone old and wise. The herb sage is high in minerals, including manganese, phosphorus, and magnesium, that help improve mental clarity and memory. Sage contains the phytochemicals, saponins, rosmarinic acid, and tannins, which make it an antioxidant, an anti-inflammatory, and an antiseptic, and it helps with colds, cold sores, flu, and sore throats. Sage leaf tea can be used as a gargle to heal sore throats and as a mouthwash to heal gingivitis. It contains volatile oils that help improve digestion. Sage contains estrogenic substances that make it useful in relieving hot flashes during menopause, relieving menstrual cramps, and promoting blood flow if periods are delayed.

NOTES: Sage may be taken safely for a week or two, after which it should be used only periodically. Long-term regular use may inhibit the absorption of iron and other minerals. Pregnant women should not take sage because it stimulates the uterus. Nursing mothers should avoid sage leaf tea as it can dry up breast milk. Epileptics should avoid sage because it contains an antiseptic oil called thujone, which can trigger seizures.

Sarsaparilla Root Tea

Sarsaparilla is a blood purifier and tones the liver. It contains the phytochemicals stigmasterol, saponin, and beta-sitosterol, which work synergistically in the tea and help with skin conditions such as psoriasis, eczema, and acne. The tea also helps heal mouth sores and ulcers. Sarsaparilla may help the body utilize calcium efficiently, and it eases rheumatic pains. Sarsaparilla has been used throughout history to treat syphilis. It is rich in iron, phosphorus, zinc, selenium, and potassium. Boiling this tea causes it to lose its healing properties. Pour hot water over the tea and let it steep for one hour.

Saw Palmetto Berry Tea

Saw palmetto berry tea comes from a small palm tree and is very beneficial in healing the prostate gland, especially if it is swollen or enlarged. It contains the phytonutrients, sterols, beta-carotene, and ferulic acid, which are powerful antioxidants that help protect cells against the harmful effects of free radicals. It contains sterols and tannins, natural antiseptics which together help inhibit the action of testosterone on the prostate that contributes to swelling. It may act to relieve the need for frequent urination caused by an enlarged prostate gland pressing on the bladder. Saw palmetto is helpful in healing urinary tract infections and impotence. It has also been shown to help reduce unwanted hair growth in women.

Senna Leaf Tea

Senna leaf tea is used to relieve constipation. The active constituents in senna are sennosides, mucilage, volatile oil, and flavonoids. It is a powerful cathartic and stimulates peristalsis in the intestinal tract. However, it should be used seldom, if ever, and never on a regular basis to avoid laxative dependency. While using senna, some people have come to depend on it for bowel function without dealing with the true cause of the constipation. When they stop taking senna, they find their bowels have become dependent on the action of the senna rather than initiating peristalsis on their own. Senna may be used for occasional constipation but for no more than a week. If constipation has not diminished after a week, consult a knowledgeable health practitioner to determine what is causing the constipation. Senna is very harsh and should be combined with ginger and cinnamon to help prevent the abdominal cramping it can cause. NOTE: Pregnant women should never ingest senna because of the pressure it imposes on the intestinal tract. Senna is a stimulant, and it can keep sensitive people awake at night. Do not take if you have insomnia, inflammatory bowel disease, Crohn's disease, ulcerative colitis, abdominal pain, or nausea, or if you're experiencing vomiting. If you are nursing, consult your doctor before taking senna. Consult a physician before giving senna to children.

Shepherd's Purse Tea

Shepherd's purse tea, made from the whole plant, is high in vitamin K and acts as an astringent to help stop hemorrhaging, especially from menopausal disorders, endometriosis, or postpartum bleeding after childbirth. It can help stop the bleeding that often accompanies colitis as well. Shepherd's purse is high in chlorophyll, a natural anti-inflammatory and is a healing herb for urinary inflammations such as cystitis.

Skullcap Tea

Skullcap nourishes and soothes the nerves because of its large content of calcium and magnesium and vitamins B-1 and B-2. It can be used for treating convulsions, epilepsy, hysteria, anxiety attacks, stress, and insomnia. It is also very helpful in relieving headaches, muscle cramps, painful menstrual cramps, and nervous stomachs. Skullcap can relieve the withdrawal symptoms of alcohol and drugs.

To prepare skullcap tea, use one teaspoonful to twelve ounces of water. Never drink more than three half-cups per day because it can cause giddiness and an irregular pulse. Use only organic skullcap to ensure that it has not been combined with toxic herbs. NOTE: Skullcap should not be used by children eight years old and under.

Slippery Elm Inner Bark Tea

Slippery elm inner bark makes a slippery, mucilaginous tea that is wonderfully soothing to a sore, irritated throat and can help stop coughing. It is delicious with a little honey. Slippery elm inner bark tea contains mucilage and certain types of lipids, called campesterol, that soothe the entire digestive tract and can help heal ulcers, colitis, and hemorrhoids. Slippery elm inner bark tea is also very nourishing, and it can be given to anyone who is having trouble keeping down food. It also can be made into a porridge. Add cardamom and cinnamon for added flavor or to reduce nausea. This gentle herb can nourish tiny babies and the elderly. It is rich in nutrients including calcium, magnesium, phosphorus, potassium, manganese, iron, zinc, selenium, beta-carotene, and vitamin C.

Thyme Leaf Tea

Thyme leaf tea contains the oil thymol and the phytonutrients, tannin and caprylic acid, which are antiseptic and antifungal. It can help fight *Candida albicans* yeast infections and helps to relieve indigestion, gas, and diarrhea. It also helps clear the respiratory tract of mucus and infections. Thyme leaves have beta-carotene and vitamin C, which are wonderful antioxidants, as well as amino acids, essential fatty acids, calcium, magnesium, selenium, potassium, and zinc.

Turmeric Root Tea

Turmeric root tea contains the phytonutrient, curcumin, known for its anti-inflammatory properties that can help relieve the muscular pain associated with fibromyalgia. It also helps cleanse the liver and dissolves gallstones. Turmeric root tea regulates menstrual cycles, improves circulation, and can help alleviate arthritis. Other phytochemicals in tumeric are beta-carotene, an antioxidant; borneal, a digestive aide; alpha-pinene, an antibacterial agent; limone, an oil that helps cleanse the liver and lungs; and eugenol, which helps calm muscle spasms. It is a good source of vitamin C as well as iron, calcium, zinc, potassium, and phosphorus.

Uva Ursi Leaf Tea

Uva ursi leaf tea helps heal urinary tract infections, including nephritis and cystitis and prostate disorders. Uva ursi contains the phytochemicals ellagic acid, beta-carotene, and quercitin, which have powerful antioxidant properties and which protect the cells from free radical damage. Other phytochemicals are myricetin, which is an anti-inflammatory, and ursolic acid, which has antifungal, antiviral, and antibacterial properties. Uva ursi contains iron, phosphorus, potassium selenium, and calcium as well as vitamins C and B. NOTE: This tea is not recommended for pregnant women or nursing mothers. Children twelve or under should avoid it as well.

Valerian Root Tea

Valerian root tea is a wonderful relaxant. It contains the phytochemicals valerenone, valepotriates, and valerenic acid, which have a mild sedative effect and help promote peaceful sleep. Because of its calming abilities, it has been known to relieve cramps, coughs, high blood pressure, anxiety, and pain. Valerian root is very bitter and may be combined with cinnamon or ginger to make it more palatable. Valerian root contains fatty acids, calcium, magnesium, potassium, zinc, B vitamins, and vitamin C. NOTE: It should not be taken with sleep medications or alcohol.

Vervain Leaf Tea

Vervain leaf tea contains the phytochemicals verbenalin and verbenin, which help soothe and calm the nerves and relieve menstrual cramping. It contains the oils geraniol and limonene, which work to cleanse the liver and sinuses, promote menstruation, and the flow of mother's milk.

NOTE: It may stimulate uterine contractions so should not be used during pregnancy.

Yarrow Leaf Tea

Yarrow leaf tea contains the volatile oils camphor and linalool, which promote sweating and can be used to reduce fevers associated wtih colds and flu. Yarrow is high in minerals including calcium, magnesium, and potassium that help stop cramping. It contains salicylic acid and tannins that are anti-inflammatory and antibacterial and has been used to treat urinary infections. Yarrow also contains flavonoids that help tighten tissue and can be used topically as a styptic to help stop bleeding.

Yellow Dock Root Tea

Yellow dock root tea is high in iron and great for anemia. It is high in the antioxidants quercitin and beta-carotene and helps cleanse the liver and blood. It has rutin, which tightens tissues, and tannins that fight bacteria so it is helpful in healing skin problems such as eczema, psoriasis, acne, and herpes.

Yucca Root Tea

Yucca root tea is anti-inflammatory as well as antirheumatic, which makes it an excellent tea for healing arthritis and rheumatism. It can be a laxative, so combine it with cinnamon and ginger. It contains the antioxidant phytonutrients, beta-carotene, tannin, and sarsapogenin. It is rich in calcium, magnesium, potassium, phosphorus, iron, and zinc. It also has some B vitamins and vitamin C.

Watermelon Seed Tea

Watermelon seed tea is a natural dieuretic. It cleans and flushes out the kidneys and bladder. NOTE: To make, grind seeds and pour a pint of boiling water over one tablespoon. Steep for fifteen minutes, strain, and drink.

Exercises and Body Treatments

Lack of activity destroys the good condition
of every human being, while movement and
methodical physical exercise save it and preserve it.
—Plato

EXERCISE IS JUST AS IMPORTANT to good health as nutrition. Without exercise, we can't properly utilize the nutrients we receive from our foods. Without exercise, our bodies lose their tone and begin to age. Our muscles begin to sag and grow weak. We must move our body to keep it strong and remain free from aches and pains. There are approximately six pints of lymph fluid in the body. The lymph fluid lines our joints and helps to keep us limber. Unlike blood, which the heart pumps, this clear fluid does not move without exercise. Exercise also helps us breathe deeply and oxygenate all of our tissues. A lack of oxygen somewhere in the body can cause pain. It is important to do some type of exercise each day.

Tool Kit for Choosing Healthy Exercises

Exercise should bring joy to our lives. Moving the body should be a natural thing that we do on a daily basis. We were designed to move. Without movement, our bodies will grow fat, flabby, and wrinkled. Our lymph fluids will not be circulated, our brains will not think as clearly, our joints will grow stiff, and our minerals will not be absorbed. Exercise helps reduce high cholesterol levels in the blood and the chance of strokes and heart attacks caused by blood clotting. It also may reduce or prevent high blood pressure and keep us fit and within a healthy body weight. Some active exercise daily can stop menstrual cramping because it strengthens and tones the abdominal muscles. As with everything else, we should also find balance with exercise. Some people are "exerciserholics," while others move only from the couch in front of the television to the refrigerator. Learn to do some form of exercise that moves the body, gives the heart a workout, and promotes sweating about half an hour to an hour daily, at least five times per week. This amount of exercise will keep you fit and in shape. Remember to exercise before eating food or wait at least a half hour to an hour after eating to allow food to digest before exercising.

The following exercises are given here because they are very therapeutic and promote health in the body. The order I have them listed in is not necessarily the most important to the least. However, I do believe that the slanting board is a must to help get blood to the eyes and brain and lift and tighten tissues or organs that are sagging due to gravity. Slanting board exercise does not give the cardiovascular system a good workout however, so slanting exercise should be done in addition to the half hour per day of sugested aerobic movement. I have included rebounding because I feel it is one of the best excercises anyone can do to move the lymph, improve circulation, strengthen the muscles (including the heart), and help the body sweat and remove toxins without ever having to beat the feet and legs on hard pavement like runners do. Swimming and water aerobics are important and helpful to anyone, but especially those who endure most any type of muscle or joint pain. Water helps the body feel almost weightless and allows for easier movement. Bike riding provides great leg exercise and outdoor biking provides fresh air and is lots of fun. Walking at a brisk pace outdoors in fresh air and sunshine is one of the healthiest exercises anyone can do; walk alone for peace and silence or listen to CDs with positive messages or beautiful music. Walking with a good, supportive friend can also bring much joy. Hiking is a bit more rigorous than walking and really strengthens the legs, back muscles, and lungs; if you are a beginning hiker, start with the more gentle slopes. Yoga and tai chi provide excellent benefits in strengthening the body as well as calming the mind. I often recommend these exercises for hyper people who need to learn to slow down and breathe properly. While yoga and tai chi movements are slower than active aerobics, they can still cause the body to sweat and give a good workout to the muscles and cardiovascular system. It's a good idea to consult your physician to make sure you are in shape before beginning any exercise. But do exercise, your health and quality of life depend on it!

RECLINING ON A SLANT BOARD

The slant board is one of the most important types of exercise equipment you can have in your home. Slant boards are built at a forty-five-degree angle, slanting toward the floor. Laying on it daily with head toward the floor and feet raised above, helps reverse the effects of gravity on the body. It takes pressure off the spine, which is especially helpful if you have pinched nerves or spinal pain. In addition, a slant board can help improve blood circulation to the brain, which in turn can improve memory and help heal varicose veins.

In *Nutrition Handbook*, Dr. Bernard Jensen writes:

> *In every fatigued and tired body, the transverse colon begins to drop. The transverse colon is made up of the softest tissue in the body. It is tied up on the extreme right and on the extreme left side to ligaments that go to the spine. I believe that 8 out of 10 people who have back troubles have a prolapsus that is basically the root of their troubles, by causing a pulling on the lower part of the back. The slant board helps correct this.*

Further, the slant board helps relieve pressure from any upper abdominal organs that have dropped and rested on the lower abdominal organs such as the prostate, uterus, rectum, and bladder. A good deal of abdominal prolapse (slippage) problems lead to hemorrhoids. Laying on a slant board daily can help relieve menstrual cramps, which are often caused by a prolapsed colon, as well as enuresis, or frequent urination.

Laying on a slant board two times daily for 15 minutes at a time will take the pressure off the lower extremities and send blood to the head, brain, sinuses, eyes, and ears. Sinus problems, problems with vision, and frequent ear infections often are a result of poor blood circulation to those areas. Blood carries nutrients to the organs and carries toxins away. Another wonderful bonus of slant board exercise is the reduction of facial wrinkles! Gravity pulls down on the skin on the face, creating wrinkles over time. Laying on a slant board lifts the facial tissues back into place.

Certain people should not use slant boards. If you have high blood pressure or internal bleeding, do not use a slant board. If you tend to faint easily or have seizures, do not get on a board. If you get on a board and feel dizzy, call for help if possible, then roll off the board gently and kneel with your head toward your knees. Breathe slowly and easy, relax, and raise up your head slowly. The dizziness should go away. Extremely obese people and pregnant women also should avoid using a slant board. If you have just eaten, do not get on a slant board. The food that needs to go down may come back up. Wait two hours after eating before reclining on a slant board. If you have any questions about whether or not you should use a slant board, ask your physician.

Slant boards come in all colors, and there is even an inflatable version. The air can be removed and the board folded up for travel purposes. Be very careful when you get on and off a slant board. To get on the board, kneel first beside the board, place your forearm on the lower end of the board for support, and use your leg to give you a bit of leverage to gently roll your body onto the board. Lie on your back with your face up at the lower end and your heels against the high end with feet facing up. Though not completely necessary, there will often be a strap at the high end that the feet can go securely under to help hold you on. To get off a board, roll to the side gently and scoot off the board. Lie on your side for a moment before sitting up. This avoids putting undue pressure on your spine. The following exercises are great when done on a slant board, but you may also do them on a mat on the floor, couch, or bed.

Slant Board Exercise 1

One of the best exercises to do on a slant board is a massage using a tennis ball. Begin with your right side at the lower abdomen inside the right hip, and gently rub a tennis ball in a circular motion up the right side of your abdomen, across the top moving from the right hip just underneath the ribs, then down the left side of the abdomen inside the left hip. This will tighten any spasticity in your colon and promote peristalsis (healthy colon muscular activity). Massaging the colon can greatly improve bowel function and help to lift and tone a prolapsed colon. Also, massaging the colon can benefit the entire body. There are reflex points in the colon much like the ones in the feet that connect to various body organs. This exercise can also be done while standing or just laying in bed, but doing it on a slant board will double the benefits.

Slant Board Exercise 2

Another great exercise to do on a slant board is meditation. Lay very still on a slant board. Breathe in deeply through your nose and out through your nose five times. Then slow your breathing. Keep breathing slowly, and relax your little toe completely. Go to the next toe, and relax it completely. Relax all your toes and then your foot. Do this for both feet. Relax your ankles completely. Continue relaxing each part of your body all the way up to your head. Then thank your body for all it does for you. This exercise is particularly good after a hard day at work. It is also great for people with musculoskeletal pain or fibromyalgia.

Slant Board Exercise 3

Lay on a slant board and relax. Breathe in deeply through your nose and out through your mouth five times. Then choose an area of your body that needs healing. Say a prayer and imagine that the air you breathe is filled with love and healing energy or healing microscopic particles. Breathe in the healing air and feel it go to the area of your body in need. Feel the healing air bathe that organ. Visualize it healed.

JUMPING ON A REBOUNDER

A rebounder is a mini-trampoline. Some fold and come with a carrying case for traveling. Jumping on a rebounder is lots of fun and can be done indoors on rainy days or outside on sunny days. Rebounder exercise is much better for you than jogging on hard pavement. Because the rebounder has springs, it prevents harsh jolts to the knees and spine. Rebounding exercises are not necessarily a substitute for jogging, nor is jogging a substitute for rebounding. Some people like jogging and it is a good form of exercise for those with strong legs, knees, spines, and the proper running shoes. While jogging is not for everyone, rebounding can be done by almost everyone. For those who feel unsteady on the rebounder, they are available with a support handle you can hold on to. Jumping on a rebounder several times a day greatly improves blood circulation. The flow of oxygen through the blood will help your brain function more effectively. The extra blood flowing through the eyes, carrying in nutrients and carrying away waste, will also help improve vision. You will feel invigorated and energized!

This exercise also greatly improves lymph circulation, ridding the body of metabolic wastes. We have about six pints of lymph in our body and ten pints of blood. The lymph fluid, which will not circulate without exercise, has many important functions. It carries nutrients to all the cells and carries off wastes. It lubricates the joints and helps prevent arthritic crystals from forming. The lymph also plays a primary role in immune function.

In addition, rebounder exercise can help tremendously with weight reduction. This exercise strengthens and tones every muscle in the body and burns fat. It even helps reduce stress!

When on your rebounder, always jump on the balls of your feet. This will strengthen the spine. You can jog in place, do jumping jacks, or just jump, bending your knees with both feet together. Have fun on your rebounder. Play some lively music or shout positive affirmations while you are jumping, such as: "I am healthy!" or "I am strong!" or "I am well!"

If you are weak from an illness, start slowly on a rebounder. Keep your feet on the mat. Just bounce gently. If you can't stand, sit on a rebounder with your feet on the floor and bounce gently.

SWIMMING

Swimming is a wonderful form of exercise. It allows the body to be weightless and, in the case of injured sore muscles, makes it much easier to move than outside the water. If you can't swim, do gentle water aerobics or just walk several laps in a pool of water up to your waist. Swimming helps strengthen and tone muscles, improve the circulation of the blood and the lymph, and alleviate pain caused by arthritis, fibromyalgia, and sciatica. Swimming greatly strengthens the lungs because one has to breathe in oxygen, hold while under water, and breath out. Swimming can enhance metabolism and aide in weight loss if one is overweight.

DOING WATER AEROBICS

Water aerobics are great for anyone, but especially for people who are overweight or have arthritis, back problems, sciatica, or fibromyalgia. It is also great for anyone who has had surgery for a cardiovascular disorder. Water exercise cushions the body providing a feeling of weightlessness while toning the tendons and muscles and providing a good cardiovascular workout.

RIDING A BICYCLE

Riding a bicycle can be lots of fun. You can ride on a stationary bike indoors or ride outside in the fresh air and sunshine. (Morning sun before 11:00 A.M. and afternoon sun after 4:00 P.M. are best to avoid getting too hot or sunburned.) If you have back trouble, raise the handlebars so you can sit up straight rather than having to bend over. There are even tricycles for the handicapped and older people who might feel safer on them. Cycling is a great exercise for people with sore feet who may not feel like walking. Biking strengthens the legs. The legs help pump blood and lymph to all parts of the body. Different leg muscles are put to use going up hill versus downhill. Cycling for half an hour is a good aerobic exercise that gives the cardiovascular system a great workout.

HIKING

Hiking is wonderful, especially if you do it in the mountains. Mountain air has lots of healing negative ions that help to balance and energize the body. Hiking builds the legs and pumps the lymph fluid. The deep breathing is also great for the lungs.

WALKING

Walking in sunshine and fresh air is one of the most wonderful exercises you can do. Swing your arms. This will help the lymph glands under the arms to move the lymph fluid. It will tone and tighten the muscles, strengthen the heart, and build the lungs. Try to walk from one to two miles five times per week.

Walking on Sand

Whenever possible, walk barefoot on the sand. Sand walking stimulates circulation in the legs and helps strengthen the leg muscles. This is an excellent therapy for poor circulation as well as for relieving sciatica. If you live near the ocean, walk in the cold water and on the sandy beach. If you do not live near the ocean, build a long sandbox in your yard that you can walk in daily.

Walking Barefoot

Just walking barefoot on the earth is immensely healing. The earth is filled with minerals and magnetic energy that help tremendously to balance our bodies. Insomnia, nervous tension, and anxiety have all been cured with this simple exercise.

DOING YOGA AND TAI CHI

Yoga and tai chi are gentle exercises that move the lymph fluid. They stretch and strengthen the muscles without hard impact on the feet, knees, or legs.

EYE EXERCISES

Whether or not you have problems with vision, exercising your eyes is a good idea for everyone to help strengthen and preserve eyesight. Most people do not realize that the eyes are vascular and carry blood, oxygen, and nutrients through them. When blood does not flow properly through your eyes, you are apt to have all sorts of eye diseases. Oxygen kills harmful bacteria that may get into the eyes, and nutrients feed the eyes and keep them healthy, thus preserving good vision.

Eye Exercise 1

I learned this exercise from Reverend LaWanna Rine, who owns and operates a beautiful health retreat called Lotus Lodge in Strasburg, Ohio. Splash your eyes each morning with cold water fifteen to twenty times. While you are splashing say, "I dedicate my eyes to seeing the beauty that God has made." Cold water helps stimulate blood flow through the eyes.

Eye Exercise 2

If your eyes are tired, look out the window as far as you can see, hopefully at a tree, lake, field, or something equally pleasant. If you live in the city, step outside and look up at the sky. This is a very relaxing exercise for the eyes.

Eye Exercise 3

Lie on a slant board or sit in a chair and look up, then down, then to the right and to the left. This is another good exercise to stimulate blood flow through the eyes and strengthen the muscles around the eyes.

Eye Exercise 4

Try rubbing the palms of your hands together until they are hot, then place them over your eyes. Do this several times per day. The energy flowing through your heated hands will help to strengthen your eyes.

BREATHING DEEPLY

Most people do not breathe properly! Many people are in a hurry and become shallow breathers as they rush around. When I was eleven years old, after spinal surgery for scoliosis, I wore a body cast that weighed twenty-five pounds for a year. It fit tightly around my neck and chest and kept me from breathing as deeply as I should have. As an adult, I took breathing exercises for two years from Professor Linda Sudermann in Switzerland, which helped me tremendously. I had fewer aches, spoke more clearly and evenly, and learned to pace myself and feel more relaxed. Breathing, which includes inhaling oxygen and exhaling carbon dioxide is vital to good health. People often have aches and pains that are caused by a lack of oxygen and a buildup of carbon dioxide in the area of discomfort.

Practice deep breathing by pausing throughout the day and allowing a breath to slowly rise from deep down within your abdomen. Then slowly release the breath. Always breathe in through your nose and out through your nose. Try putting some reminders around your living area, such as red dots from an office supply store, to help you remember to breathe fully. Deep breathing greatly benefits the adrenal glands and can be especially beneficial to people with muscle aches or fibromyalgia.

Tool Kit for Choosing Rejuvenating Body Treatments and Beauty Aids

A healthy person with good muscle tone, clear eyes, strong teeth, glowing skin, shiny hair, and a positive attitude about life is a beautiful person. Even models and movie stars are beginning to realize that heavy makeup and expensive clothes over a malnourished, exhausted body does not make a beautiful person. Here are some tools for helping your body stay healthy and truly beautiful.

REJUVENATING BODY TREATMENTS

Over the years, people have become aware of rejuvenating body treatments. Spas have sprung up everywhere and going to a spa and getting the various treatments available is not only enjoyable but also promotes good health and well-being. We feel pampered and rested when we have just come from the spa. Now you can incorporate many of these delightful treats for the body in the privacy of your own home. Realize that your body deserves to be nurtured and try some of these treatments on a daily basis. Practicing good body care as part of your lifestyle will not only make you feel better and look more youthful, it will also help you to form a genuine appreciation and love for yourself. Learn to carve out the time to light a candle and soak in a nice relaxing bath, soak your feet, do some skin brushing, or apply a facial mask. The mere act of taking some time for youself, will give you a great feeling inside.

Skin Treatments

The skin is the body's largest organ, and it has often been called the third kidney because it releases some of the same toxins the kidneys do. The skin covers a two-square-yard area on the average adult and weighs about six pounds. It protects us from the destructive effects of harmful bacteria and excessive sunlight.

The skin mirrors our general well-being. When the skin is not working properly, pores can become congested, and acne or boils may appear. Uric acid builds up in the body when the skin is underactive. Also, when the other channels of elimination such as the kidneys, bowel, and lungs are not eliminating properly, many of the toxins from those organs are routed to the skin.

Skin Brushing

The skin can eliminate uric acid crystals, catarrh, and various other acids more easily when the top layer of dead skin cells has been removed. Skin brushing is the most efficient way to remove dead skin cells. Use a natural bristle brush with a long handle.

Brush your skin for two to three minutes each morning when it is dry, before you shower. Move the brush over your body in a circular motion, starting with the soles of your feet. The feet have reflex points that connect with most of the body's organs, and brushing them can stimulate those points. Continue brushing up your legs in a circular motion and move upward toward your heart. When you have reached your chest area, continue to brush in a circular motion. Then begin brushing at the palms of your hands, using a circular motion, and progress toward your heart again. Men and women should avoid brushing the nipples. Brush your back as best you can stroking from top to bottom with the long handle attached to your brush. A smaller, softer brush can be used to brush your face. Skin brushing is excellent for circulating the blood and lymph fluid, preventing wrinkles, and tightening and softening the skin. It also releases uric acid crystals and other toxins in the skin, and helps break up cellulite, and prevents moles, warts, and skin tags from forming. So brush your skin each day to ensure good skin health and add a special glow to your skin.

Bathing

The skin is a vital organ with living pores. Therefore, it is important to use filtered water without chlorine in it when you bathe or shower. Chlorine is a poison; most cities add cholorine to their water to kill harmful bacteria. However, chlorine can also kill beneficial bacteria that live on the skin. Chlorine is also an irritant and can cause skin rashes, and it can dry out the healthy oils that keep our skin soft and pliable.

When bathing or showering in chlorinated water, the body absorbs some chlorine and carries it into the bloodstream, where it can damage friendly organisms. The blood then carries the chlorine to the liver, placing an extra burden there.

Taking a shower with filtered water or water filtered through a magnetic filter, alternating hot and cold water, greatly improves circulation and can relieve aches and pains. Hot water sends blood rushing through our veins and opens our pores to release toxins. Cold water slows down the blood and closes the pores.

Soothing Baths

Relaxing in a soothing bath filled with warm water and therapeutic ingredients has many health-promoting benefits. It makes you take time to relax and release the stresses of the day. It calms the nerves. It gives you time out from work, friends, and family to put your thoughts in order, read an enjoyable book, or ponder and work out something that may be disturbing to you. Baths can have various different ingredients added to them that can release tight muscles or heal the skin. Some baths can promote blood circulation, induce sweating, or break a fever. Other baths are just for the feet in order to help them relax or provide healing to various foot disorders. Historically, hydrotherapy (the use of water to heal the body) has been used by many cultures including ancient Rome, China, and Greece. Try some soothing baths, you'll be glad you did!

Lemon Juice, Red Clover Tea, and Baking Soda Bath. If you have skin problems such as psoriasis, eczema, dry skin, fungus, or ringworm, or would just like to cleanse your pores and have silky-smooth skin, try this bath. This bath also helps abolish halitosis (bad breath).

Chop four lemons into eighths and place them into a cheesecloth or mesh bag. Knot the ends so they don't fall out, and put the whole thing into a tub of very warm filtered water. Add two cups of red clover tea and two cups of baking soda, and soak for half an hour. The water may turn blue, green, or gray from toxins your body emits.

Foot Bath for Fungus. Use a foot bath to get rid of fungus on feet and toes, such as athlete's foot fungus. Pour two gallons of hot water into a basin. Add two tablespoons food-grade hydrogen peroxide. Soak your feet for twenty minutes to half an hour. NOTE: Food-grade hydrogen peroxide is very different from most peroxide. Food-grade peroxide is 35 percent peroxide while most peroxide is only 3 percent. Food grade peroxide is a stronger, more pure peroxide and more effective in healing baths. Never spill it directly on the skin. If you do, the skin will foam, lighten, and tingle. Wash it with cold water immediately. All food-grade peroxide should be diluted before using. It is difficult to find food-grade peroxide in a local pharmacy or health food store. See resources in the back of this book to learn where to order.

Circulatory Treatments

The following baths are used specifically for improving circulation or breaking a fever. Hot baths relax and soothe the muscles. Baths should be comfortably hot, never hot enough to scald. Ginger in a hot bath will relax and soothe but also promote circulation and help break a fever. Cold baths invigorate the body and encourage the flow of blood. NOTE: If you have heart disease, high or low blood pressure, multiple sclerosis, or diabetes consult your doctor before you try any of the following baths. Pregnant women should avoid long hot baths as well as cold baths. Children and elderly people should bathe only in warm water; baths that are too hot may tire them. Otherwise, baths that promote circulation are very healing for the body.

Epsom Salts Bath

If your muscles are tired and sore from tension after a long day or because you have strained or pulled them, try an Epsom salts bath.

Add three cups of Epsom salts to a tub of hot water. Make the water as hot as you can physically stand it. Soak for a minimum of fifteen minutes. Rinse off thoroughly. The magnesium in the Epsom salt helps relax muscles and relieves pain. The hot salt bath also helps the body release toxins. You may feel a little weak when you get out of the bath, so step out carefully or have someone nearby you can call on for help. This bath is not recommended if you are pregnant, have high blood pressure, or have open wounds.

Ginger Bath

If you have chills from a high fever or suffer from numbness and cold hands or feet due to poor circulation, try a hot ginger bath.

Place two tablespoons of powdered ginger into a tub of warm, filtered water, and soak for at least fifteen minutes. Rinse well afterward. Ginger warms the body and can substantially improve circulation. You will feel warm and tingly all over after a ginger bath. Dry off well and dress warmly or snuggle under some flannel blankets.

Kneipp Leg Baths

Father Sebastian Kneipp of Woershofen, Germany, developed this treatment, which has healed thousands of people with aching legs, poor circulation, and numbness and tingling in the limbs. Father Kneipp had people walk in cold water up to their knees for thirty feet and then walk on grass or sand until they were dry. You can walk in cold water in your bathtub for a count of thirty, but do not towel off; if possible, go out and walk in the grass. Allow the air to dry you to receive the bath's full benefits.

This therapy can also be accomplished with a garden hose. Run the water over your feet and ankles first—the body parts furthest from your heart. Then let the water run over your toes all the way up one leg to the groin, around to the back of your leg and back down the front of your leg. Do this five or six times on both legs for best results. Walk or run until your legs dry.

Another good Kneipp therapy is to place your arms in cold water up to your shoulders. Move your arms in a circular motion through the water for five or ten minutes. Let them dry naturally. This is a great therapy for the blood circulating through the heart.

Cold Sheet Treatment

The famous American herbalist John R. Christopher originally developed the cold sheet treatment, and it's very effective in helping the body sweat out toxins and reduce persistent fevers. Do this only when a capable person or skilled practitioner is available to assist through the entire process.

Make some peppermint tea and have two cups ready within reach of your bathtub. Take a square, porous cotton cloth and add one tablespoon of powdered ginger, one tablespoon of powdered mustard, and two teaspoons of cayenne pepper. Take the opposite two corners of the cloth and tie them together into a knot. Do the same with the remaining two opposite corners. Prepare a bucket of ice-cold water. Place a white cotton sheet in the cold water, and place the bucket near your bathtub. Cover the bed where you will be sleeping with plastic wrap, and save enough plastic wrap to cover yourself. Have a lot of warm blankets available as well. Drop the herbal "tea bag" into a tub of hot water.

Cover any tender areas such as under the arms, nipples, genitals, or any wounded areas where there may be a cut or scratch completely with Dr. Christopher's Complete Tissue and Bone cream (see resources) before getting into the tub, to prevent burning. While in the tub, drink the two cups of peppermint tea. Try to stay in the tub for fifteen minutes to half an hour. When you step out of the tub, have someone wrap the sheet soaked in cold water around you and help you get into the plastic-wrapped bed.

Lie with the cold wet sheet around you on the plastic-wrapped bed and have someone wrap plastic over the top of you and the cold sheet. Then have your assistant cover you with warm blankets. Stay in this cocoon overnight. You may get up the next morning and take a shower. There may be colorations on the sheet from areas where you sweated profusely.

Warming Bath for Circulation

A warm bath is great for improving the circulation. It promotes sweating, which releases toxins from the skin and can be used at the first signs of fever or flu. Place one tablespoon each of yarrow herb, peppermint leaf, elder flowers, and ground or powdered ginger in a gallon-size pot. Pour two quarts of boiling water over the herbs, and let it simmer for ten minutes. Strain the mixture and pour it into a warm bath. Soak in the bath at least twenty minutes. Rinse with cool water, dry off well, and get into bed with lots of warm covers and stay for at least an hour. If you have taken your bath at night, you can go to bed for the night.

Foot Bath for Sore Feet

For tired, aching, sore feet, pour two gallons of hot water into a basin. Add one-half cup of sea salt and ten drops of lavender oil. Soak feet for twenty minutes to half an hour.

Facial Treatments

The face and head are areas that are exposed to the air, heat, cold, and elements more than any other part of the body. If the face is unhealthy with acne or any skin infection, we often feel self-conscious because it is the part of the body we show most to the world. Having headaches is no fun either and can keep us from enjoying our family and friends or from getting our work done. Taking care of our face, head, and scalp is an important part of an overall lifestyle to promote a healthy body. The following are treatments to help address headaches, facial acne or infections, and take care of the hair and scalp.

Facial Exercises

It is important to exercise your face in order to keep the skin healthy and to avoid getting wrinkles and bags under the eyes. Facial exercises also help eliminate headaches by stimulating blood circulation throughout the face and head.

On each hand, place your pointer finger and middle finger together. Place both sets of fingers at the center of your forehead so they are touching. Press your fingers gently against your temple. Maintaining a slight pressure, move the fingers of your left hand to the left and the fingers of your right hand to the right. Lower your fingers slightly until they are just outside your eyes. Then gently move your fingers back to where you started. Do this three times. Now gently move your fingers up from the edge of your eyes toward your hairline. Do this several times. Then place the two fingers of each hand at the crease between your nose and the cheeks on each side. Press in three times. Then move your fingers up from each side of your nose toward the outer edge of your eyes up to the hairline, three times. Now place the first two fingers of both hands together at the center of your chin and move them outward along your jawline and toward the tips of your ears, three times. Start again with the two fingers of both hands in the center of your chin, and press in and move down your throat, three times.

If you have a headache, do all these facial exercises and continue onto the back of your head. Place the two fingers of both hands together right in the center of the back of your head, and press in and move down your head, three times. Separate all the fingers of each hand, and place them on top of either side of your head and press in, three times. Return to the front of your head, and place the tip of each middle finger at the beginning of each eyebrow, and move toward the nose. Press in three times. Place your fingertips in the middle of your brows and press in three times. Finally, place the tip of each middle finger at the end of each brow near the outer edge of the eyes and press in three times. I have known people whose headaches have disappeared completely with these exercises alone. No aspirin required!

Honey and Ginger Facial Mask for Cleansing Pores

Cleansing the pores of the face removes the dirt and grime that has accumulated in them. Here is a wonderful mask to help you do so. The honey and ginger facial mask will also tighten and tone the skin, and bring good circulation to the face.

Heat two tablespoons of raw organic honey until it is warm, but not boiling. Add one teaspoon of ground oat flour and one-eighth teaspoon of powdered ginger and stir. Apply the mask carefully to your forehead, cheeks, jaws, chin, and neck. Avoid your eyes and the area just under your eyes. Let the mask dry. You will feel a pleasant tightening and tingling. To remove the mask, place a steaming-hot wet washcloth over your face or hold your face over a bowl of steaming water. When you have removed the mask, massage some almond oil into your face. It will feel clean and refreshed!

Facial Treatment to Maintain Youthful Skin

Blend half a cucumber and half an avocado in a blender. Massage onto your face and leave on for fifteen to twenty minutes. The cucumber is very cooling and soothing, and the avocado helps nourish the pores with essential fatty acids. This treatment helps reduce wrinkles and dryness, making your skin look young and supple.

Facial Treatment for Acne

Boil two quarts of water. Pour it into a large bowl. Add ten drops of tea tree oil and five drops of lavender oil. Place a towel over your head, and hold your face over the steam. This will open and cleanse your pores. When you are finished, apply a paste made of oregano oil and goldenseal root powder to your face. (Break open four to six capsules of goldenseal. Add three drops of oil of oregano and just enough distilled water to make a paste. If your face tends to be dry, add olive oil to the goldenseal mixture instead of water.) Spread the paste onto any acne, and leave it on for at least an hour. Then rinse your face with warm water, and when it is clean, rinse with cold water to close the pores. Spray the face with colloidal silver of 10 parts per million several times per day. Use natural collagen cream to tighten the pores. NOTE: This treatment has also been known to improve conditions of rosacea.

Scalp Treatments

The scalp or the skin under our hair is teaming with thousands of pores and hair follicles. When these become congested with hardened oil, dirt, or bodily toxins, it can affect the health of our hair. Here are a few scalp treatment that have helped many to get rid of dandruff or scalp itching and to increase hair growth.

Scalp Treatment for Hair Loss 1

Warm one-fourth cup of sesame oil in a small stainless steel pan. Do not boil it. Massage the oil into your scalp, and wrap a hot wet towel around your head. Warm the towel again when it cools by dipping it into hot water. Leave the towel around your head for a half hour. Then wash your scalp with a biotin or keratin shampoo (found at health food stores). Do this three times per week. This treatment helps slow hair loss and in some cases has strengthened and thickened the hair.

Scalp Treatment for Hair Loss 2

Blend one egg yolk with three tablespoons of juice from a freshly squeezed lemon. Massage the mixture into your scalp. Leave it in while you are taking a shower, then wash your hair with a biotin or keratin shampoo. The protein from the yolk helps nourish the hair follicles. I don't know of any research on this but have used it with my clients for years with good success in slowing hair loss and strengthening and thickening existing hair.

NOTE: For more treatments on hair loss, I would highly recommend the book called, *Grow Hair and Stop Hair Loss* by Riquette Hofstein. Riquette uses natural therapies that have worked for many celebrities in bringing new hair growth to the scalp where there was none before. (See resources.)

Scalp Treatment for Dandruff

Gather ten leaves of fresh spearmint, wash them well, and place them into a blender. Add a quarter cup of organic, raw apple cider vinegar, one tablespoon of jojoba oil, and five drops of tea tree oil or five drops of oil of oregano. Blend the mixture well, then massage into your scalp. Wash your hair with a pine tar shampoo.

BEAUTY AIDS

Beauty aids are so readily available everywhere we go but are often full of chemicals that may not be that good for us. Remember, whatever we put on the outside of our bodies often soaks in to the inside and is picked up by the blood and carried through the liver. More and more, companies are coming out with more natural ingredients for our skin, hair, and nails. Read ingredients. If the words are long and complicated, they are probably not that good for you. The following are some great beauty aids for coloring the hair that contain only botanical ingredients from nature. They will bring highlights to the hair and nourish and strengthen it as well.

Hair Coloring

Some people maintain their natural hair color up until the day they pass away, while others become gray in their early twenties. The length of time that hair retains its original color is often based on genetics. Good nutrition and a clean, healthy colon may also affect hair color. Studies have shown that minerals, including zinc, and the B vitamins, especially PABA (para-aminobenzoic acid), can help prolong the length of time hair maintains its original color. The tiny villi that line the intestinal tract absorb these nutrients. If the colon is congested, prohibiting absorption, the body cannot utilize them.

Rice bran syrup is high in the B vitamins and blackstrap molasses is high in the minerals necessary for hair color. Hypoglycemics have difficulty breaking down the natural sugars found in blackstrap molasses and rice bran syrup; liquid ionized trace minerals and a good B-complex food supplement are an alternative.

Most hair dyes contain ammonia and other chemicals that are very toxic to the human body. Please remember that whatever we put on our skin or scalp is absorbed through tiny living pores and passed on to the blood. The brain is close to the scalp, and it is the first organ to be affected by the chemicals in hair dyes. If you like to color or highlight your hair, don't be discouraged. There are natural hair colors available that do not contain ammonia. Check with your health food store for information about these. Henna is a wonderful natural hair color made from a plant that has been used to color the hair for ages. It actually feeds and nourishes the hair and scalp with healthy nutrients and gives the hair red highlights. Additional hair rinses made from herbs follow.

Hair Rinse for Blondes

Prepare chamomile tea by placing a tablespoon of chamomile leaves in sixteen ounces of boiling water. Let it steep until it is warm, then add the juice of one raw organic lemon. Stir the mixture well, then strain it. Pour the rinse through your hair and let it sit for about ten minutes while you take a shower. Then wash your hair with a natural shampoo and rinse it well. Natural shampoos that bring out blonde highlights are available in health food stores.

Hair Rinse for Brown or Chestnut-Colored Hair

Bring one cup of raw organic apple cider vinegar to a boil. Add two teaspoons of sage leaves and one-half teaspoon of decaffeinated black tea. (Avoid caffeinated tea, for even on the scalp the caffeine is absorbed and can cause sensitive people to feel wired!) Steep the tea until it is warm, then strain it. Pour the rinse through your hair, and let it sit for approximately ten minutes while you bathe or shower. Wash your hair with a natural shampoo and rinse it.

Hair Rinse for Brunettes

Bring one cup of raw organic apple cider vinegar to a boil. Add two teaspoons of decaffeinated black tea and let it steep until warm. Pour the rinse through your hair, and let it sit for ten minutes. Shampoo your hair with a natural shampoo, then rinse it. Natural shampoos for brunettes are available in health food stores.

Hair Rinse for Redheads

Bring one-half cup of raw organic apple cider vinegar to a boil. When it has cooled but is still warm, add a half cup of fresh beet juice, juiced in your juicer. Stir the mixture well, then pour the rinse through hair. Let it sit for ten minutes. Shampoo your hair and rinse it. Natural shampoos that bring out red tones are available in health food stores.

NATURAL TOILETRIES

Look in your bathroom cabinet and read the labels on all the bottles there. They should all contain natural ingredients that would not be harmful to swallow. Try to avoid using any toiletries that contain aluminum or synthetic chemicals. These are all toxic to the human body. Do not use spray deodorants in an aerosol can. They are as harmful to breathe as they are to put into the open pores under the arms. They are also contributing to the thinning of Earth's ozone layer. Make sure the toiletries contain nourishing nutrients that will "feed" the skin.

Lotions

It is best to use lotions that have nutrients that nourish and feed the skin. Look for lotions containing natural herbs, vitamins, and aloe vera. Avoid lotions that contain dyes, artificial fragrances, and chemicals.

Mouthwash and Toothpaste

The mouth is like a small ecosystem, containing saliva, enzymes, and friendly bacteria that help combat harmful bacteria. If you use mouthwash and toothpaste with flouride, dyes, and chemicals, you can cause a disturbance in the natural balance maintained inside your mouth. In addition, you will absorb and swallow a portion of these chemicals each time you use them. Use natural toothpastes and mouthwashes that are high in minerals and healthy ingredients that can actually nurture your mouth and gums.

Mouthwash for Gum Infections ————————————

- 2 capsules of goldenseal
- 1 cup distilled water
- 1/2 teaspoon tea tree oil or 2 drops oil of wild oregano
- 1 dropper of colloidal silver, 10 ppm

Break open the capsules of goldenseal, and use the contents only, not the capsule. Mix all the ingredients together. Swish the mouthwash through your mouth four to six times per day.

Soaps and Shampoos

Most soaps and shampoos contain harmful chemicals. Use soaps and shampoos made from natural ingredients, which can actually nourish the skin. Aubrey Organics, for example, makes soaps and shampoos with excellent ingredients that can feed the skin with vitamins and minerals. I am sure there are other companies that use only all natural ingredients, but I have done quite a bit of research on Aubrey and can safely say that all of their products are completely pure and natural. You can buy Aubrey products at any good health food store.

Deodorants

Remember that whatever we use on our skin is absorbed into the bloodstream through our pores. Most deodorants that we rub on our skin contain aluminum, propylene glycol, artificial colors, artificial preservatives, and artificial fragrances. These chemicals can be poisonous and dangerous. There are some very nice deodorants available now that are free of these harmful ingredients. Natural deodorants often contain witch hazel, grapefruit seed extract, and lavender oil, which are antibacterial. Some have wonderful natural fragrances such as jasmine, mint, and lemon. Our body needs to sweat in order to remove toxins. A healthy body will naturally have different odors than a toxic body. A healthy body will have very little smell while a toxic body can smell very foul like bad breath. Soaking in a baking soda bath can remedy excessive body odors. To keep your underarms dry, try some natural powders that work as antiperspirants from your health food store.

CLOTHING

The clothing we wear has a tremendous effect on our skin. Synthetic clothing can keep our skin from breathing properly, and it can prevent our skin from eliminating as it should. Often synthetic clothing is made with very strong dyes and preservative chemicals, which can cause skin allergies. Wear clothing made of natural fibers such as cotton, hemp, silk, or wool. It is especially important for you to wear comfortable clothing made of natural fibers during a cleanse to allow your skin to receive fresh air through the clothing and be better able to release toxins through your pores.

SLEEP

Getting a deep, restful sleep each night is crucial to good health, so the body can mend and repair itself. Every sick person is fatigued, and there are many reasons people suffer from insomnia. If you have a major sleep disorder you could be suffering from sleep apnea, which is dangerous and should be checked by a physician. According to Norman Ford in *How to Get a Good Night's Sleep*:

> *Obstructive Sleep Apnea (OSA), a disorder that exists only during sleep and cannot be diagnosed while awake. Apnea is caused by accumulations of fat around the upper respiratory tract at the back of the throat. As muscle tone relaxes during sleep, the surplus fat falls back and chokes the airway, completely blocking intake of air to the lungs. The body's vital oxygen supply may be cut off for a full minute or more at a time. Apnea, a frequent and potentially deadly disorder, affects 20 million Americans, mostly overweight middle-aged males. Records show that one of every 4 males over 35 has some degree of apnea, while apnea afflicts one of every two males over 65. All these people suffer from dangerously low levels of oxygen in the bloodstream and brain while asleep. And the constant stress created by deprivation of slow-wave and REM sleep leads to high blood pressure in 60 percent of apneics.*

Dr. Dave Carpenter further explains this in his article, "Healthy Sleep Habits" from the website www.path-to-health.com:

> *To have a basic understanding of the sleep cycle and how it works, let's talk about the pineal gland and what it does. This tiny gland produces two hormones that are key to sleeping and waking. Melatonin is produced as it gets dark and helps us sleep while seratonin is produced by light stimulation and wakes us up. Studies show that even when you are sleeping soundly in the middle of the night, headlights from a passing car shining into your room or someone turning on the light in the bathroom and temporarily lighting your room, will cause the pineal gland to stop producing melatonin and begin to wake you up.*

There are many causes for insomnia. One is a bad mattress. If you are sleeping on a soft, lumpy mattress, your body may ache the next morning. There are many wonderful mattresses on the market today. Go to the store and lay on several to see which one supports your body and feels best to you. Some mattresses have been well researched. They support the body with air rather than metal coils. These mattresses allow the body to completely relax. There are also great memory-foam mattresses that support and move with the contours of the body. They are firm and support the spine, but wonderfully soft at the same time so no part of the body feels pressure. Hard mattresses may support the spine but can be very uncomfortable to the muscles as they don't give with the shape of the body. For those who don't want to invest in an entire memory-foam bed, they also make memory foam pads that can be placed on top of any mattress. Futons are another option in bedding. They were originally designed in Japan stuffed with cotton or synthetic batting. They were made to be folded away during the day and stored in a closet. American futons usually have a bit more padding and are placed on a frame that can fold into a couch during the day. All futons lack the springs and synthetic casings of true mattresses. Futons in this country are usually made of cotton and are very "earth friendly." Search around, try them all and see what works best for you.

Another robber of sleep is worry. If you feel worried when you lie down at night, write down all your troubles or make a list of what you want to accomplish the next day. Once you have recorded your concerns on paper and your subconscious mind knows the issues will be taken care of, you can fall asleep much more easily.

Eating late in the evening can also keep the body from resting. If the body is having to digest food, it can't fully relax and go to sleep. Eating foods high in sugar or drinking caffeine or alcohol in the evening can keep you awake as well; you may fall asleep, but you will wake up hungry between 1:00 and 3:00 A.M. when your blood sugar drops. The liver cleanses around the same time, and fried foods, sugar, and alcohol in your system can cause the liver distress when it begins to process them, causing further restlessness. Eat a light meal at night, and don't eat after 7:00 P.M. Have a glass of raw vegetable juice around 9:00 P.M. to hold your blood sugar steady through the night and promote a restful sleep. If needed, take some calcium and magnesium in liquid form to help your body relax.

Sleeping late in the morning and a lack of exercise can keep you from sleeping at night. Try to get up by 7:00 A.M., and get some fresh air and exercise each day. Walking barefoot on the earth has proven to be a wonderful sleep promoting therapy. Avoid watching violence on TV before you go to bed. Allow your body and subconscious mind to be calm. Be thankful for all the good things in your life. Take a warm bath. Write in your journal. Listen to relaxing music. Have a cup of chamomile tea. Remove all electrical devices from around your bed, such as radios, telephones, televisions, electric clocks, and electric blankets. Studies have shown that these can interfere with sleep.

Try to be in bed by 10:00 P.M. If you are ill, go to bed by 9:00 P.M. Our bodies were designed to sleep when the sun sets and wake with the sunrise. Sleep is crucial to healing, good health, and long life. Do everything you can to allow your body to receive deep, restful sleep.

Tool Kit for Preparing Poultices and Salves

Natural poultices are soft moist concoctions that can be made from oils, vegetables, or herbs. They are often heated and wrapped in a cotton cloth or gauze and placed on an aching, painful, inflamed or sore area of the body. They can also be used to heal wounds where a buildup of pus needs to be drawn out. Some poultices provide nutrients to the area or herbs that promote circulation and blood flow. Other poultices might be drawing in nature to help pull toxins from the body. Cold poultices may be used to decrease inflammation or heat in an area. Natural salves are ointments made from herbs and oils that can be applied directly to the affected area to help heal a wound, cut, or burn. Salves may have antibacterial ingredients that fight infection. Poultices and salves can be purchased premade, but these often contain synthetic chemicals and may not be as effective as natural ones that you make yourself. If you do decide to buy a poultice or salve, natural ones are available in health food stores. Read ingredients. Following are some poultice and salve recipes that may be helpful during times of need.

CABBAGE POULTICE

Cabbage poultices help heal varicose veins because they improve circulation and act as an astringent to tighten and heal the stretched tissue in the vascular walls.

1 cup cabbage, chopped
1 to 2 tablespoons marshmallow root or slippery elm bark powder
$^1/_3$ cup raw apple cider vinegar

Place the cabbage and herbs in a blender with the raw apple cider vinegar, and blend the mixture into a thick paste. Smear the paste on any varicosities (swollen areas on your leg), and wrap the area with plastic wrap. Keep your legs propped up through the night on a pillow while wearing this poultice. Rinse your legs well the next day.

CASTOR OIL POULTICE

Castor oil is a natural anti-inflammatory and has been used for centuries to heal and repair various parts of the body. Someone in the Middle Ages was so impressed by its healing abilities, they called the castor bean plant the *Palma Christi,* or the palm of Christ. The castor bean plant is indeed a beautiful plant with large palmate leaves. Heritage Products and Home Health make the best castor oil. Castor oil should be pure, cold-pressed, hexane free, and certified. It can be purchased in any good health food store. It has been known to be helpful in aiding the detoxification processes in the body.

Castor oil has many wonderful topical uses. As William A. McGarey, MD, writes in *The Oil That Heals:*

> *We still have no explanation why castor oil placed in the ear canal will be so helpful to a child with a hearing problem, or why a pack using this oil will help restore normalcy to a hyperactive child, or speed up the healing of hepatitis, or help to get rid of gallstones or even help heal abrasions and infections. Perhaps it is to be found in the human body and the secret healing capabilities of the substances God gave us here on the earth for our use and benefit.*

Castor oil has been beneficial in treating warts, reducing the size of bone spurs, healing scar tissue, reducing fibroids and healing endometriosis, cleansing the liver, and reducing tumors. It has also been used over the abdomen in cases of nonmalignant ovarian cysts, liver disorders, abdominal pain, diarrhea, constipation, menstrual cramping, and gallbladder inflammation and stones. It has been used on the forehead to reduce headaches, on the spine to reduce backache, and on painful joints and sprained ankles. NOTE: Castor oil should not be used during pregnancy on any part of the back or abdomen, and it should not be used on an active ulcer or bleeding wound. People with chemical sensitivities should use it with caution or under the care of a physician, as the packs can draw more chemicals from the tissues of the body into the blood.

   1 tablespoon to ¹/₂ cup castor oil

Put enough castor oil in a cup to cover the affected area. For example, a tablespoonful may be enough to cover a small scar, while a large scar might require one third of a cup. If you are going to cover your entire back or your entire abdomen, it may take half a cup to saturate enough of the cloth to cover those areas. Put the cup in a pan of water. Simmer the water, but do not let it boil. Dip a cotton flannel cloth or wool flannel cloth into the warm oil. Lay it on the affected area, put plastic wrap over the cloth, and cover that with a towel. Place a heating pad on top set on a low to medium heat. Do not use high heat. Keep the poultice in place for one hour.

CHICKWEED AND CALENDULA OIL SALVE

Use this salve on rashes, psoriasis, eczema, or burns.

   2 tablespoons of dry or 3 tablespoons fresh chickweed
   2 tablespoons of dry or 3 tablespoons fresh marigold blossoms
   2 cups olive oil

Mix the chickweed and marigold into two cups of olive oil and let it sit for two weeks, shaking the container daily. Strain the oil through a cheesecloth, then apply it directly to the damaged skin. Store it in a dark bottle in a cool place.

COMFREY POULTICE

Comfrey poultices are wonderful for sprains and bruises. Comfrey is so powerful in mending and repairing that it has been called knitbone. It is also very helpful in clotting blood during heavy bleeding.

1 ounce dried comfrey root powder
$^1/_2$ cup distilled water
1 cup fresh comfrey leaf, chopped, or 2 tablespoons dried comfrey leaf, soaked
1 tablespoon pure virgin olive oil
10 drops tea tree oil
12 drops birch or lavendar oil

Soak the comfrey root in the distilled water overnight. Then simmer the mixture for fifteen minutes. Strain the mixture, and blend in the fresh comfrey leaf or dried comfrey leaf that has been soaked overnight and simmered for one minute and strained (just use the herb). Add the olive oil, tea tree oil, and birch or lavender oil. Spread the poultice onto the sprain, and cover it with plastic wrap.

EYE POULTICE

This poultice is very soothing for tired, sore, inflamed, swollen, or aching eyes.

$^1/_2$ cucumber
3 tablespoons distilled water

Place the cucumber and water in a blender. Blend into a mush. Divide mixture in half and spoon onto two 6-inch-square pieces of cheesecloth. Fold edges of cloth over the mixture, and place a poultice over each closed eyelid. Leave on for 30 minutes.

HERBAL POULTICE

This herbal poultice can be used anywhere on the body to draw out infections. It is especially good for a gum infection.

4 capsules slippery elm bark (break open and use contents only)
4 capsules white oak bark (break open and use contents only)

plaintain or comfrey powder (amount equivalent to slippery elm bark
   powder)
10 drops myrrh oil
10 drops thyme oil
5 drops clove oil
2 drops oil of wild oregano
10 drops Roman chamomile oil

Mix all the ingredients to form a paste. Cut a piece of cheesecloth to
form a two-inch by one-inch swatch. Spread the paste on the cheesecloth,
and roll it into an oblong poultice. Use dental floss to tie off each end. Place
the poultice between your gum and cheek, and leave it there from one to
eight hours. Use it during the day or at night. For infections on the body,
apply the paste directly, cover it with gauze, and tape it in place. Store these
poultices in a plastic zipper bag in the refrigerator.

ONION POULTICE

Onion poultices help draw out the poisons of colds, bronchitis, flu, and
pneumonia.

   2 to 4 onions, peeled
   2 tablespoons warm olive oil

Peel the onions, and bake them in the oven until well done. Mash
them in a bowl with two tablespoons of warm olive oil. Wrap the mash in
cotton cloths, and tie them onto your feet. You can also place an onion
pack on your chest. Cover the pack with plastic wrap, a thin towel, and a
warm heating pad.

PAIN RELIEF OIL SALVE

This oil helps relieve the pain of arthritis, aching joints, and sore muscles.
It stimulates blood flow and brings oxygen to the tissues, thereby promoting healing.

   8 ounces extra virgin olive oil
   1 cup dried calendula blossoms
   1 ounce eucalyptus oil
   1 cup dried arnica flowers
   2 ounces peppermint oil

2 tablespoons powdered cayenne pepper
8 ounces wintergreen oil pepper
3 tablespoons gingerroot, grated

Place all the ingredients in a quart jar. Let the mixture soak for three weeks. Strain the mixture, and keep it in a sterile glass airtight container. Use as needed. Be careful not to ingest this salve or get it into your eyes!

PLANTAIN POULTICE

1 cup fresh plaintain, chopped
4 ounces olive oil
2 ounces honey

Blend all the ingredients. Apply the mixture to insect bites, bee stings, or animal bites. This is also a wonderful poultice for burns.

SLIPPERY ELM AND MARSHMALLOW POULTICE

Use this poultice on bedsores, boils, blisters, burns, and wounds.

2 tablespoons slippery elm powder
2 tablespoons marshmallow root powder
2 tablespoons comfrey root powder
1 tablespoon goldenseal root powder
1 tablespoon myrrh powder
distilled water

Mix the powders together. Add enough warm distilled water to form a paste. Cover the wound with the paste, then wrap it with a bandage. Change the bandage once or twice daily.

TOMATO POULTICE

Tomato poultices are great for softening nursing mothers's caked breasts. They also may be used to soften hardened scabs on wounds.

1 cup tomatoes, chopped
1 tablespoon raw apple cider vinegar

Blend the ingredients together. Apply the poultice to the stiffened area.

WHEATGRASS POULTICE

These poultices are good for healing wounds of any kind. They are also excellent for any type of gum disease. Wheatgrass juice acts as a natural antiseptic and antibiotic.

After juicing wheatgrass, take enough of the pulp to cover the affected area and add a little of the juice (enough to saturate the pulp without dripping) back into it. Place the poultice directly on a wound such as a cut or burn. It will not burn and healing will be rapid. For gum problems, place the poultice inside your mouth between your gum and jaw.

WHEATGRASS JUICE EYE WASH

This wash is a great treatment for eye infections, sties, and bloodshot eyes, and it may even help cataracts.

1 teaspoon wheatgrass juice

Fill an eye cup with the wheatgrass juice. Tilt your head back and flush your eye. You can put an old towel around your shoulders in case of spillage.

WHEATGRASS JUICE VAGINAL DOUCHE

Wheatgrass juice will help heal vaginal infections, deodorize, and sanitize the vaginal tract.

3 to 4 ounces wheatgrass juice

Fill a three- to four-ounce syringe with wheatgrass juice, and insert it vaginally.

Tool Kit for Choosing Healing Therapies

In this tool kit, you will find the tools you need to help heal the organs, nerves, muscles, and bones of the body. For each body part, you will be given a nutritional plan and specific physical exercises as well as emotional therapies to follow. Remember, the body works as one whole unit. While working with any one particular body part, you will be helping the rest of your body as well. For example, when we heal the adrenal glands, it helps improve the work of the heart and nervous system as well. Each part of the body needs the specific nutrients it requires to be strong. It needs exercise and movement to promote circulation and strengthening, it also needs for you to work with any emotions that may be keeping it from healing. We are physical, emotional, and spiritual beings, and we need to attend to all these areas in order to know health as our birthright.

ADRENAL GLANDS

The two adrenal glands are small yellow masses of tissue that are triangular in shape and, true to their name (*ad* means near and *renal* means kidney), are situated on top of each kidney in the lower back. They are part of the endocrine system, which is made up of glands that secrete hormones directly into the bloodstream. Each adrenal gland is divided into two parts. The outer region is called the adrenal cortex. The inner core is known as the adrenal medulla. Although they are together anatomically, the cortex and the medulla are made of different types of tissue and function as distinct glands. Both help the body deal with stress and both help regulate metabolism.

The Adrenal Cortex: Vital to Life

The adrenal cortex's functions are vital. The adrenal cortex is divided into three zones which can be seen under a microscope. The outer zone secretes a hormone called aldosterone, which helps maintain blood pressure and blood volume by inhibiting the amount of sodium excreted in the urine. When there is a disturbance in the adrenal glands' functioning, too much sodium is excreted into the urine. This causes water to leave the body in large quantities, and the blood volume can become so low, a person could die of low blood pressure.

The middle and inner zones of the adrenal cortex work together and secrete several important hormones, including hydrocortisone, corticosterone, and androgen. Hydrocortisone, or cortisol, regulates metabolism and controls the way the body utilizes carbohydrates, proteins, and fats. Cortisol promotes production of glucose from amino acids and fats in the liver. This ensures adequate fuel supplies for the cells when the body is under stress. Hydrocortisone and corticosterone help suppress inflammatory reactions and regulate the immune system. They will act to suppress the immune system if it becomes overly reactive. Hydrocortisone counteracts inflammation, pain, and swelling of the joints due to arthritis and bursitis. Adrenocorticotropic hormone, or ACTH, produced by the pituitary gland in the brain, controls the secretion of hydrocortisone. Hydrocortisone is secreted in varying amounts throughout a twenty-four-hour cycle. A minimal amount is secreted at midnight, rising to a peak at 6:00 A.M., then falling slowly throughout the day.

The adrenal cortex produces a small amount of female hormones in men and male hormones in women. A tumor in this gland can cause an excessive amount to be produced, causing feminine characteristics in males and masculine characteristics in females. Androgen hormones found in the adrenal cortex help stimulate the development of male sex characteristics. When the adrenal gland is unhealthy, it can produce an excessive amount of androgen, which can cause acne. In women, an excessive amount of androgen can also cause the growth of body hair on the face, arms, chest, or abdomen.

The Adrenal Medulla: Important for Fight or Flight

Within the inner core of each adrenal gland is an adrenal medulla. The adrenal medulla's tissue develops from nerve tissue and it is controlled by the sympathetic nervous system, the body's first line of defense against stress. The adrenal medulla secretes the hormones epinephrine, or adrenaline, and norepinephrine, or noradrenaline, in response to sympathetic nerve stimulation. Epinephrine is also released in response to hypoglycemia. These hormones are secreted when a person is physically injured, frightened, angry, or under stress. The adrenal medulla prepares a person physiologically to deal with threatening situations. Epinephrine and norepinephrine bring about all the responses necessary for fight or flight. People have been known to perform amazing feats, such as carrying a heavy piece of furniture out of a burning house or lifting a car to free a child trapped underneath.

The adrenal medullary hormones cause blood to be routed to those organs necessary for emergency action. Blood vessels to the skin become constricted, thus protecting the body from blood loss in case of lacerations. This explains why people often look pale when they are afraid or angry. Blood vessels to the brain and muscles are dilated; increased blood flow to the brain allows the person to become instantly alert, while more blood flow to the muscles causes a person to have more stamina. Glucose and fatty acid levels rise in the blood, assuring that we have the necessary fuel for energy. All the airways become enlarged so we can breathe effectively. Epinephrine and norepinephrine are secreted daily in small amounts.

Thus, we can see how important it is to care for our adrenal glands and keep them healthy. Our ancestors used adrenaline to fight wild animals to protect their families. In today's world, people produce adrenaline while sitting at stoplights when they are late for a meeting or preparing for an examination. However, they often are not exercising to use up the adrenaline. Some stressors, such as unhappy marriages or job situations, can go on for years. Prolonged chronic stress is harmful because there are negative side effects to long-term elevated levels of cortisol. Excessive amounts of cortisol can lead to ulcers, high blood pressure, arthritis, fibromyalgia, and atherosclerosis. Excessive amounts of epinephrine can lead to exhaustion.

Emotional Therapies

- If you are in a job or marriage that is unhappy, seek counseling.
- Explore ways to make positive changes so you are not always under stress.
- Let go of fear and worry, and practice joy in your life.
- Find things to do that make you happy and nurture your soul.
- Give yourself credit after having accomplished a goal.
- Learn to trust the universe for your highest good in life. Trusting creates miracles while fear attracts fearful situations.

Exercise

- Practice deep, relaxed breathing—especially at those stoplights!
- Exercise on a regular basis. Yoga, walking, and swimming are wonderful for releasing stress.
- Get a massage on a regular basis.
- Take time to listen to music or read a positive book.
- Nurture friendships with positive people.
- Avoid television programs with violence.
- Eat in a relaxed atmosphere, and chew your food well. Eat dinner before 7:00 P.M., and go to bed by 10:00 P.M.
- Ensure a good night's sleep by resting on a comfortable mattress.
- Practice living in harmony with your body's natural rhythms.

Nutritional Suggestions

- Avoid stimulants such as caffeine, sugar, and nicotine.
- Take chlorella and spirulina, which are high in RNA and DNA, amino acids, and chlorophyll. They rejuvenate and cleanse the adrenal glands.
- Eat raw nuts and seeds. Soak the nuts and seeds for twenty-four hours; they will be easier to digest and the nutrients will be more fully available. Blend them to make dips and salad dressings.
- Eat licorice root, dulse, and kelp.
- Ingest ionic trace minerals.
- Take vitamin B complex, pantothenic acid, calcium, magnesium, and zinc keep the nervous system calm and support the adrenal glands.
- If you are suffering from exhaustion, take tablets of raw bovine adrenal.
- Herbs that calm and strengthen the adrenals are Chinese corticeps, ashwaganda, and schizandra.

APPENDIX

The appendix is a narrow tube attached to the cecum, or first part of the large intestine. It is located on the lower right side of the abdomen. N. W. Walker, DSC, writes in *Become Younger*, "The function of the appendix is to provide a secretion which prevents the feces from remaining stationary in the colon; at the same time its secretion neutralizes excessive putrefactive bacteria, in much the same way that the tonsils protect the throat." Appendicitis results when bacteria get into the appendix and it becomes swollen and inflamed. This is why it is so important to eat healthfully and keep our colons clean!

Nutritional Suggestions

- Eat cabbage and drink cabbage juice.
- Eat foods that are rich in sodium, such as celery, mineral whey, strawberries, and okra.
- Eat foods that are high in fiber, such as ground flaxseeds, oat bran, rice bran, whole grains, raw vegetables, alfalfa tablets, and chlorella.
- Include slippery foods, such as aloe vera juice, slippery elm tea, and flaxseed tea in your diet.
- Eat foods that are high in friendly bacteria, such as yogurt and raw sauerkraut.

- Include antiparasitic foods, such as garlic and onions, in your diet.
- Practice colon cleansing once or twice a year, and take parasite-fighting herbs, such as wormwood, cloves, black walnut, and garlic. The cecum is often called a "worm nest" because it's where parasites tend to lodge.
- Work on preventing constipation. When the colon becomes backed up with old fecal matter, it can become impacted and block the opening of the appendix into the cecum.

Emotional Therapies

- Release anxiety. Trust. Relax. Breathe.
- Allow rhythm in your life. This means allowing time for work, time for play, time for exercise, and time for rest and sleep so that you don't feel pressured or hurried at any time.

BLOOD

The blood is the stream of life that flows through the human body. Not a single part of the body can live without this red fluid. It picks up oxygen from the lungs, where it combines with iron molecules in the hemoglobin, and then carries the oxygen to every cell in the body. The blood also collects simple nutrients that have been broken down during digestion and distributes these within the cells, where they are used to build new tissue and produce energy. The blood also picks up waste products and carbon dioxide from the cells, and carries them away. The liver and kidneys remove most of the wastes, while the lungs remove carbon dioxide. In addition, the blood fights germs that cause disease when they enter the body. Blood has an amazing ability to clot and form a protective seal over a wound, keeping more blood from escaping the body. There are about ten pints of blood in a person who weighs 160 pounds.

Red Blood Cells

A cubic millimeter of a person's blood contains about five million red blood cells! Red blood cells are manufactured in bone marrow. When fully grown, they leave the marrow. They circulate in the bloodstream for about four months, until they use up their supply of energy and are destroyed. To constantly replace these cells, the body must manufacture about two million new blood cells every second. When the body fails to make enough new blood cells or when the amount of hemoglobin falls too low, anemia results.

White Blood Cells

White blood cells are called leucocytes, and there are between five thousand and ten thousand in a cubic millimeter of blood. There are three main types of leucocytes: granulocytes, monocytes, and lymphocytes. Granulocytes are developed in bone marrow and devour bacteria that enter the body. Monocytes are produced in both bone marrow and the spleen, and they also destroy bacteria. Lymphocytes are formed in the lymph glands, and they produce antibodies that fight bacteria.

Nutritional Suggestions

· Eat foods that are high in chlorophyll, such as green leafy vegetables, green vegetable juices, and wheatgrass juice.
· Eat foods that are high in organic iron, such as green vegetables, red beets, black cherries, black berries, figs, and prunes.
· Take chlorella, blue-green algae, green kamut, and barley grass.
· Use red clover, chaparral, and Pau d'Arco teas to cleanse the blood.

Emotional Therapies

· Consider your will to live. Are you happy in your life? If not, change what is causing sadness and bring in thoughts, feelings, and activities of joy!

BONES

Bones form the framework for our bodies, and they are tied together by ligaments that form the joints. About two-thirds of a person's bone weight is made of minerals, especially calcium and phosphorus. The rest comes mostly from collagen, a fibrous protein. When collagen is boiled, it yields gelatin. When bones are exposed to acidity, they begin to dissolve and eventually become so soft they can be bent or tied in a knot.

There are two types of tissue in bones. The hard, outer part of the bone is called compact tissue. The inner part is spongy and called cancellous tissue. Bone tissue is very active in the body. It cleanses the blood of harmful substances, including radioactive products. New blood cells are made in bone marrow. The bones store calcium, flouride, sodium, and phosphorus.

Exercise

- Exercise daily, low-impact activities are best.
- Lift light weights. Resistance strengthens the bones.

Nutritional Suggestions

- Include almonds, sesame seeds, kale, millet, celery, raw goat's milk, and raw vegetable juices in your diet.
- Take calcium, magnesium, sodium, sulfur, silicon, potassium, and phosphorus.
- Combine boneset, horsetail, and oatstraw into a mineral-boosting tea. You can also find them in capsule form if you prefer. Follow directions on the bottle.

Emotional Therapies

- Feel strong! Let go of heavy burdens.
- Stand tall. Affirm that life supports you.

EYES

The eyes are our most important organs for learning about our world. They help us see our friends and family, our surroundings, and the beauty of nature. We can even view the stars, which are trillions of miles away!

The human eyeball is about an inch in diameter. It is seated in fat, inside a space, or orbit, in the skull, surrounded by bone. Each eyeball has six muscles attached, which move it and control the size of the pupil. The conjunctiva (a mucous membrane) covers the front of the eyeball, except for the cornea. Nerves within the conjunctiva warn us if a foreign object, like a particle of dust, enters the eye.

The cornea is a clear dome of tissue over the iris, the colored part of the eye. The iris is like a thin curtain of tissue in front of the lens. The crystalline lens is about the size of a small lima bean. The pupil, which looks like a black hole, is located in the center of the iris. Light passes through the cornea, the iris, and the pupil.

The center of the eyeball holds a clear jellylike substance called the vitreous humor. The retina is located in the inner layer of the eyeball. It contains light-sensitive cells called rods and cones. Cones help us see in daylight, and rods help us see at night. Nerve fibers come together in front of the rods and cones from all parts of the retina to form the optic nerve, which goes to the spinal cord.

Eye Color

Heredity determines iris color. For example, Asian, African, and some Hispanic babies are born with brown eyes. Their eyes remain brown, though they may darken. Caucasian babies and some Hispanic babies are born with blue eyes. Some of these babies begin to develop eye pigment soon after birth. The eyes usually become their true color between six months and seven years of age. Eye pigments may continue to develop throughout one's life.

Eye Defects

Hyperopia, or farsightedness, occurs when the eyeball is too short. Focus falls behind the retina, and the person has difficulty seeing close objects clearly.

Myopia, or nearsightedness, occurs when the eyeball is too long. Focus falls in front of the retina, and distant objects appear blurred.

With astigmatism, the shapes of the cornea and lens are abnormal. Light rays focus on, in front of, and in back of the retina. This results in blurry vision for both near and distant objects.

People who are color blind cannot distinguish between certain colors. This is an inherited trait.

Strabismus, or crossed eyes, mainly occurs in children. Imbalanced eye muscles cause one eye to turn out or in. Exercises may help strabismus. A patch over one eye may also help. Glasses or surgery may be required if all other techniques are unsuccessful.

Nutritional Suggestions

· Eat lots of green leafy vegetables, including spinach and raw juices from these vegetables, as well as carrots and carrot juice.
· Eat blueberries, celery and celery juice, cabbage, and egg yolks.
· Include soaked nuts and seeds and mineral whey in your diet.
· Take bilberry (320 milligrams per day to improve night vision) and eyebright.
· Take vitamins A, B complex, C, ionic trace minerals, and zinc.
· Eat whole grains, especially brown rice.
· Take latein.

- Eat egg yolks soft-boiled or raw in shakes.
- Eat plenty of fish, kale, raw goat's milk, and brewer's yeast.
- Do a liver cleanse once or twice a year.

Exercise

- Do eye exercises (see page 118).

Emotional Therapies

- Try to "see" clearly and understand each situation in your life.
- Be confronting!
- Don't hide your head in the sand or avoid issues you need to see and face.
- Breathe deeply.
- Trust.
- Relax.

HEART

The heart lies in the center of the chest between the lungs. The upper, wider portion of the heart points toward the right shoulder, while the lower part points toward the left side of the body. The heart beats in the lower section. This is why many people believe incorrectly that the heart is entirely on the left side of the body. The heart is a very busy pump linked by a hundred thousand miles of pipeline. It is about the size of a fist and weighs less than a pound. It beats seventy times each minute and pumps five quarts of blood through its chambers every sixty seconds. By the end of each day, the heart has pumped more than a hundred thousand times. The heart is essential to life. As long as it pumps blood, the body receives the oxygen it needs. When the heart stops, the oxygen supply is cut off and the body dies. A buildup of fatty deposits and calcium in the arteries causes a heart attack. We must keep the heart's pipeline clean and healthy.

Nutritional Suggestions

- Avoid foods fried in fat or hydrogenated oils.
- Cook only with olive, grape seed, or coconut oil.
- Eat only oils that have been cold-pressed.
- Include flaxseed oil in your nutritional program.
- Avoid heavily processed cheeses and creams.

- Avoid margarine, and eat organic butter sparingly.
- Eat lots of raw and steamed vegetables, raw nuts and seeds, and whole grains.
- If you eat meat, eat only lean meat sparingly, baked or broiled fish, chicken, and turkey.
- Eat foods high in potassium (see "Tool Kit for Selecting Healthy Minerals" in chapter 5).
- Drink hawthorne berry tea.
- Take vitamin E, magnesium, A-flow (it chelates plaque from arteries), and policosanol (which lowers cholesterol). Also take CoQ10 or Co-enzyme Q10 which is found in every cell of the body and which acts as an enzyme and facilitates the activities of other enzymes. CoQ10 is a powerful antioxidant and acts as a catalyst to promote energy production in the cells. The heart and the liver contain and need the highest amounts of it.

Exercise

- Exercise daily to keep the blood circulating and keep the heart muscle strong.

Emotional Therapies

- Nurture your soul.
- Reduce stress in your life.
- Practice deep breathing.
- Practice expressing love and feelings to those you care about.
- Love yourself!
- Laugh and be happy.
- Release emotional pain.

IMMUNE SYSTEM

The immune system protects us from illness and is composed of highly specialized fighter cells called lymphocytes or white blood cells produced by a complex of lymphoid organs that contain lymph tissue. These organs include the bone marrow, lymph nodes (located near the joints), spleen (located in the upper left abdominal cavity), thymus (located just above the heart), tonsils, adenoids, and appendix. These fighter cells generate antibodies that defend and protect us from harmful invading viruses, bacteria, fungi, and even body cells that have gone astray such as cancer cells. Lymph vessels and lymph nodes carry a clear lymph fluid containing lymphocytes to every tissue of the body and eventually back into the blood. Two major classes of lymphocytes are the T-cells that grow to maturity in the thymus, and B-cells that mature in the bone marrow. T-cells alert B-cells to begin making antibodies. Other T-cells attack and destroy infected cells. B-cells secrete antibodies that neutralize bacteria, viruses, and fungi and prepare them for destruction by phagocytes (cells generated in the bone marrow that destroy foreign matter). A large part of our immune system is located in the intestinal tract. Peyer's patches are lymph tissue located in the walls of the small intestines that produce lymphocytes. We also have friendly bacteria called acidophilus and bifidus in our intestinal tract that fight harmful bacteria. Our immune system is vital to our health and most important to take care of.

Nutritional Suggestions

- Drink raw vegetable juices.
- Take vitamins A, B, C, E, zinc, and selenium.
- Take coenzyme Q10, a powerful antioxidant that fights free radicals.
- Take propolis.
- Take acidophilus and bifidus if you have had a round of antibiotics.
- Take colostrum.

If you feel a cold or flu coming on, the following may be taken until you are well:

- Goldenseal to fight infection.
- Echinacea to boost the immune system and cleanse the lymph.
- Grapefruit seed extract (in capsule form) to fight viruses, fungi, and bacteria.
- Colloidal silver, 10 parts per million, to fight viruses, fungi, and bacteria.

Exercises

Be sure to exercise to move the lymph. Lymph fluids will not flow properly without exercise. Rebounding is one of the finest exercises to keep the immune system healthy.

Emotional Therapies

· Breathe deeply to release stress each day.
· Get plenty of deep rest.
· Meditate.
· Choose not to be a victim or martyr in life.
· Stand strong for what you believe.

KIDNEYS

The kidneys resemble large purplish brown beans and lie above the small of the back on either side of the spine. The right kidney is slightly lower than the left to allow room for the liver. They are about four to five inches long and weigh about six ounces apiece. Blood moves into each kidney through the renal artery and returns to the heart through the renal vein. There are about a million tiny coiled tubes called nephrons in the kidneys. Nephrons filter out urea, uric acid, creatinine, and other wastes from the blood and pass them into the ureters. The ureters take the urine into the urinary bladder, below the pelvis, where it is expelled through the urethra. The body expels about a quart and a half of urine each day.

Kidney problems can cause elevated blood pressure. If there is a shortage of blood supply to the kidneys, they produce a chemical called angiotensin. This chemical constricts blood vessels throughout the body and raises blood pressure. Arteriosclerosis (hardened arteries) can decrease blood flow to the kidneys. Kidney and bladder infections can be extremely painful. Nephritis is an inflammation of the kidneys. When nephritis is severe, wastes accumulate in the blood, a situation that can result in death. Take care of your kidneys and bladder to prevent infections from occurring.

Nutritional Suggestions

· Drink lots of purified water with ionic trace minerals, at least eight glasses per day. If you are not used to drinking water, start with one or two glasses and build up.
· Drink eight ounces of water with a tablespoon of raw apple cider vinegar to cleanse the kidneys.
· Eat cucumbers, watermelon, carrots, green leafy vegetables, parsley, lemons, limes, grapefruits, apples, pears, and pomegranates.

- Avoid high-protein diets. Uric acid crystals build up in the kidneys from processed foods and high amounts of animal proteins.
- Avoid processed milk. The body is unable to absorb the calcium, and the calcium goes into the kidneys via the blood and creates stones.
- Drink raw vegetable juices such as carrot, celery, cucumber, and parsley.
- Drink herbal teas such as juniper berry, uva ursi, corn silk, alfalfa, and shavegrass.
- Avoid caffeine and alcohol. Caffeine pulls calcium out of the bone and causes it to pass through the kidneys.
- Eat foods high in magnesium, potassium, and natural sodium to keep the urine's pH alkaline and to hold calcium in the bone. (See "Tool Kit for Selecting Healthy Minerals" in chapter 5.)

Emotional Therapies

- Learn to release anger and fear.
- Practice creative self-expression.
- Learn to praise yourself and allow yourself to grow and bloom. Remember, a flower deprived of sunlight will die.
- Practice feelings of self-worth.
- Do whatever it takes to bring happiness to your life.

LIVER AND GALLBLADDER

The liver and gallbladder are miraculous organs indeed! They work together with the bile ducts as a team to perform the functions of the biliary system, which helps the body rid itself of wastes and processed fats. Weighing from two to three pounds, the liver is reddish brown and shaped like a cone. It occupies the upper-right abdominal cavity just beneath the diaphragm and has two main lobes. Its base touches the stomach, right kidney, and intestines. The gallbladder—a small sac, shaped like a pear—is tucked underneath and attached to the liver.

The remarkable liver has many vital functions. About one-quarter of the heart's output of oxygenated blood flows into the liver via the hepatic artery. In the liver, the artery divides into many branches to provide oxygen to all the liver cells. Blood, carrying such nutrients as fats and glucose from the intestines and spleen, enters the liver through the portal vein. Blood exits the liver through the hepatic vein, carrying away carbon dioxide and plasma proteins. Bile is produced in the liver and passed to the gallbladder where it is stored by means of a tube called a cystic duct.

The liver produces important proteins for blood plasma. One of these is albumin, which regulates the exchange of water between blood and tissues. Another is globin, which is a part of the oxygen-carrying pigment called hemoglobin. Others complement a group of proteins that play an important part in the body's defense system against infection. The liver also produces cholesterol and special proteins that help transport fats around the body. The liver regulates blood levels of amino acids, the building blocks of proteins. After a meal, some amino acids are converted to glucose, some to protein, and others to urea, which is passed out of the body through the kidneys and excreted in the urine. If not required immediately by the body's cells, the liver stores glucose (a form of sugar) as glycogen. When the body needs heat or energy, the liver converts glycogen back to sugar and releases it into the bloodstream.

Working together with the kidneys, the liver helps cleanse the blood of drugs, nicotine, caffeine, chemicals, and preservatives. A healthy liver absorbs these poisonous substances, changes their chemical structure so they are water-soluble, and excretes them into the bile. The bile carries waste products away from the liver and stores them in the gallbladder. The gallbladder contracts and expels bile into the duodenum (the first part of the small intestine) when the stomach sends food there.

The liver also processes estrogen. When estrogen is not processed properly, women may have an excess in their body. This can cause PMS symptoms, such as bloating, water retention, weight gain, irritability, headaches, anxiety, hypoglycemia (causing sugar cravings), an increase in prolaction (a hormone that can cause depression), an increase in inflammatory prostaglandins (which can cause pain), and cramping of the uterus's smooth muscles. Caffeine, alcohol, nicotine, sugar, fried foods, fast foods, and foods high in hormones, such as beef and milk, can hinder the liver in its job of processing estrogen and create premenstrual symptoms.

Nutritional Suggestions

- Eat lots of bitter greens such as kale, beet tops, cilantro, and arugula.
- Eat beets, raw or steamed, or take beet tablets.
- Drink raw juices such as wheatgrass, parsley, spinach, and beet.
- Take digestive enzymes with meals.

- Take chlorella.
- Use olive oil and lemon juice as a salad dressing.
- Take milk thistle, burdock, and yellow dock.
- Avoid heated oils, hydrogenated oils, rancid oils, and fried foods.

Emotional Therapies

- Learn to forgive.
- Express passion.
- Learn to release anger and fears.
- Build self-esteem.

LUNGS

The lungs are organs of external respiration. Human beings have two lungs located in the chest cavity. These large spongy pyramid-shaped organs provide the blood with oxygen and remove carbon dioxide. The right lung has three lobes, and the left lung has two lobes. There are approximately six hundred million alveoli, or air sacs. If the walls of the air sacs were spread out flat and placed side by side, they would cover about six hundred square feet. Each air sac is lined with a network of tiny capillaries that carry blood. The blood is cleansed and purified of toxic carbon dioxide, brought in from all the cells to the lungs, and the toxins are released when we exhale. This is why proper deep breathing is vital to our health! All the cells in our bodies depend on the oxygen we breathe in. And if we did not breathe out, they would die from carbon dioxide poisoning. If we do not breathe deeply, we will become fatigued and exhausted.

Nutritional Suggestions

- Avoid dairy products, wheat, and sugar.
- Eat turnips, peppers, radishes, onions, and garlic to cleanse mucus from the lungs and promote blood circulation.
- Drink mullein tea to cleanse mucus from the lungs.
- Take echinacea, poke, and lobelia in small amounts and only when needed to relieve lung congestion.
- Avoid smoking. Tar and nicotine irritate the lungs and create congestion.

Emotional Therapies

- Love your lungs; don't feed them poison.
- Resolve the emotional blocks that create negative habits in your life.
- Learn to love yourself and develop a sense of self-security.
- Practice building self-esteem.
- Nurture yourself and others.
- Sing!
- Practice deep breathing.
- Hug a tree.
- Hug a friend.

LYMPH FLUIDS AND LYMPH NODES

The lymph, formed from blood plasma, is a colorless fluid. It contains much less protein than plasma and, unlike plasma, no red blood cells. Lymph fluid bathes and nourishes every cell of the body. Organic sodium carried within the lymph helps hold calcium in solution. An adult has about six pints of lymph fluid, which consists of water, white blood cells, digested foods, and wastes excreted by the cells. Lymph fluid moves through tiny vessels called capillaries and larger vessels called lymphatics. Muscle contractions keep the lymph fluid moving. Therefore, we must exercise in order to pump the lymph fluid.

Lymph nodes or glands are plentiful around the neck, under the arms, and in the groin. The nodes produce lymphocytes, which help defend the body against harmful bacteria and disease. They help regulate the amount of poisonous substances or microorganisms that enter the blood.

Nutritional Suggestions

- Avoid table salt.
- Eat foods high in natural sodium such as okra, green leafy vegetables, and mineral whey.
- Drink celery juice.
- Drink potato peeling broth.
- Drink raw green vegetable juice, which is high in chlorophyll.
- Take mullein, blue violet, chaparral, and echinacea.

Exercise

· Walk and swing your arms.
· Jump on a mini-trampoline.
· Practice water aerobics.

Emotional Therapies

· Allow harmony and peace in your life.
· Enjoy counseling others.
· Learn to say "no!"
· Learn to speak about and deal with your feelings instead of repressing them.

MUSCLES

There are more than six hundred muscles located throughout the body that make movement possible. Muscles are grouped into two types, the skeletal and the smooth. Skeletal muscles are attached to the bones and assist them in movement. They must be stimulated by nerves to operate. Therefore, injury to the nerves can result in paralysis. Smooth muscles are in the blood vessels and internal organs, including the digestive tract. They can be stimulated by nerves and hormones. The cardiac, or heart muscle has tissue that resembles both skeletal and smooth muscles.

Muscles, which depend on food for their energy, produce a waste product called lactic acid. When the muscles are overworked, lactic acid accumulates and causes muscle fatigue and pain. Rest allows the muscles to relax and the body to remove the wastes. Fear or anger can cause the release of epinephrine (adrenaline), which affects muscle movements of the autonomic nervous system.

Nutritional Suggestions

· Eat foods that are high in potassium, such as olives, bananas, green leafy vegetables, and potato peeling broth.
· Eat foods that are high in protein, such as soaked nuts and seeds, beans, eggs, goat's milk, goat cheese, fish, chicken, and turkey.
· Eat whole grains and root vegetables, both release carbohydrates that create energy for muscles.
· Include ionic trace minerals, calcium, magnesium, and potassium in your diet.

Exercise

- Exercise on a regular basis to keep the muscles strong. Keep in mind that too much aerobic exercise at once can cause muscle fatigue.
- Incorporate slow stretches after a workout to help your body cool down and rid the muscles of lactic acid.

Emotional Therapies

- Be flexible! If you have made a decision and receive new information, be willing to change your mind.
- Cultivate inner peace and release tension.

NERVES, BRAIN, AND SPINAL CORD

The nervous system is divided into two separate systems. The central nervous system is composed of the brain and spinal cord. The peripheral nervous system consists of the nerves of the autonomic nervous system as well as twelve pairs of cranial nerves that extend from the brain and thirty-one pairs of spinal nerves that extend from the spinal cord. Cranial nerves control sensations and actions, including sight, smell, taste, chewing, and swallowing. The thirty-one pairs of spinal nerves—including eight cervical, twelve thoracic, five lumbar, five sacral, and one pair of cocygeal—control the muscles. The autonomic nervous system acts independently of the central nervous system and regulates involuntary processes. It is made up of the sympathetic and parasympathetic nervous systems.

Nutritional Suggestions

- Eat whole grains, especially brown rice.
- Eat egg yolks soft-boiled or raw in shakes because they are high in lecithin.
- Eat soaked nuts and seeds because they are high in essential fatty acids necessary for nerve function.
- Eat plenty of fish, kale, raw goat's milk, and brewer's yeast.
- Take vitamin B complex.
- Herbs that soothe the nerves are kava-kava, valarian root, blue verrain, and lady's slipper.

Emotional Therapies

- Breathe deeply.
- Trust.
- Relax.

OVARIES AND UTERUS

The uterus is a pear-shaped reproductive organ located in the lower-central abdominal area in women. An ovary (ovum-producing gland) is located on each side of the uterus and connected to it by fallopian tubes. Each ovary holds as many as four hundred thousand potential egg cells. Usually only one egg cell is produced each month, about eight or nine days after menstruation stops. The egg travels slowly to the uterus. If fertilization occurs, the egg-sperm combination attaches to the uterine lining, which becomes thick with blood vessels and fluids to nourish the embryo. If fertilization does not occur, the uterine lining sloughs off and results in menstrual bleeding.

The pituitary gland in the brain produces a follicle-stimulating hormone, which causes eggs to ripen each month. The ovaries produce estrogen and cause the uterine cells to divide and create a new lining each month. After an egg is released, the ovaries produce progesterone to continue building the uterine lining. For most women, menstruation begins around age twelve and ceases between the ages of fifty and fifty-five.

Nutritional Suggestions

- Eat soaked nuts and seeds, almond cream, and seed sauces.
- Use flaxseed, borage, and olive oils.
- Take vitamin E and evening primrose oil.
- Include magnesium, calcium, silicon, and trace minerals.
- Take black cohosh.
- Drink red raspberry leaf tea to reduce menstrual cramping and tone the uterus.

Emotional Therapies

- Practice self-respect and believe in your self-worth.
- Trust yourself to attract others whom you can trust.
- Release fears of intimacy.

· Practice introspection. Spend time in nature. Have a pet to love.
· Let go of fear.
· Allow yourself to birth and grow new ideas.

PANCREAS

The pancreas is an elongated gland about six to eight inches long and one and a half inches wide. It is pinkish yellow. It lies in the back of the abdomen just behind the stomach. The duodenum, or first part of the small intestine that joins to the stomach, loops around it. The pancreas consists of both exocrine and endocrine tissue. The exocrine tissue secretes enzymes, including pancreatin, into the duodenum by way of a duct called the ampulla of Vater. These enzymes break down and digest proteins, carbohydrates, fats, and nucleic acids. The pancreas also secretes bicarbonate to neutralize the stomach acid entering the duodenum.

The endocrine tissue is composed of more than a million small clusters of cells known as the islets of Langerhans, scattered throughout the pancreas. About 70 percent of these cells are beta, or B-cells, which produce the hormone insulin. The remainder of the endocrine cells are alpha, or A-cells. They secrete the hormone glucagon. Both the alpha and the beta cells are regulated by the amount of glucose in the blood. If there is a low level of glucose, glucagon will be released to help increase blood glucose. High levels of glucose will stimulate the release of insulin to help decrease blood glucose. Together, these hormones regulate the blood's glucose levels.

When there is an abundance of sugar or glucose in the blood, B-cells secrete insulin directly into the bloodstream. The blood carries the insulin to cells throughout the body to help them utilize glucose, their main fuel. Insulin stimulates the liver, fat tissue, and muscle cells to take in glucose and metabolize it. It also stimulates the liver to store some glucose as glycogen, and it promotes the storage of fats and proteins to be used during leaner times.

When there is too little insulin, the cells cannot utilize glucose effectively. If glucose goes unused, it accumulates in the blood and tissues and is then carried out in the urine. Sugar in the urine is a major symptom of hyperglycemia or diabetes mellitus.

If the pancreas produces too much insulin, blood sugar is utilized too rapidly and can cause dizziness, frequent hunger, craving of sweets, and fatigue. These are the symptoms of low blood sugar or hypoglycemia.

Hypoglycemia can be a precursor to diabetes because the pancreas is in the first stages of improper release of insulin.

A-cells secrete glucagon between meals when the blood sugar is low. Glucagon stimulates the liver to convert glycogen back to glucose, and it raises the blood sugar level. It causes the adipose tissue to release its stores of fatty acids into the blood. Adipose tissue is located just beneath the skin and helps provide insulation from the heat and cold. It is found around the internal organs and acts as a protective padding. In addition to providing protection and padding, its primary purpose is to reserve nutrients and store energy in the form of fat.

Nutritional Suggestions

- Avoid refined white sugar, high fructose corn syrup, and hydrogenated oils.
- Use natural sugars in moderation.
- Chew on licorice root if you don't have high blood pressure and drink blueberry or dandelion leaf teas.
- Eat whole grains and soaked nuts and seeds—foods that metabolize slowly.
- Eat raw honey, dates, molasses, and maple syrup in small amounts.
- Use stevia to sweeten herbal teas.
- Take chromium picolinate with trace minerals.
- Take gymnema sylvestre to regulate insulin and blood sugar levels.
- Other herbs that help the pancreas are bitter melon, agrimony, and cinnamon.

Emotional Therapies

- Practice generosity, build self-esteem, love yourself, and share yourself with others.
- Learn to allow things to be as they are.
- Learn to let go.
- Give and receive love.
- Enjoy the sweetness of life.

PROSTATE AND TESTES

The prostate gland is about the size of a walnut and is composed of muscular and glandular tissue. It is located below the urinary bladder and secretes a substance that transports sperm cells. The tube that empties the bladder, called the urethra, passes through the prostate. If the prostate becomes large and swollen due to disease or infection, it can press on the urethra and block the passage of urine. Cancer of the prostate gland is becoming more prevalent in the United States and is now the second leading cause of death among men in this country. The testes, the glands that produce sperm, are located near the prostate.

Nutritional Suggestions

· Eat soaked nuts and seeds whole or blended into creams, nut butters, and some nuts and seeds that have not been soaked. Grind unsoaked nuts and seeds or chew them really well in order to digest them properly. There are benefits to eating soaked nuts and seeds because soaking takes out about half the fat, makes them twice as nutritious because they have started sprouting a new plant inside, and makes them easier to digest. Nut butters and whole nuts and seeds are also nutritious because of the good essential oils they contain. We need smaller amounts of these than nuts and seeds that have been soaked.
· Take magnesium, calcium, silicon, zinc, vitamin E, lecithin, B complex, and B6.
· Use saw palmetto for the prostate, and damiana and ginseng for the testes.
· Use flaxseed and borage oil.
· Drink red raspberry leaf tea.
· Take pygeum, gravel root, and hydrangea.
· Drink herbal teas made from buchu, corn silk, and juniper berry.

Emotional Therapies

· Practice self-respect and believe in your self-worth.
· Trust yourself to attract others whom you can trust.
· Release fears of intimacy.
· Practice introspection. Spend time in nature; have a pet to love.
· Let go of fear.
· Allow yourself to birth and grow new ideas.

SKIN, HAIR, FINGERNAILS, AND CONNECTIVE TISSUE

The skin is the body's largest organ and weighs about six pounds. If the skin of an adult were stretched out on a flat surface, it would cover nearly eighteen feet. The skin regulates body temperature and releases perspiration through the pores. Amazingly, a piece of skin about the size of a quarter contains four yards of nerves and twenty-five nerve endings, a yard of blood vessels, a hundred sweat glands, and over three million cells!

The skin is made up of two parts: the epidermis, or surface, and the dermis, or lower part. The epidermis contains nerves, but no blood vessels. Melanin pigment is located there and determines skin color. Epidermis cells are regularly pushed up to the skin's surface and sloughed off. The dermis, or lower portion, of the skin is made up of a closely woven connective tissue. Nerve glands, blood vessels, lymph vessels, and hair follicles are located in the dermis.

The skin also has two kinds of glands: one secretes perspiration and the other secretes oil. Two million sweat glands are distributed throughout the skin. They secrete liquid wastes and regulate body temperature. When sweat evaporates, the body is cooled. Sebaceous, or oil, glands open mostly into hair follicles. Oil from these glands keeps the skin moist and the hair shiny. Blackheads form when the oil becomes oxidized, or hardened, in the pores.

Nutritional Suggestions

· Eat foods that are high in silicon, such as oatstraw tea, horsetail herb, and bell peppers.
· Take bioflavonoids including rutin to build connective tissue and help heal varicose veins, hemorrhoids, and hernias.
· Include ionic trace minerals, calcium, and zinc in your diet.
· Include cabbage and cabbage juice and white pulp from grapefruits and oranges in your diet.
· Use oils rich in essential fatty acids, such as flaxseed and borage oil.
· Take juniper berry, parsley, and corn silk teas.
· Eat watermelon.

Exercise

· Do skin brushing.
· Consider a bowel cleanse and a kidney cleanse.

Emotional Therapies

· Release skeletons from your closet.
· Decide on a purpose in life that you can fulfill.

· Enjoy the journey toward a goal.
· Let small things be purposeful.

SPLEEN

The spleen is located to the left of and a little behind the stomach, below the diaphragm. It is about five inches long and three inches wide, and it weighs approximately seven ounces. The cells are similar to those in the lymph glands. The spleen filters and destroys foreign substances in the blood and destroys worn-out blood cells. It also stores blood cells and releases them during injury when the body requires extra blood.

Nutritional Suggestions

· Eat foods that are high in iron, such as green leafy vegetables and red beets.
· Eat foods that are high in chlorophyl, such as raw green juices.
· Eat foods that are high in sodium, such as mineral whey and celery juice.

Emotional Therapies

· Allow yourself to do what you love.
· Allow life to flow along gently.

STOMACH AND INTESTINAL TRACT

The stomach is a large baglike organ shaped like a J, which lies between the esophagus and small intestine. It is positioned in the upper-left side of the abdomen. The top part of the stomach joins with the esophagus at the cardiac sphincter. The lower end of the stomach empties into the duodenum, or beginning of the small intestine, at the pyloric valve. Glands that secrete mucus to lubricate food and other glands that secrete hydrochloric acid and pepsin, which partially digest food, are found in the stomach wall.

Foods that are spicy, too hot, or too cold irritate the stomach. Unchewed foods irritate the stomach as well. Fear, anger, or constant tension can produce excessive secretions of stomach acids that burn the stomach or duodenum. This can cause ulcers. Poorly combined foods can cause fermentation in the stomach. Excessive gastric juice can be forced back up into the esophagus. When this happens on a regular basis, a hiatal hernia may develop.

The small intestine is a tube about twenty feet long and one inch wide, narrower than the large intestine. Most of the digestive processes take place here. Enzymes are secreted from the walls of the intestines as well as from the liver and pancreas. Digestion is completed in the small intestine, and the digested food is absorbed by fingerlike projections called villi. Blood and lymph fluid pick up the nutrients from the villi and distribute them to the cells.

The large intestine is about five to six feet long and two and a half inches wide. It consists of the ascending colon on the right side of the abdomen, the transverse colon that stretches across the top of the abdomen, and the descending colon that runs down the left side of the abdomen to the sigmoid colon and then the anus. The large intestine joins the small intestine at the cecum. The area where the colon bends from ascending to transverse is near the liver and is called the hepatic flexure. The point where the colon bends from transverse to descending is near the spleen and is called the spleenic flexure.

Nutritional Suggestions

- Eat cabbage and drink cabbage juice.
- Eat foods that are rich in sodium, such as celery, mineral whey, strawberries, and okra.
- Eat foods that are high in fiber, such as ground flaxseeds, oat bran, rice bran, whole grains, raw vegetables, alfalfa tablets, and chlorella.
- Include slippery foods that contain mucilage, such as aloe vera juice, slippery elm tea, and flaxseed tea in your diet.
- Eat foods that are high in friendly bacteria, such as yogurt and raw sauerkraut.
- Include antiparasitic foods, such as garlic and onions, in your diet.

Emotional Therapies

- Release anxiety. Trust. Relax. Breathe.
- Allow rhythm in your life. Include time for work, time for play, time for rest, and time to sleep.

THYMUS

The thymus is located under the breastbone in the upper part of the chest. It is considered an endocrine gland because it has no ducts. The thymus plays a major roll in the processes of the immune system. Important fighter cells, called T-cells, grow to maturity in the thymus. The thymus selects the T-cells that are strong and sends them into the bloodstream to protect the body from invading germs. It also eliminates the weaker T-cells. The thymus is most active before puberty and begins to shrink in size, slowing its activity, when we grow older.

Nutritional Suggestions

- Eat carrots, cabbage, green vegetables, and seaweeds.
- Include red clover tea, vitamins A and E, zinc, and selenium in your diet.

Exercise

- Tap your thymus daily to keep it healthy and youthful.

Emotional Therapies

- Live life fully!
- Boost your will to live by doing things you are passionate about.
- Enjoy small things.
- Partake in hobbies that bring you joy.

THYROID

The thyroid gland is an endocrine, or ductless, gland located in the neck. It has two lobes, located on either side of the windpipe. The thyroid absorbs iodine from the blood. Iodine combines with other chemicals in the thyroid to form thyroxine. This hormone is released into the blood vessels located within the thyroid and distributed to the body's cells. As needed, thyroxin is then changed into several more hormones that regulate the rate at which oxygen and food are changed to heat and energy. This is why thyroid hormones are necessary for metabolism, body growth, and even mental development and function. Goiter, or enlargement of the thyroid gland, develops when the body doesn't have enough iodine. (See "Thyroid Disorders" in chapter 4.)

Nutritional Suggestions

- Eat plenty of green leafy vegetables.
- Eat seaweeds that are high in minerals and iodine, such as dulse (and dulse tablets), kelp capsules, and powder for seasoning.

- Include trace minerals in your diet.
- Include herbs such as Irish moss, watercress, and sarsparilla.

Emotional Therapies

- Speak your truth. Say what you need to say.
- Sing!
- Practice public speaking.

TONSILS AND ADENOIDS

Tonsils and adenoids are both located in the back of the throat, with the adenoids positioned upward behind the nose. They are both made of lymphoid tissue. White blood cells called lymphocytes are formed in the lymphoid tissue. These germ fighters are the body's first line of defense, trapping poisons before they progress into the body. Do all that you can to avoid having them removed.

Nutritional Suggestions

- Avoid dairy products, wheat (gluten), and sugar.
- Follow the mucus cleanse program.
- Eat lots of fiber and vegetables to keep the bowels moving. When the bowels are constipated, the tonsils and adenoids must work harder to collect and filter poisons from the blood.
- Drink mullein tea. Take propolis and echinacea (only when you have a sore throat).

Emotional Therapies

- Speak up! Deal with your anger and release it.
- Sing!
- Use your voice to help others.

chapter 4 ∞

Remedies

Nature will heal when given the opportunity.
−Dr. Bernard Jensen

WHEN I WAS A CHILD, my mother and grandmother would bake onions and mash them warm into a cotton cloth and lay them on my chest or tie them around my feet when I was sick with lung congestion. When I grew up, my grandmother got pneumonia and I took care of her for few weeks. She was so sick everyone thought she might die. I remembered the onion poultices and faithfully put them on her chest and tied them around her feet. When I started doing this, her fever broke and her coughing stopped. When I worked with my father-in-law, Dr. Bernard Jensen, at the Hidden Valley Health Ranch, I saw miracles occur with natural remedies. I used to walk with him in his organic orchards and gardens and he would say, "Darling, nature will heal when given the opportunity." And indeed I have seen miracles take place time and again when people change unnatural lifestyles from rushing, worrying, and eating packaged, processed foods to relaxing, walking barefoot on the earth, thinking happy thoughts, and eating vegetables pulled from the garden. Thousands of people came to Dr. Jensen's Health Ranch to learn the art of healthy living. They would come on walkers and canes, with terrible skin conditions, severe constipation, and all sorts of illnesses. With organic foods, herbal remedies, natural vitamins, exercise, water therapies, and proper rest, they healed beautifully. In my practice today, I continue to see nature and natural remedies help people get well. The following are natural remedies that I have had experience with. Go to a knowledgeable physician when you are ill or have questions about any of the remedies provided here.

Tool Kit for Choosing Natural Home Remedies for Everything from A to Z

Natural remedies have been used successfully throughout time to relieve pain, heal wounds, combat illnesses, and even save lives. Natural healing techniques empower us to be ready during times of crisis. These remedies are not meant to take the place or the advice of a knowledgeable physician. If a problem persists, go for professional testing and treatment.

ACNE

Follow the facial treatment for acne presented in chapter 3. Cleanse your colon as described in chapter 6. Take twenty-five thousand international units of vitamin A and fifty milligrams of zinc each day, and take two capsules of oregano oil twice a day. Drink yellow dock root tea three times per day.

ANEMIA

Drink a glass of black cherry juice daily. Drink a glass of raw vegetable juice made from carrots and parsley; carrots, beets, and parsley; or carrots, beets, and spinach. Be sure to get into the fresh air and sunshine daily, walk, and do some deep-breathing exercises. Oxygen attracts and holds iron in the body. Yellow dock root and dandelion leaf teas are also great blood builders. Chlorophyll is like the blood of the plant and builds the blood of the body.

ARTHRITIS

According to Dr. Ruth Yale Long of the Nutrition Education Association, "Arthritis is a nutritional deficiency disease. If we all eat the nutrients we need, we can live out our lives without the misery of arthritis."

Take an Epsom salts bath four to five times per week. Rinse off and place castor oil poultices on your arthritic areas. Drink eight ounces of celery juice three times per day. Celery juice is made simply by juicing four to six whole sticks of celery to make eight ounces of juice. You can add two ounces of carrot juice made with one large or two small carrots to the celery juice to improve the taste and receive the benefits of the carrot. Celery juice is high in organic sodium, which helps neutralize acidity in the body, dissolve bone spurs, and allow the calcium to go back into solution or back into your bones. Black cherry juice is also great for breaking up crystals in the joints. It helps relieve and heal arthritis as well as gout. Buy only natural black cherry juice that contains no added sugars or preservatives. For the best results, grow or purchase your own black cherries and juice them. It takes about two cups of cherries with stems and seeds removed to make one eight-ounce glass of black cherry juice. People with diabetes or hypoglycemia will need to dilute the black cherry juice (use three ounces of black cherry juice and five ounces of water) because of the fruit sugars it contains.

Vegetables and fruits contain an organic, biochemical, absorbable form of sodium. According to Dr. Bernard Jensen in *The Chemistry of Man*:

Organic sodium keeps calcium in solution in the human body. Sodium was named the "youth" element due to its properties of promoting youthful, limber, flexible, pliable joints. Joint troubles need not manifest in the individual who has a good reserve of sodium, the "youth" element in the stomach walls and the joints. Goat milk and goat whey are rich in natural sodium.

Dr. Jensen raised goats at his ranch. Rather than having to raise goats, you can drink a wonderful goat's milk whey drink daily; see chapter 1.

Other important nutrients that help relieve and heal arthritis include alfalfa tablets, which are high in absorbable minerals. Include essential fatty acids in your diet to relieve inflammation. Glucosamine sulfate helps form and repair bones and cartilage. Liquid minerals and trace minerals ensure absorption into the bone. Take a good multivitamin containing all the B vitamins to help nourish the body overall and reduce free radicals. Take turmeric, which has anti-inflammatory properties. White willow bark can relieve inflammation and ease pain. This can be taken as an herbal tea or in capsule form.

ASTHMA

Asthma is a disease that causes the bronchi or air passages in the lungs to become inflamed, congested with mucus, and constricted, blocking the flow of air and oxygen. Symptoms of asthma include wheezing, tightness of the chest, inability to breathe, and coughing. Children, teens, and adults can have asthma and it is usually caused by allergies and weakened immune system. Several triggers cause asthma including dust, mold, mites, pets, feathers, air pollution, cigarette smoke, food additives including MSG and sulfites, perfume, chemicals in cleaning solutions, and hair spray.

People with asthma may also have reactions to wheat, dairy products, and sugar, and should avoid them. Wheat and dairy products are gluey and pasty and might contribute to the mucus in the lungs. Wheat also can paste down the small villi in the intestinal tract. Many asthmatics are allergic to dairy products and notice improvement when they leave them out of the diet. Sugar and all artificial sweeteners can weaken the immune system. The nutritional plan and cleanse in this book have helped many asthmatics gain relief and begin healing because toxins are cleansed from the body and the immune system is strengthened. Consult with your doctor or health practitioner before you begin a cleanse. Eat foods that help release mucus from the body, such as turnips, lemons, limes, radishes, garlic, and onion. Add cayenne and ginger to your diet.

A good home remedy that has been known to help open up the bronchial passages is to breathe over a pot of steaming water in which you have put a few drops of eucalyptus and peppermint oil. Rub five drops of eucalyptus oil and three drops of peppermint oil mixed with one tablespoon of cold-pressed almond or safflower oil on the chest and around the nasal passages to promote blood flow and oxygen supply to the bronchial tubes. And here are a few other suggestions for improving conditions:

Get a good air filter. The Alpine Air Filter of America purifies the air in the home and kill mites and mold (see resources).

This lobelia solution can help to open up the bronchial tubes and help to release mucus.

Lobelia Solution:

five drops lobelia tincture
six ounces distilled water

Mix the lobelia tincture in the distilled water. Take it three times per day as well as at the time of an asthma attack.

Take two propolis tablets, two times per day to strengthen the immune system and soothe the lungs.

Take ten tablets of chlorella that has had the cell wall shattered with the
Dyno Mill two to three times per day. I like to recommend Sun
Chlorella because of the tremendous amount of research backing it.
(see resources). Chlorella can help to cleanse the liver and pull mucus
out through the stools.

Take two thousand milligrams of vitamin C with bioflavonoids per day.

Take fifty milligrams of B complex per day to help calm and strengthen the
nervous system.

Take one-fourth to one-half teaspoon of liquid ionic trace minerals in water
each day. I recommend those by Trace Mineral Research because they
contain highly absorbable minerals and trace minerals that come from
plant settlement from the Great Salt Lake of Utah (see resources).

Take two plant enzymes just before each meal to make sure all food is
digested properly.

Take two grapefruit seed extract capsules two times per day for four days,
and leave off for three days each week for six weeks. Grapefruit seed
extract also boosts immunity.

Drink a cup of mullein tea several times per week.

Add five drops of lobelia to a cup of mullein tea to help stop an asthma
attack.

Use onion poultices and castor oil packs on the chest several times a week
(see "Tool Kit for Preparing Poultices and Salves" in chapter 3).

Practice relaxing and breathing slow and easy on a daily basis. Do whatever
you can to let go of fear, worry, stress, and anger. Any of these feelings
can bring on an asthma attack.

ATHEROSCLEROSIS

In *Hardening of the Arteries, Heart Attack—Stroke*, Raj Pal, PhD, RNC,
states:

*Cardiovascular disease is the number one killer in the country. Deaths
surpass those from all other causes combined. Atherosclerosis, or hardening of the arteries, is a contributing factor not only in heart attacks
and strokes, but also in high blood pressure. It causes poor circulation,
which in turn restricts the disbursement of nutrients to other parts of
your body organs, tissue and skin. It contributes to providing less oxygen to the brain, thus slowing down your thinking process and memory.*

Atherosclerosis allows arteries to become filled with fat and the arterial walls to harden. The heart has to pump harder to move the blood through these blocked arteries, and blood pressure goes up.

One of the main causes of atherosclerosis is damage to the arteries by free radicals. Another cause is diets high in fried foods, margarine, partially hydrogenated oils, saturated fats, and rancid oils. Smoking causes tremendous damage to the arteries.

To prevent and heal atherosclerosis, consume antioxidants that fight free radicals, such as vitamins A, B, C, and E, as well as absorbable minerals and trace minerals. Make sure you ingest essential fatty acids such as flaxseed oil. Coenzyme Q10 is a powerful antioxidant, and garlic is a wonderful agent that helps regulate fat and cleanse the arteries. Lecithin and citrus pectin emulsify fat in the arteries as well. There is a wonderful natural oral chelating agent product called A-Flow. It contains most of these nutrients and several others in a balanced ratio. It is natural, safe, and effective, but still a good idea to consult with your physician before taking. A-Flow helps to remove arterial plaque and fights the causes of plaque. It is also high in antioxidants that disarm free radicals. See the resources section at the end of this book to learn where to find it.

Good nutrition on a daily basis is crucial to healing atherosclerosis! Follow the nutritional plans presented in chapter 1. Cleansing and exercise are also tremendously beneficial for healthy arteries.

ATTENTION DEFICIT DISORDER (ADD) AND ATTENTION DEFICIT HYPERACTIVITY DISORDER (ADHD)

ADD and ADHD are growing disorders among children in the United States, affecting more boys than girls. Adults suffer from this disorder as well. Individuals with ADD have difficulty focusing and concentrating. Children in classrooms may appear to be lethargic or daydreaming. They have difficulty concentrating on one topic at a time for very long. Individuals with ADHD have the same troubles with concentration and are also hyperactive. These children are very busy, talkative, and into everything. Adults with this disorder seem impatient, in a hurry, on the go, and talkative. They may hardly finish one idea before skipping to another and another.

ADD/ADHD has been linked to many factors. Smoking; drinking caffeinated soft drinks, tea, or coffee; or taking certain drugs during pregnancy may affect a child's nervous system during development in the womb. Oxygen deprivation during childbirth or an infection, injury, or high fever at an early age can affect the brain and nervous system. Mercury causes toxicity in the brain and nervous system especially in fetuses and small children whose brains are still developing. Mothers that have consumed large amounts of fish contaminated with mercury can affect their infants in the womb. High mercury types of fish are swordfish, king mackerel, and shark. Other sources from which children and adults have received mercury are from thimerosol, a preservative in vaccinations as well as from dental mercury fillings. Discuss these with your doctor and dentist before taking. There are always alternatives. Research has shown that a large percentage of people with ADD/ADHD also have blood sugar disorders. They may suffer from allergies, including food allergies, especially to wheat, dairy products, and sugar. They may be sensitive to preservatives, additives, and food coloring. Household cleaners, perfumes, dry-cleaning fluids, insecticides, newspaper inks, cigarette smoke, and gasoline exhaust can cause allergic reactions and upset the brain and nervous system. Many children and adults with ADD/ADHD eat foods that are far from nutritious and are loaded with salt, fat, or sugar. Many crave sugar and caffeine. Their bodies lack the nutrients necessary to nourish their brain and nervous systems.

To improve conditions,

Carefully follow the nutritional plans described in chapter 1.

Take one or two tablespoons of flaxseed oil, borage oil, or primrose oil daily to nourish the nervous system.

Take three teaspoons of coconut oil to improve nerve function.

DHA, taken according to the directions, provides an essential fatty acid that plays a major role in brain and nerve function.

Include ionic trace minerals in your diet to balance the flow of electrolytes through the body, neutralize acidity, and have a calming effect on the body.

Take a good multivitamin with fifty milligrams of the B complex vitamins; A multivitamin provides nutrients needed for health. The B vitamins help nourish and calm the nervous system.

Take one or two digestive enzymes with each meal to assure nutrients are absorbed from foods.

Phosphatidylserine, taken according to the directions, is essential for healthy brain functioning.

Ginkgo biloba aids brain function, concentration, and memory.

Chlorella helps cleanse the liver and blood, provides protein, chlorophyll, RNA/DNA and a wide range of vitamins and minerals that nourish the brain and nervous system, and helps balance blood sugar.

Consider having a competent health practitioner do a hair and mineral analysis. People with ADD or ADHD test for heavy concentrations of mercury, lead, or copper.

HMD or Heavy Metal Detox (see resources) has proven under scrupulous research to gently and safely remove mercury and heavy metals from children and adults.

BEDSORES

A bedsore is caused by repeated friction on the skin from bedsheets when someone is confined to bed for an extended period of time. Here is a healing paste that has worked well in the treatment of bedsores.

Soothing Herbal Paste

2 parts slippery elm powder
1 part marshmallow root powder
1 part goldenseal root powder

Mix the powders with hot distilled water, enough to form a paste. Spread the paste on bedsores and cover with a bandage.

BED-WETTING, OR ENURESIS

Wetting the bed is common in children under the age of five. Their bladders are often too small to hold all the urine through the night, and they sleep too soundly to wake up. Never scold your child for bed-wetting! This can create emotional disorders and make the problem worse. Get up during the night, take your child to the bathroom, and put them on the toilet.

Parsley, corn silk, plantain, and oat straw are herbs that can strengthen the bladder and stop bed-wetting. These can be taken in capsules or tea form before 5:00 P.M. Bioflavanoids, calcium, and magnesium can also help strengthen the bladder, as can Kegel exercises. Kegel exercises are easy and painless. These exercises were discovered by Dr. Arnold Kegel in order to help strengthen the pelvic floor muscles of the body to prevent urinary incontinence. Women and men can do these exercises by squeezing this lower pelvic muscle. If you are squeezing the correct muscle, you will draw in the perineum, which is the muscle and tissue just between the vaginal opening and anus in a woman and between the testicles and anus in a man. Practice squeezing this muscle for five minutes, two times per day morning and night. This will strengthen the pelvic muscle and help to prevent enuresis, or bed-wetting, as well as incontinence. Children can be taught to do Kagel exercises as well. Avoid caffeine and do not drink fluids within three hours of going to bed.

BEE STINGS

If you are severely allergic to bee stings, go to the hospital immediately if you are stung. Otherwise, use raw, organic honey or bentonite clay on the sting. If it is available, use natural mud. The plaintain poultice mentioned in chapter 3 is also great for bee stings.

BLEEDING

Place cayenne pepper in the wound. Cayenne will stop external bleeding. For internal bleeding, bleeding with colitis, and vaginal bleeding that is not from menstruation, take two cayenne capsules, three times per day. Shepherd's purse, horsetail, and stinging nettle teas or capsules will also help stop the bleeding. Midwives often use it to help stop postpartum bleeding.

BOILS

A boil usually begins with a painful red area on the skin due to some type of infection. After a while, a boil will swell with fluid and pus. This is caused by white blood cells that move in to fight the infection. Eventually a "head" will form on the boil. Sometimes doctors will lance a boil to surgically remove the liquid. Teenagers can get cystic acne, which is an infection that forms in a pore clogged with oil. Some boils are caused by the staphylococcus germ. These are called furuncles or carbuncles and can have one or several openings and cause chills and fever. Boils usually occur around hair follicles—on the face, neck, under the arms, pubic area, buttocks, or thighs. All boils can be quite painful. Many boils can be drained through the surface of the skin using natural methods. However, if you have a severe boil causing fever, see a competent physician. The following are some natural home remedies for boils.

Disinfecting Solution

> 6 drops tea tree oil or 4 drops oregano oil
> 1 cup hot distilled water

Mix the oil and the water. Wet a cloth with the solution, and hold it on the boil. Keep wetting the cloth with the solution until the boil breaks open. Then put a salve on the boil made from one-half teaspoon olive oil, six drops oregano oil, and one capsule goldenseal. Open the capsule and pour goldenseal into the oil, and mix well. Apply to the affected area, and bandage well. There is also a colloidal silver herbal salve that works great as well. See the resources section for where to find it.

BREAST AILMENTS

For nursing mothers whose breasts are caked from milk, blend organic tomatoes and make a tomato poultice (see chapter 3).

To promote milk flow in nursing mothers, make a tea with nettles and blessed thistle. Drink at least a few cups each day. Also, eat plenty of green leafy vegetables. Almond cream, sesame sauce, and sunflower seed sauce also help to promote a rich milk flow. Here are a couple of other recipes that help increase mother's breast milk.

Atole

> 4 cups purified water
> 3 heaping tablespoons of cornmeal
> 1 cinnamon stick
> 1 cup almond milk
> $^1/_2$ cup natural maple syrup or 5 to 10 drops of stevia

Boil 4 cups of purified water with a cinnamon stick. Take 1 cup of the boiling water and add 3 heaping tablespoons of cornmeal. Stir until smooth. Add this cup of mixture into the pot of boiling water. Stir until smooth. Boil for 10 minutes on low. Cool. Mixture will get thick. Add one cup of homemade almond milk or almond milk from the health food store and natural maple syrup or stevia to taste. Refrigerate. Drink at least twice a day.

To supplement breast milk, the following is a nice formula to give to babies.

Natural Baby Formula

    1 ounce goat milk powder
    3 ounces distilled water
    $^1/_2$ ounce pure cream
    1 teaspoon milk sugar

Combine all the ingredients and stir well.

When the mother is not producing enough of her own milk, fresh raw goat milk is the best substitute. It is the nearest in composition to human milk and is very healthy for the baby. If there are no goats in the area, the natural baby formula above is also a very good substitute.

Breasts often become sore just before menstruation due to excess estrogen. When the liver has not processed the estrogen properly, the breasts can swell and ache. To help the liver process estrogen, avoid fried foods, caffeine, sugar, alcohol, and meats and milk that are high in hormones. Take four hundred international units of vitamin E three times daily, a good multivitamin/multimineral with all the B vitamins, and evening primrose oil. Get plenty of exercise, eat lots of vegetables, and make sure the bowels are moving.

BRONCHITIS

Bronchitis is an infection that causes inflammation in the bronchi, the pipes that carry oxygen and air into your lungs. Bronchitis is usually caused by a virus in the lining of the bronchi that causes swelling and the production of mucus. Mucus is made to help protect the bronchi from the inflammation and carry off the germs. However, the mucus causes congestion and makes it very difficult to breathe. Many times, a person will begin to cough in order to rid the body of the mucus and infection. We get viruses when the body is worn down, exhausted, and the immune system is weak. People that smoke or live in areas where there is lots of pollution are more likely to get bronchitis because the bronchi and lungs are already weak. Here is a home remedy that has helped in many cases to relieve and heal bronchitis. If the condition persists, see a physician.

Oregano Solution

10 drops oregano oil
4 ounces warm distilled water

Mix the oil and warm water, then drink it four times daily. Mix twenty drops of oregano oil or twenty drops of garlic oil with three tablespoons of olive oil and rub on the chest and feet. Cover the chest with warm onion poultices (see chapter 3). If coughing is severe, take valerian root to relax the throat. Gargle with one tablespoon of raw apple cider vinegar in six ounces of water. Take two propolis, twice daily and one echinacea or goldenseal twice daily. Grapefruit seed extract is also very beneficial in helping break up the mucus and stop a cough. Recommended dose is two capsules, twice daily with food. If the throat is sore, spray with a colloidal silver solution of ten parts per million.

BRUISING

If you tend to bruise easily, take five hundred milligrams of bioflavonoids and one hundred milligrams of rutin three times per day. If you have a severe bruise, use arnica cream or salve on it. Arnica cream can be found in any health food store and contains the arnica herb that has proven to be beneficial in healing bruises. It contains the essential oil called thymol that helps reduce inflammation and flavonoids that knit tissue back together. The comfrey poultice in chapter 3 is also very healing for severe bruises. See also Dr. Christopher in resources for Complete Tissue and Bone Cream.

BURNS AND SUNBURNS

Raw organic honey mixed half and half with fresh organic wheat germ oil will heal a burn quickly. Place the honey and oil on the burn, and keep a sterile white cotton cloth over it. Aloe vera juice and gel are also wonderful for healing burns. According to Anne McIntyre in *Herbal Medicine*:

> *The University of Pennsylvania Radiology Department has found that the juice of this plant [aloe vera] is more effective in treating radiation burns than any other known product. It is now one of the most*

popular herbs used commercially in face creams, hand and body lotions and shampoos.

In treating severe burns, be careful when changing the bandages. The bandages may stick and cause severe pain or, worse, pull off the healing skin. John W. Keim writes about this in *Comfort for the Burned and Wounded*. He discovered that placing clean, moist plantain leaves over the salve worked well. The leaves should be wrapped with gauze and a towel. This wrapping allows air to get through to the burn. In addition, the leaves are very healing. If plantain leaves are not available, Mr. Keim found that burdock and dandelion leaves work well also. Soaked dried leaves may also be used. The bandage can be changed every twelve hours and will not tear or pull the skin or tissue. With this type of treatment, there should be no infection and little or no scarring.

BURSITIS

Bursitis occurs when the bursae have become inflamed. Bursae are small sacs filled with fluid that are located between the tendons and bones throughout the body. Bursitis is treated much the same way tendonitis is. Avoid alcohol and caffeine. Soak in Epsom salts baths and apply castor oil poultices (see chapter 3). Apply arnica cream or Complete Tissue and Bone Cream (see resources) and wear an ace bandage. Take marshmallow herb, turmeric, calcium, magnesium, trace minerals, B complex, and vitamin C to reduce inflammation. Rest the injured tendon.

CALLUSES

Rub castor oil on calluses on the hands or feet. They will soften and come off beautifully.

Calluses are composed of several layers of skin produced to protect an area from wear and tear. Wearing shoes that are too tight, for example, can put daily pressure on a specific area on the foot. Some people stand or walk in such a way that the same area of the foot is stressed daily. Over time, calluses can become hardened and painful.

To prevent calluses, change your shoes and wear different pairs. Wear shoes that are made of leather or cloth and allow the foot to breathe. Wear shoes that are supportive but do not put extreme pressure on specific areas. Notice how you stand and walk. If you are putting undue pressure on a certain area, practice standing and walking so that you are no longer causing that pressure. If you have a severe problem with your feet, see an expert. If you are overweight, this can cause extra pressure on the feet as well. Follow the healthy eating plans presented in chapter 1, and drop those extra pounds.

Soak the affected foot each day in hot water with a half cup of baking soda for twenty minutes to an hour. Rinse your foot, then scrub the callus gently with a pumice stone. Apply castor oil and put on an old cotton sock before going to bed. Rinse your foot in the morning with warm water and baking soda. Baking soda removes castor oil from your body as well as from your clothes. If the callus is painful, put a bit of castor oil or Complete Tissue and Bone Cream (see resources) on a bandage and keep it bandaged during the day.

CHOLESTEROL, HIGH

Cholesterol plays a vital role in cellular health. It is necessary for the brain and nervous system to function properly and for the manufacture of sex hormones. Cholesterol is a fat and is manufactured in the liver.

There is a lot of confusion right now about cholesterol. Many people believe that margarine is good for them and that butter is bad. This is far from the truth! Chemicals that harden margarine can also harden the arteries! A little real butter is better for you. Butter contains vitamin A, which is great for your eyes, and some protein. Hydrogenating oils keep margarine solid, even in your blood and arteries. Avoid hydrogenated oils and polyunsaturated oils. Read labels.

Many people also believe that artificial eggs are better for maintaining healthy cholesterol levels than real eggs from healthy chickens. This is not true. Fertilized eggs from healthy chickens are high in lecithin, which emulsifies cholesterol.

Refined white sugar can cause high cholesterol. The liver converts excess sugar into fat in your blood! These fats are then deposited in the arteries, creating plaque.

To lower cholesterol, eat foods high in fiber, such as whole grains—including oats, barley, millet, and quinoa—beans, steamed vegetables, and salads. Use apple pectin or citrus pectin, which binds to plaque and fat and pulls it out of the body. Use lecithin on soups, in vegetable juice, or on salads to help cleanse plaque and lower cholesterol levels. Eat lots of garlic or take garlic capsules. Policosanol, a natural food substance (see chapter 5), has proven to be tremendously successful in lowering cholesterol. Eat beets or take beet tablets. Beets help cleanse the liver and gallbladder. Eat raw grated beets and steamed beets and drink raw vegetable juice, such as carrot, celery, parsley, beet, and ginger. Carrot juice flushes fat from the bile in the liver and helps control cholesterol, and ginger improves circulation.

Food supplements that help reduce cholesterol include alpha lipoic acid and lipotropic factors, which help prevent fat deposits. A-Flow, an oral chelation formula, and essential fatty acids, such as black currant seed, flaxseed, borage, and primrose oils, help raise the good fats or high-density lipoproteins and lower the bad fats or low-density lipoproteins. Cayenne, coenzyme Q10, and niacin help improve circulation, and glucomannan and gugolipids also reduce serum cholesterol.

Follow these nutritional suggestions for one month. Then do a seven-day colon cleanse followed by a liver cleanse (see chapter 6). Exercise is also very important.

COLDS AND COUGHS

Dr. Jensen had wonderful results treating coughs with the following recipe.

Cough Syrup

    6 yellow onions, chopped, or 6 lemons, chopped
    1 cup raw organic honey

Place the onions or lemons over water in a double boiler. Cover them and bring to a boil. Lower the temperature to a simmer. Cook the mixture for one hour. Remove the mixture from the heat and add the honey. Blend the mixture and then strain it. Take one teaspoon of warm syrup every hour. It will soothe your throat, help stop a cough, and cleanse the bowels.

Your health food store may also have some good cough syrups. Look for wild black cherry bark syrup or horehound syrup. Zinc lozenges or Swiss Herbal lozenges can be helpful. Also, gargle with one tablespoon of apple cider vinegar to a half cup of warm water. Use onion poultices on the throat and chest. The steam from a vaporizer with eucalyptus oil can soothe irritated throats. Propolis tablets, liquid, or tincture, elderberry tea, echinacea and goldenseal, vitamin C, and Dr. Christopher's antiplague formula can all help to heal the body.

CONSTIPATION

For occasional constipation, take cascara sagrada capsules or tea before bed-time.

Cascara Sagrada Tea

$^1/_3$ teaspoon cascara sagrada bark powder
$^2/_3$ teaspoon cardamom powder
a pinch of ginger powder
1 teaspoon honey
1 cup boiling water

Pour the boiling water over the herbs. Add the honey and stir. Cover for five minutes, then drink slowly.

If constipation is a chronic problem, you may need to change your lifestyle. Make sure you are drinking eight glasses of distilled water daily with fifteen drops of ionic liquid trace minerals in each glass. Constipation is often related to a magnesium deficiency. Peristalsis, or movement of the colon, depends upon minerals and trace minerals in order to function properly.

The colon must have adequate fiber each day to work well. Fiber comes from fruits, vegetables, whole grains, nuts, and seeds. Have a tablespoon of ground flaxseeds each morning on a bowl of cooked millet. Flaxseed tea is mucilaginous and also beneficial in promoting healthy elimination. Eat papayas, pineapple, and apples in between meals. These fruits are high in enzymes. Apples contain pectin, a wonderful natural fiber. Chewing alfalfa tablets works wonders for some people. People who are sensitive to alfalfa tablets fare better with chlorella tablets. The fiber is finer in chlorella tablets (you must get the shattered-cell wall type of chlorella in order to utilize the storehouse of nutrients). Take five to eight chlorella tablets just before each meal with two teaspoons of flaxseed oil. This combination makes an oily bolus that lubricates and sweeps the colon clean. Raw beet juice and spinach juice promote peristalsis in the intestinal tract.

Grated raw beets and steamed beets are great for the colon. Watermelon eaten first thing in the morning helps encourage good bowel movements. Dried fruits help tremendously as well, but you must pour boiling water over all dried fruit in order to kill parasites. Remember it is best to eat fruit alone. Combining your foods properly, as well as taking digestive plant enzymes just before meals, helps improve digestion.

Make sure you have plenty of good bacteria, such as acidophilus, lactobacillus, and bifidus, in your digestive tract. Eating yogurt is a good choice for people who do not have allergies to milk. Many people with milk allergies can tolerate yogurt because it has been predigested and is high in friendly bacterial cultures. It is best to make your own yogurt with raw organic goat's or cow's milk. If this is not possible, try to find certified organic yogurt in your health food store.

Exercise is crucial to ensure good daily bowel rhythm. In addition, your emotions play a large role in bowel activity. If you are under a lot of stress daily, this can cause constipation. Practice deep breathing throughout the day. If you feel suppressed in general and do not feel you can talk out your problems, you may subconsciously be suppressing your colon. Try to talk to a good friend or go for a walk and talk to a tree, but get those feelings out. If you avoid going to the bathroom when nature calls, your colon may become blocked. Always go if you feel the slightest urge!

If you have had children, are overweight, or have frequent urination, there's a good possibility that your colon has prolapsed and is pressing on your bladder. For this, you should lie on a slant board for fifteen to twenty minutes twice daily. Massage your colon with a tennis ball while you are reclining on the board as described in chapter 3. This helps to tighten and tone the colon and is a great exercise for promoting peristalsis.

DANDRUFF

Do a colon cleansing and kidney cleansing, as described in chapter 6. Take two tablespoons of flaxseed oil, fifty milligrams of zinc, and six hundred international units of vitamin E daily. Drink two cups of oatstraw tea daily, and take horsetail herb. Use the scalp treatment for dandruff treatment described in chapter 3. Rubbing a bit of eucalyptus oil mixed half and half with olive oil has also helped many get rid of dandruff.

DIABETES MELLITUS

Diabetes mellitus is a disorder that results when the pancreas stops producing sufficient amounts of insulin. Insulin is a hormone that regulates the absorption of glucose, which produces energy in the cells; it also stimulates fat cells and the liver to store reserve glucose. When there is an insufficient amount of insulin, glucose builds up in the blood, causing hyperglycemia.

High levels of glucose in the blood lead to frequent urination because of the increased volume of urine required to carry sugar out of the body. One side effect of an increase in urination is constant thirst. Excessive levels of sugar in the urine can impair the body's ability to fight infection. Sugar can even cause infections, including yeast, bladder, and skin infections. People with diabetes become weak with fatigue because their cells lack glucose (an important source of energy), which has been carried away with the constant urination. Diabetics often lose weight as their bodies strive to obtain energy by breaking down stored fat. Hyperglycemia can eventually cause damage to the blood vessels and nerves, leading to numbness of the limbs and diseases of the heart, eyes, and kidneys.

According to the American Diabetes Association:

There are 20.8 million children and adults in the United States, or seven percent of the population, who have diabetes. While an estimated 14.6 million have been diagnosed, unfortunately, 6.2 million people (or nearly one-third) are unaware that the have the disease.

There are two major types of diabetes. Type 1 diabetes, or insulin-dependent diabetes mellitus (IDDM), is the more severe type and affects 5 to 10 percent of people with diabetes. It develops rapidly, usually occurring in young people between the ages of ten and sixteen. In this type, the insulin-secreting beta cells have been destroyed (often from a virus or overactive immune response), and insulin can no longer be produced.

Type 2 diabetes, or noninsulin dependent diabetes, affects 90 to 95 percent of diabetics and usually occurs in people over the age of forty. However, there recently has been an alarming increase among teenagers and children. In this type, insulin is produced but not enough to manage the sugar levels in the blood. There are several risk factors for developing type 2 diabetes. These include a diet rich in refined carbohydrates, hydrogenated oils, processed foods, soft drinks, high fructose corn syrup, and sugar; excess weight; and lack of exercise.

Type 2 diabetes claims about a hundred million victims worldwide each year. In the United States, it is the sixth-leading cause of death and one of the primary causes of blindness, kidney disease, and amputations.

Avoid refined white sugar. Use natural sugars such as maple syrup, honey, dates, and molasses sparingly. Use stevia or agave to sweeten your food and drinks. These sweeteners actually balance the pancreas and have very few calories. Take chromium picolinate and trace minerals to help balance the pancreas and reduce sweet cravings.

Gymnema sylvestre, a wonderful herb from India, lowers high blood sugar levels and greatly reduces excessive secretion of glucose in the urine. It also increases beta cells that produce insulin, and may reduce the need for insulin treatments. Recent studies have shown that cinnamon can actually balance blood sugar levels as well. Fenugreek seeds were used in ancient Italy, Greece, and India to treat blood sugar disturbances in the body. Fenugreek seeds can help reduce insulin requirements by lowering blood glucose levels. Soak fenugreek seeds, sprout them, and put them in salads and on soups. The high fiber content delays glucose absorption. Exercise and stress management are crucial for people suffering from diabetes or hypoglycemia. Walk at least twenty minutes to a half hour daily to balance sugar levels and keep the body metabolizing at optimal levels. Practice deep breathing.

Add some "sweet" activities to your life. Make a list of all the things you love to do and do them! Too many people eat sweets because their lives are empty and without joy. Practice generosity, build self-esteem, love yourself, and share happy times with others. Learn to allow and let go. Listen to pleasant music, call a friend, go to a play, take walks in nature. The next time you crave a candy bar, be creative and do something fun! Life is sweet! Enjoy the sweetness of life.

Become informed about diabetes. Read *Sugar Blues* by William Dufty, *The Diabetes Improvement Program* by Patrick Quillin, and *The pH Miracle for Diabetes* by Dr. Robert Young. Take care of you! It's your life!

DIARRHEA

When you have diarrhea, there is usually a poison in your system that needs to be released. Taking medicine to stop it prevents the toxicity from getting out of the body. Instead, stop eating regular meals. Prepare some barley or brown rice gruel, cooking the barley or rice really well until it is almost a mush. Eat several small bowls of it throughout the day. You also may eat a very ripe banana at separate times from the gruel.

Alternate between drinking red raspberry leaf tea, thyme tea, cinnamon tea, and ginger tea. These help check diarrhea and relieve nausea.

Diarrhea also can be the result of an inflammation of the intestinal tract caused by bacteria, viruses, or parasites. Viruses are spread through close human contact. Bacteria and parasites are transmitted through contaminated water or food. A rainforest herb called Sangre de Drago has proven to be very beneficial in healing intestinal inflammation and stopping diarrhea. Colloidal silver can kill viruses and bacteria, so it's very useful in stopping diarrhea caused by any of these micro-organisms. Black walnut, wormwood, and cloves are helpful if diarrhea is caused by parasites. In all cases of diarrhea, you should take acidophilus and bifidus to reinstate friendly bacteria into the colon. If diarrhea persists more than three or four days, you can become dehydrated and need to seek medical advice. Symptoms of dehydration include dry mouth, little urination, and intense thirst. If you have a fever of 100°F, abdominal pain, or black or red blood in the stools, go to the doctor. Call your doctor if your child has diarrhea for more than twenty-four hours. Children can dehydrate much more rapidly than adults. A doctor will be able to test your blood and run a stool test to determine the cause of the diarrhea.

EAR INFECTIONS

Ear infections are common in children and swimmers. They are caused by germs, including bacteria and viruses, that get into the ear and middle ear (just inside the ear canal). These germs can also get into the eustachian tubes, which are passages between your middle ear and throat. These tubes are important because they allow air to move in and out of your middle ear, killing germs and preventing pressure from building up. Little children have very tiny eustachian tubes and they are less able to keep germs out. Allergies and colds can cause mucus to become trapped in the eustachian tubes and middle ear allowing infection to grow. Water from swimming can become trapped in the middle ear forming damp breeding grounds for germs. Ear infections are not spread from person to person. They occur when germs grow in the middle ear due to congestion. Ear infections can be extremely painful and cause fever. You might even have difficulty hearing. If you get an ear infection, the following oil has proven to be very helpful time and again for healing the ears.

Garlic-Mullein Ear Oil

1 part garlic oil
3 parts mullein oil

Combine the oils. Put the mixture in a dropper bottle, and place it in a cup of hot water. Put one to two drops of warm oil in each ear. This oil helps reduce inflammation and swelling, fight infection, and soften hardened earwax. Avoid dairy products, wheat, and sugar, and make sure the bowels are working well. Keep the immune system strong by taking two propolis tablets daily.

Swimmers should use the following: one ounce colloidal silver at 125 parts per million with ten drops of tea tree oil added. Natural Path/ Silver Wings carries a great colloidal silver with herbal tincture of Swedish bitters and tea tree oil that I also highly recommend for ear infections (see resources).

EDEMA

See "Swollen Ankles, Fingers, or Wrists" later in this chapter.

ENURESIS

See "Bed-Wetting" earlier in this chapter.

EYE DISORDERS

Included below are a few simple eye remedies and suggestions. If you are experiencing any eye problems, see your ophthalmologist immediately. For nutritional suggestions for strengthening the eyes and a recipe for an eye poultice, see chapter 3. For more in-depth eye information, read *Smart Medicine for Your Eyes* by Dr. Jeffrey Anshel.

If the eyes become dry in the wintertime, vessels in the sclera can become irritated, swollen, and red. Bioflavonoids, which strengthen blood vessels, can help prevent this condition. The fluid of the eyes is part of the lymph system, so feed your lymph with the mineral whey drink described in chapter 1, and drink plenty of celery juice. Oils are an important lubricant too, so incorporate flax seed oil, borage oil, and pumpkin seed oil into your diet. The eye poultice in chapter 3 can also soothe irritated eyes.

The eyes are vulnerable to several types of infection. A sty results when one of the small glands attached to an eye becomes infected. Iritis, an inflammation of the iris, can be caused by allergies or infection. Conjunctivitis, an inflammation of the conjunctiva, can be caused by allergies, infection, chemical burns, or injury. Pink eye is a type of conjunctivitis. A compress can be prepared that may help soothe and heal infected eyes.

Goldenseal Eye Compress

¹/₃ teaspoon goldenseal powder
1 ounce fresh cabbage juice

Boil two ounces distilled water. Turn off the heat, let cool, and add the goldenseal and juice. Goldenseal contains the alkaloid berberine, which helps fight infection; cabbage juice is high in vitamins C and A and can help fight bacteria and viruses. Stir with a sterile spoon and strain through a cheesecloth. Dip two pieces of gauze, large enough to cover each eyelid, in the solution and place over the closed eyelids. Leave for fifteen minutes to a half hour.

Cataracts are an opacification or cloudiness that occur in the lens and which block light from reaching the retina and impair vision. Most cataracts begin after age forty-five and are often caused by free-radical damage, heavy metals, eye injury, smoking, or diabetes. Vitamin B, eyebright tea, which is also rich in vitamins C and A, and bilberries and blueberries, which are rich in bioflavonoids, may help prevent cataracts. Splashing the eyes with cold water each morning also helps because it stimulates the circulation of blood through the eyes. A diet rich in vegetables, especially spinach and carrots, help maintain eye health.

Glaucoma results when fluid pressure increases inside the eyeball. This occurs when either the eye is producing too much fluid or the drainage system in the eye has broken down or is blocked. Glaucoma has many causes including eye injury, eye surgery, nutritional imbalances, and some medications such as steroids. It may also be related to high blood pressure and diabetes. To help prevent glaucoma, follow the nutritional plans in chapter 1, the cleansing program outlined in chapter 6, and the eye poultice in chapter 3. Include plenty of cold-pressed oils including flax, borage, and olive oils in your diet, as well as liquid trace minerals and zinc. Vitamin A, beta-carotene, B complex, B6, and bioflavonoids may be helpful. Vitamin C can possibly help to reduce the pressure.

Blepharitis is an inflammation of the outer edges of the eyelids that can occur when the glands in the eyelids and hair follicles become blocked with mucus and inflamed. A bacterial infection may be involved and burning, swollen eyelids can result. The eyes may also become pasted together during sleep. Drink raw juices of green leaves and carrots. Rinse your eyes with warm water and use the compress above. Include bilberry and eyebright herbs in your diet. Vitamin A, beta-carotene, vitamin C with bioflavonoids, liquid trace minerals, and zinc (no more than 50 milligrams) have traditionally been used to improve conditions. Use an air filter to remove dust, mold, and pollen from your home.

FEVER

To relieve a fever, soak in a hot ginger bath, then rinse in cool water. Take an enema with two quarts of cool distilled water, two tablespoons of chlorophyll, one tablespoon of white willow bark powder, and one cup of catnip tea. Aspirin was originally made from willow bark, which is like a natural aspirin without the side effects. Take two capsules of white willow bark three times daily. Children should take half that amount. A small enema can be made for children with one cup of cool distilled water, two teaspoons of chlorophyll, and one teaspoon of white willow bark powder.

FUNGUS

Fungus usually appears on the feet and toes. Soak your feet in a footbath, as recommended in chapter 3. Rinse your feet and apply tea tree oil or oil of oregano. People who chronically have fungus on their feet usually have low thyroid function. The thyroid helps manage the body's metabolism and circulation. When the thyroid function is low, blood does not circulate to the extremities as it should so they lack nutrients and oxygen. Nutrients feed the feet and toes, and oxygen kills the microorganisms that cause fungus. If you have chronic fungus, test your thyroid with the thyroid basal temperature test at the end of this chapter. If you have low thyroid function, study the information under "Thyroid Disorders" later in this chapter.

FIBROMYALGIA

Fibromyalgia is a rheumatic disorder that causes severe aching in the muscles, much as if one has been beaten or bruised. Approximately ten million people in the United States have been diagnosed with fibromyalgia, and that figure is rising. The etiology is still unknown and there is no known cure. Most people who have fibromyalgia have often had some type of trauma, injury, or severe stress. The immune system may be weak, and there may be a disturbance in the brain's chemistry. The Epstein-Barr virus or other viruses may be involved. People with fibromyalgia may have *Candida albicans* (a fungus) or parasites. They may be anemic and have low thyroid function and hypoglycemia. However, people can have any of these disorders and not have fibromyalgia.

The common denominators in patients with fibromyalgia are stress and sleep disturbance. Studies have shown that people deprived of sleep have muscular pain. People who have chronic stress produce high amounts of adrenaline, which can cause insomnia, poor digestion, rapid heartbeat, and even sore muscles. Nobel prize winner Hans Seyle found that stress can cause calcium leak from the bone and become deposited in tissues. He explains his research in *Stress Without Distress*. Nancy Selfridge, MD, conquered fibromyalgia and has worked with many others to do the same. She has written a wonderful book called *Freedom from Fibromyalgia: The 5-Week Program Proven to Conquer Pain*. Two other very informative books are *New Hope for People with Fibromyalgia* by Theresa Foy DiGeronimo, MEd and *From Fatigued to Fantastic* by Jacob Teitelbaum, MD.

People with fibromyalgia suffer from insomnia and when they don't sleep, the muscular pain is more severe. They often feel exhausted with chronic fatigue, never reaching a deep restful sleep due to the pain. Other symptoms of fibromyalgia include headaches, digestive disorders, feelings of disorientation, difficulty concentrating, depression, and bruxism (tooth grinding).

Several herbal remedies can be very effective in healing *Candida albicans* and viruses. These are, Pau d'Arco, grapefruit seed extract, and caprylic acid (made from coconut). People with fibromyalgia who have *Candida albicans* should start with small dosages and build up gradually, or they might feel much worse.

Ionic trace minerals are essential for keeping the body alkaline. Turmeric and white willow bark, two anti-inflammatory herbs, can ease discomfort. Malic acid, found in apples, assists the cells in producing energy. CoQ10 improves tissue oxygenation. Ginkgo biloba improves brain and nerve function, and cayenne improves circulation. Glucosamine sulfate is a naturally occurring precursor for proteoglycan synthesis. Glucosamine sulfate can strengthen joints as well as connective tissue. Bioflavonoids are important components of vitamin C that help to build connective tissue. Acidophilus and Eugalan Topfer Forte (a powdered form of *Lactobacillus bifidus*) are good probiotics that soothe the digestive tract and provide friendly bacteria that keep the colon healthy. Flaxseed tea and aloe vera juice also soothe the digestive tract. Take enzymes before each meal to assist the body in breaking down and absorbing nutrients. Flaxseed oil and borage oil help provide the essential fatty acids necessary for healthy nerve functioning. Magnesium, calcium, and potassium help relax the muscles and in some cases are all a person with fibromyalgia will need to help them relax and sleep. If not, 5-hydroxytryptophan (5HTP) is a natural supplement that helps promote proper sleep cycles. Skullcap and valerian root can also help promote deep restful sleep.

A good multivitamin/multimineral with a high amount of B vitamins for the nervous system is very important. Chlorella is most effective in cleansing the colon, liver, and blood. Vitamin E improves circulation and is a powerful antioxidant. NOTE: There is a wide selection of supplements that can help with fibromyalgia. However, all people with fibromyalgia will not need to take all mentioned supplements. For specifics, it is important to work with a doctor to determine first if you have fibromyalgia. Then find out for sure if you have have *Candida albicans* or a virus. If not, you will not need the remedies suggested for these. You need to find out if you have hypoglycemia, low thyroid function, or exhausted adrenal glands. If so, bringing these areas into balance will help strengthen the body so it can rest properly. Relaxing the muscles, improving nerve function, and getting proper sleep is paramount for those suffering with the pain of fibromyalgia. Cleansing the colon and liver can also be very beneficial.

People with fibromyalgia must avoid caffeine and alcohol. Their livers often work more slowly than those of healthy people. They also should follow the nutritional program outlined in chapter 1 and stay away from household chemicals and cigarette smoke.

Baths with a quarter cup of gingerroot tea can greatly improve circulation and reduce pain. Epsom salts baths relax the muscles. Essential oils such as thyme, oregano, birch, eucalyptus, and lavender (with a pinch of cayenne to improve circulation) are very soothing and healing when rubbed into the muscles. Rub these oils up and down the spine as well. Viruses often live in the spinal cord.

Gentle exercise and deep breathing are crucial for a fibromyalgia patient. Avoid strenuous exercise, which will produce lactic acid and cause more pain. Walking, jumping on the rebounder, cycling, yoga, tai chi, and swimming or water exercises are excellent. You must get oxygen to all the body's cells to help decrease pain. Massage is also important. Walk barefoot on the earth as often as possible. This can help reconnect you to the earth's natural circadian rhythms, thus helping you to achieve a deeper sleep.

Learn to release anger and tension. Be gentle with yourself. If you follow this program, you will soon have more pain-free days than painful ones.

GUM DISEASE

Gum disease, or periodontal disease, is common throughout the United States. People with gum disease have bad breath. Gum disease is caused by bacteria, plaque (mucus and bacteria), and particles of food and sugar that deteriorate on the gums. Gingivitis, or gum inflammation, is the beginning of periodontal disease. In the advanced stage, called pyorrhea, gums become infected, swollen, and red, and they bleed easily. Too much bleeding can cause anemia. Eventually, the teeth may fall out.

Avoid sugar and white flour. Use a water pick to loosen plaque. Floss your teeth gently, and brush with a soft brush. Rub clove oil or thyme oil directly on your gums to kill bacteria and relieve any pain. Rinse your mouth with food-grade peroxide (one-half teaspoon mixed with eight ounces distilled water).

HAIR LOSS

Eat two organic raw egg yolks laid by free range hens daily. Wash the eggs well before cracking them open. You may add black cherry juice to the egg yolks for better flavor and blend them into a Good Morning Health Shake or Avocado Pudding (see recipes in chapter 1). Drink two cups of oatstraw tea per day and one cup of rosemary leaf tea per day. Follow the advice under scalp treatment for hair loss (see chapter 3). Poached eggs and soft-boiled eggs are also helpful. If the problem is chronic, balance the adrenal glands by taking raw organic adrenal, ashwaganda, or licorice root capsules and meditating and relaxing each day. Taking B complex and biotin has also proven to be very helpful. Put rice bran on your cereal or salads.

HEADACHES

Many headaches are caused by poor circulation to the head. Follow the facial exercises in chapter 3. Rub peppermint oil mixed half and half with safflower or lavender oil on the temples, but be sure not to get it in the eyes. Peppermint oil contains menthol and promotes blood circulation as well. Lavender oil has relaxing properties that can promote rest and reduce headaches. Take fifty milligrams of niacin together with B complex to promote blood flow to the head and ease a headache. Rosemary tea is helpful in treating headaches. Feverfew is often useful in stopping migraines. Follow the directions on the bottle. If headaches persist, consult a knowledgeable physician.

HEMORRHOIDS

Hemorrhoids are actually swollen veins in the anus and rectum, similar to varicose veins. The tissue of the veins has weakened, often due to prolonged constipation and straining. Grind flaxseeds and use one teaspoon daily for three days, then increase gradually to three teaspoons daily. Too much fiber at once can cause gas. Use one tablespoon of flaxseed oil three times daily to lubricate the colon and soften stools. Flaxseeds are high in fiber, which helps the colon function well. A cup of flaxseed tea, taken three times daily, can soothe the intestinal tract and promote good peristalsis. Slippery elm tea and capsules also soothe the alimentary tract and rectum.

Drink a cup of oatstraw tea daily. Oatstraw is high in silicon, which can strengthen the walls of the veins and arteries. Take two thousand milligrams of vitamin C with bioflavonoids three times daily. Bioflavonoids help to strengthen connective tissue. If hemorrhoids are persistent, take extra rutin, fifty milligrams three times daily. Rutin is one of the bioflavonoids that has proven to be very effective in reducing hemorrhoids.

Soak in a warm sitz bath of two quarts of water and one cup of calendula tea and one tablespoon of witch hazel (which can be found in liquid form at your health store). Calendula tea soothes hemorrhoids. Witch hazel acts as an astringent and can help relieve bleeding. Rinse off and apply castor oil to the anus and rectum. If hemorrhoids are bleeding, take one capsule of cayenne mixed with ginger three times daily to help stop the bleeding. Be sure to eat foods high in iron (dark green leafy vegetables, beets, figs, and blackstrap molasses) if you have been bleeding.

HERPES SIMPLEX 1 (HSV-1) AND HERPES SIMPLEX 2 (HSV-2)

Herpes simplex 1 is a virus that usually causes cold sores on the mouth, skin eruptions, and eye infections. As many as 80 percent of the United States population have been infected by this virus but not all have noticeable symptoms.

Herpes simplex 2 is a virus that can cause genital blisters. Approximately thirty-five million Americans have been infected but not all are symptomatic.

Both herpes viruses are contagious. People who have these viruses should follow a healthy eating regime for two weeks, as outlined in chapter 1, then do the colon and liver cleanse.

Take five hundred milligrams of L-lysine with water twice daily on an empty stomach. L-lysine is one of the eight essential amino acids found in protein that the body does not produce on its own. It helps strengthen the immune system and has the ability to fight and prevent the herpes virus. Food sources include brewer's yeast, eggs, fish, and lima beans. Take a good multivitamin high in B complex three times daily; two thousand milligrams of vitamin C three times daily; sixty milligrams of quercetin (a bioflavonoid and powerful antioxidant) three times daily; fifty milligrams of zinc two times daily; acidophilus four times daily on an empty stomach; HPVS (an effective herbal formula) according to directions; one dropperful of colloidal silver twice daily; and oregano oil capsules three times daily. Apply oregano oil or tea tree oil to any cold sores. Apply three parts olive oil mixed with one part oregano or tea tree oil to genital blisters. The Monastery of Herbs carries very effective herbal remedies called HPVS #1 and HPVS #2.

HIATAL HERNIA

A hiatal hernia occurs when the cardiac sphincter muscle, which is the sphincter that opens from the esophagus into the stomach, becomes weak and fails to keep food, acids, and gases from entering the esophagus. This condition, called gastroesophageal reflux, causes burping, irritation of the esophageal tissues. and heartburn. Sometimes people even cough up mucus and blood, and the esophagus becomes ulcerated. Hiatal hernias can be a result of trauma, injury, or many years of overeating. It may also be a result of a genetic weakness in the sphincter muscle. Digestive enzymes help tremendously, as does combining food properly and eating small meals. Papaya and papaya tablets, flaxseed tea, and aloe vera juice are all very soothing. Bioflavonoids and silica in horsetail herb or oatstraw tea help strengthen and repair the tissue.

HYPOGLYCEMIA

Hypoglycemia means the blood sugar or glucose levels are low. This usually occurs when the pancreas is producing too much insulin. Insulin helps manage blood sugar levels by facilitating the transport of sugar to the body's cells. It is also responsible for glucose synthesis in the liver. When there is too much insulin, blood sugar is utilized too rapidly, causing a person to feel light-headed, weak, shaky, tired, dizzy, anxious, depressed, short-tempered, nervous, and hungry. These people are often hungry and crave sweets. However, if they eat sweets, they may feel better for a short while only to have their blood sugar level crash again, feeling worse than ever.

Sugar intake prompts the pancreas to produce a surge of insulin. Eating small meals of foods that break down slowly throughout the day will normalize insulin production. Eat lots of raw and steamed vegetables, beans, soaked nuts and seeds, nut butters, brown rice, lentils, baked or broiled fish, chicken, turkey, yogurt, and cottage cheese. Eat no more than two fruits per day. In addition, ground flaxseeds, oat bran, and rice bran are high in fiber and slow a hypoglycemic reaction.

Avoid sugar, fruit juice, soft drinks, caffeine, nicotine, alcohol, and refined white flour. Supplements that are very helpful include glucose tolerance factor (GTF), chromium picolinate, digestive enzymes, chlorella, spirulina, B complex, brewer's yeast, amino acids, trace minerals, and vitamin E.

Blueberry leaf, huckleberry leaf, dandelion root tea, and stevia can help balance the pancreas. Licorice root tea supports the adrenal glands. Do not use licorice root on a daily basis. Every other day or every third day is best. Do not use it at all if you have high blood pressure.

INDIGESTION, BURNING STOMACH, AND GAS

Indigestion, burning stomach, and gas usually occur after eating a large meal with poor food combinations. Eugalan Topfer Forte is a wonderful product that contains a natural culture of live lactobacillus bifidus in a special food base that enhances their proliferation. It does contain some milk powder, but even people who have allergies to dairy products can usually tolerate it because of the high content (thirty million live lactobacillus bifidus organisms per one-ounce serving) of beneficial bacteria, which aid digestion. To prepare, place five level teaspoons (one ounce) of Eugalan Topfer Forte in five ounces of warm water. Stir the mixture well and drink it slowly. Children should take one teaspoon two times a day, and infants may take a half teaspoon daily. This delicious drink soothes the entire digestive tract and usually relieves indigestion, burning, and gas almost immediately. It can also benefit people with stomach ulcers.

If you have a tendency to get indigestion with your meals, take a few plant-based digestive enzymes with some water just before eating. The enzymes will help facilitate proper food digestion. Most Americans over the age of forty have lost a lot of their digestive ability, having consumed many meals of processed foods throughout their lives.

Papaya, papaya juice, and papaya tablets can help relive indigestion, burning in the stomach, and gas. I had a client with a stomach ulcer that he believed was a result of years of chronic beer consumption. Papaya juice helped him heal the ulcer. Charcoal tablets absorb excess gas in the gut. However, they should not be used on a regular basis. Charcoal may absorb healthy nutrients from the digestive tract as well. If you are taking medications, pregnant, or nursing consult your doctor before taking charcoal.

Combine your food properly, take digestive enzymes, aloe vera juice, acidophilus, and lactobacillus bifidus to correct the problem. If indigestion and burning persist or if nausea develops, seek the advice of a knowledgeable physician.

INFECTIONS, TOPICAL
Antibacterial Herbal Paste

$^1/_3$ ounce tea tree oil or oregano oil

1 ounce olive oil

4 capsules of goldenseal root powder (broken open and poured into paste)

2 capsules of marshmallow root or slippery elm (broken open and poured into paste)

Mix the oils goldenseal root powder and marshmallow root or slippery elm powder to form a paste. Apply the paste to the infected area, and cover it with a bandage.

INFLUENZA

Influenza is commonly called the flu. Symptoms include fever, chills, aching all over, headaches, and coughing. Some people develop diarrhea, nausea, and vomiting. Influenza is caused by a highly contagious viral infection, of which there are more than two hundred varieties! Antibiotics are not effective against viruses. Follow all the recommendations under colds and coughs listed above, unless diarrhea, nausea, and/or vomiting are present. With these symptoms, follow the recommendations for diarrhea. Take Eugalan Topfer Forte or acidophilus. Sip ginger tea. Take the warming bath described in chapter 3. Drink lots of fluids. Follow the exercise for headaches described above.

KIDNEY AND BLADDER INFECTIONS

When suffering from a kidney or bladder infection, avoid all dairy products except natural yogurt. Avoid caffeine, alcohol, salt, pork, and red meat (which is high in uric acid). Eat lots of raw vegetables, such as asparagus, parsley, celery, cucumber, green leafy lettuce, watercress, and garlic. Drink raw vegetable juices with carrot, cucumber, and parsley. Drink parsley tea. Eat watermelon but not with other foods. Eat steamed vegetables, brown rice, quinoa, millet, lentils, and beans.

Take acidophilus, propolis, and goldenseal. Take or drink as a tea: juniper berries, corn silk, and uva ursi. Take a dropper of colloidal silver or six drops of grapefruit seed extract three to four times per day. Take lots of acidophilus between meals on an empty stomach. Drink eight glasses of distilled water with four drops of ionic trace minerals in each glass. Keep the colon clean by taking chlorella and flaxseed oil.

NOTE: When taking grapefruit seed extract, do not get it on your teeth because it can be wearing on the enamel. Put it in water and drink it with a straw.

KIDNEY STONES

For kidney stones, follow the program for Kidney and Bladder Infections (above). Avoid red meat and dairy products. Drink eight ounces of water with one tablespoon of raw apple cider vinegar added to it, four times per day. Drink water with freshly squeezed lemon juice. Use lemon juice and olive oil or apple cider vinegar and olive oil salad dressings. Drink raw apple juice. Apples, lemons, and asparagus are helpful. Hydrangea, gravel root, and marshmallow root tinctures, teas, or capsules can help dissolve stones and relieve pain.

Soak in hot Epsom salts baths. Use castor oil poultices on the kidneys.

LICE

Wear rubber gloves and apply tea tree oil or oil of oregano mixed half and half with lavender oil to a lice-infected area, three to six times per day. Wash scalp with pine tar shampoo and hands with pine tar soap. Tea tree oil shampoo and soap may be used as well. Avoid eating sugar.

MENSTRUAL CRAMPING

Cramps can occur when the transverse colon has prolapsed and is pressing on the uterus. They can also occur when the liver does not process estrogen well or when minerals—especially calcium and magnesium—which keep muscles in the abdomen relaxed, are lacking. Also, clotting can occur during menstruation and cause cramping. Vitamin E and red raspberry leaf tea greatly reduce clotting and cramping. Avoid caffeine, sugar, and dairy products. Castor oil poultices will relieve the pain. Colon and liver cleansing have often eliminated menstrual cramping. Daily exercise is most important such as brisk walking or jumping on the rebounder. Chiropractic adjustments and accupuncture can be very helpful as well.

MENSTRUATION, IRREGULAR

Take two hundred international units of vitamin E three times per day to facilitate blood flow and circulation. Make sure the vitamin E is natural and the label says d-alphatocopherol rather than dl-alphatocopherol. Dl-alphatocopherol is the synthetic form of vitamin E. It is not utilized as well by the body and its potency is reduced compared to that of natural vitamin E. Herbs, such as dong quai, red raspberry leaf tea, and vitex can help regulate the menstrual cycle.

MORNING SICKNESS

Pregnant mothers may take ginger tea or peppermint leaf tea to relieve morning sickness. Vitamin B6 taken with a B complex can also be very helpful as well as eating small meals throughout the day.

MOSQUITO BITES

To repel mosquitoes, rub lemon grass oil on the skin or eat lots of garlic and brewer's yeast.

NAUSEA

Nausea can be caused by a stomach virus, vertigo, or car sickness.

To relieve nausea, drink ginger tea, red raspberry leaf tea, or peppermint leaf tea.

OSTEOPOROSIS

Osteoporosis, which means "porous bones," is a common bone disease. In old age, porous bones are brittle, and they break easily. After a fracture or break, they are slow to heal. A deficiency of vitamin D causes bones to soften. This condition is called osteomalacia in adults and rickets in children. The term used to describe a lowered bone mass which can be a precursor to osteoporosis is osteopenia. One of the best treatments for bones is raw organic vegetable juice because it is so easily absorbed. One glass of carrot juice is equal in calcium to a glass of milk and is much more absorbable. Most juices from green leafy vegetables are even higher in calcium than carrot juice.

Avoid caffeine in coffee, tea, sodas, and chocolate. Excessive caffeine contributes to osteoporosis by leaching calcium from bones and increasing urinary output of calcium. Douglas Kiel conducted a study and found that drinking two cups of coffee each day greatly increased the risk of bone fractures. A diet high in animal protein, sugar, salt, and processed foods creates acidity in the body, leading to calcium loss. An article in the *American Journal of Clinical Nutrition*, 6, summarizes a study conducted at the University of California in San Francisco, on 9,704 postmenopausal women. It showed that those women who ate a diet high in animal foods and low in vegetables had increased acidity levels and a resultant greater risk for lowered bone density than women with normal pH levels. When the body is acidic, it will pull calcium from the bones to help neutralize acids.

The phosphoric acid found in soft drinks inhibits the body from absorbing calcium properly. Vitamin D, boron, zinc, magnesium, calcium, sodium, and digestive enzymes will assist in calcium absorption. Raw vegetables and raw vegetable juices contain organic sodium, which neutralizes acids and holds calcium in the bone. Goat whey is high in absorbable minerals as well as organic sodium, and it is a great acid neutralizer.

Exercise is also crucial for anyone with osteoporosis. A lack of exercise accelerates bone loss.

RINGWORM

Ringworm is a fungus that occurs on the skin and looks like a rounded, slightly raised red patch. Make a paste with goldenseal root powder and tea tree oil. Place the paste on the infected area and keep it bandaged. Ringworm can be contagious!

SHINGLES

Shingles is caused by the varicella zoster virus, which also causes chicken pox. The virus can live in the body for years before being triggered by stress. Symptoms include a rash and severe pain. Soak in a tub of warm water and four cups of calendula tea. Use calendula cream on the sores to promote healing and reduce the pain. Echinacea, olive leaf, garlic, and colloidal silver minimize replication of the virus. Take lots of vitamin C, vitamin E, and beta-carotene, and cleanse the colon.

SKIN RASHES

For skin rashes, soak in a bath of warm water and two cups of raw apple cider vinegar for twenty minutes. Raw apple cider vinegar will often help stop itching. Rinse off, then rub on a salve made of chickweed, marigold (calendula), and olive oil. If rash does not improve within two to three days, colon cleansing can be most helpful. Also, you may need to see a qualified dermatologist to tell you what type of rash you have and make suggestions for healing. If it is coming from an allergy, you may have to avoid all foods that could be causing it, wear only cotton clothing, use natural soaps with no perfumes and dyes, and make sure your home is free from mold.

SNORING

To relieve snoring, lie on your back. Place a castor oil poultice over your abdomen so it covers the top side of the areas where the adrenal glands are located—in the back above the kidneys and the liver. Losing weight and cleansing the colon and liver will often solve problems with snoring. Rubbing peppermint oil mixed half and half with lavender oil on the bridge of the nose and just beneath the nostrils will help open up air passages and reduce snoring. If snoring continues, go for a sleep apnea test.

SORE THROAT

To soothe a sore throat, try the gargle below.

Apple Cider Vinegar Gargle

    1 tablespoon apple cider vinegar
    6 ounces distilled water

Mix the vinegar and water. Use it to gargle several times a day.

Get plenty of rest. Keep the colon clean. Take propolis, echinacea, grapefruit seed extract. Colloidal silver can help heal a sore throat as well. Avoid sugar, dairy products, and wheat.

SWOLLEN ANKLES, FINGERS, OR WRISTS

Some people are "lymphatic types" and have a tendency to swell. Avoid salt and foods that contain salt. Use the salt substitutes suggested in chapter 1. Vitamin B6 is a natural diuretic and helps the body release fluids. Never take extra B6 unless you are taking a B complex. Fluids build up in the body when the kidneys are not releasing fluid properly as urine. Herbal teas can flush the kidneys and help improve their function. Drink juniper berry tea. Eating watermelon is also very cleansing for the kidneys. Watercress is a natural diuretic

TENDONITIS

Tendonitis is the inflammation of a tendon. Symptoms include pain, numbness, tingling, and tenderness. Avoid alcohol and caffeine. Have some spinal adjustments and massages. Soak in Epsom salts baths and apply castor oil poultices (see chapter 3). Apply arnica cream and wear an Ace bandage. Take tumeric, calcium, magnesium, trace minerals, B complex, and vitamin C to reduce inflammation. Rest the injured tendon.

THYROID DISORDERS

The thyroid is a major gland and part of the body's endocrine system. The endocrine system is made up of ductless glands that secrete hormones directly into the bloodstream. These glands consist of the pituitary, thyroid, parathyroid, testes, ovaries, adrenal cortex, and pancreas. If any one of these is not working properly, it affects all the others.

The thyroid gland has two lobes and is located in the front of the neck just below the larynx (voice box) with one lobe on each side of the trachea (windpipe). The thyroid is a master gland, and it helps control the body's metabolism and temperature.

A thyroid gland that produces too much thyroid hormone is a condition known as hyperthyroidism. This condition speeds up bodily processes, and the metabolism is overactive. People with hyperthyroidism may become hyperactive, nervous, jittery, irritable, and fatigued. They have trouble sleeping at night, sweat more, and have increased bowel movements, rapid heartbeat, protruding eyeballs, and goiter. Grave's Disease is a common type of hyperthyroidism.

Follow the nutritional plans presented in chapter 1 and strictly avoid all stimulants. A good digestive enzyme taken just before each meal, along with a multiple vitamin high in B complex and liquid trace minerals, will help the body digest at a normal pace and absorb nutrients. Lemon balm (also called Melissa) and motherwort taken as teas or in capsule form (follow directions) have traditionally been used to help people with a hyperactive thyroid function because they act to calm and soothe the nervous system and help ease the jittery, nervous feeling that often accompanies hyperthyroidism. Also, it is crucial to make sure your pH is alkaline. A half-teaspoon of liquid trace minerals taken in eight ounces of water daily can help neutralize pH. Vegetables known to help suppress thyroid hormone production are kale, mustard greens, broccoli, cabbage, turnips, and brussels sprouts. Eat some of these daily. According to James Balch, MD, and Phyllis Balch, CNC, in *Prescription for Nutritional Healing:*

> *Be wary of treatment with radioactive sodium iodine (iodine B1, or I-B1), which is often recommended for this condition. Severe side effects have been known to accompany the use of I-B1. Also, do not rush into surgery. Try improving your diet first.*

Hypothyroidism occurs when the thyroid gland is not producing enough thyroid hormone. People with low thyroid function are often tired, sluggish, and cold. They suffer from constipation, dry skin, infections, depression, goiter, and obesity. Broda Barnes, MD, studied hypothyroidism during his thirty years of medical practice and wrote *Hypo-Thyroidism: The Unsuspected Illness.* In this book he explains how hypothyroidism can cause many different illnesses and health disorders. Because he was unsatisfied with results gained from blood tests, he developed a wonderful test, based on basal temperature, which the layperson can take at home. A worksheet for taking the test follows.

If your temperature is lower than 97.8°F for more than two days and you have several of the symptoms listed above, you should read Dr. Barnes's book. Nova Scotia dulse and kelp are high in natural absorbable iodine and other minerals and can strengthen the thyroid gland. Nori and hijike are also good choices. A product containing raw thyroid from animal sources has helped many, especially if the thyroid function is really low and dulse does not help raise the temperatures enough. These items are available at health food stores. Armour Thyroid tablets also contain raw thyroid and are natural, but they must be prescribed by a physician. People with low thyroid function should follow the nutritional plans presented in chapter 1 and eat cruciferous vegetables in moderation. These may suppress the funtion of the thyroid gland.

Thyroid Basal Temperature Test

Your basal temperature test is accurate when tested in the axilla (armpit) each morning for a period of six days. The normal reading when taken this way is between 97.8°F and 98.2°F. If your temperature is consistently low, your thyroid is underactive. Be sure to record the reading accurately. It is your accuracy that determines the value of the test. If the temperature is consistently high, there is a possibility your thyroid is overworking or you may have an infection somewhere in the body. See your doctor and ask for further testing to determine the causes.

At night, before retiring, shake down a thermometer and lay it beside your bed on a night table or chair. Immediately upon awakening, place the thermometer in your armpit, pressing your arm against your body with no clothing in between. Keep still and be quiet. Any motion can upset your temperature reading. Leave the thermometer under your arm for ten minutes. Record your result below.

Date _____ Temperature _____
Date _____ Temperature _____
Date _____ Temperature _____
Date _____ Temperature _____
Date _____ Temperature _____
Date _____ Temperature _____

For menstruating females: Start taking your temperature on the second day of your period.

Thyroid Appraisal Indicator

Following is a list of symptoms that accompany low thyroid function. If you have the problem now, draw a check mark in the blank. If you had the problem in the past, draw an X. If you have checked three or more of these and have a low underarm temperature, your thyroid is not functioning at an optimal level. Follow the suggestions for hypothyroidism and always check with your health practitioner to confirm treatment.

_____ Low energy
_____ Excessive fatigue
_____ Repetitive infections

_____ Chronic headaches

_____ Circulatory disturbances

_____ Chronic skin condition

_____ Poor memory

_____ Poor concentration

_____ Depression

_____ Coarse hair

_____ Brittle nails

_____ Extreme sensitivity to cold

_____ Chronic boils

_____ Eczema

_____ Winter itch

_____ Fish skin

_____ Psoriasis

_____ Frequent colds

_____ Frequent episodes of tonsillitis

_____ Frequent sinus infections

_____ Frequent ear infections

_____ Migraine headaches

_____ Tension headaches

_____ Irregular menstrual periods

_____ Painful menstrual periods

_____ Excessive bleeding with periods

_____ Infertility problem (male or female)

_____ Neurotic tendency

_____ Irritability

_____ Nervousness

_____ Emotionally explosive

_____ Cold skin

_____ Sensitivity to cold at temperatures conformable to others

_____ Skin pallor

_____ Hair loss

_____ Labored or difficult breathing

_____ Hoarseness

_____ Swelling of feet

_____ Swelling of eyelids

_____ Decreased sweating
_____ Constipation
_____ Palpitations
_____ Poor equilibrium
_____ Muscle aches and weakness
_____ Hearing disturbances
_____ Burning and prickling

ULCERS

A peptic ulcer is an open wound in the stomach lining or anywhere along the intestinal tract. People with peptic ulcers have intense burning or severe pain. Some may suffer from nausea and vomiting. Pain is more intense when the stomach is empty, and eating or drinking lots of water relieve the pain.

Ulcers occur as the result of ongoing stress, which causes the release of excess stomach acids. Taking antacids and certain medications such as aspirin and even vitamin C over a long period of time can contribute to ulcers. A diet high in sugar, caffeine, and processed foods can produce too much acidity and cause ulcers. Food allergies can cause an imbalance in intestinal flora. Heavy smokers and people who abuse alcohol often get ulcers as well.

To heal ulcers, avoid alcohol, caffeine, cigarette smoking, heavy use of antacids, ascorbic acid in some types of vitamin C, and many types of drugs. Food allergens must be identified and avoided. Avoid wheat, salt, sugar, fried foods, and processed foods. Eat papayas and drink papaya juice. Follow the food plans presented in chapter 1. Raw cabbage juice has been tremendously successful in healing ulcers. Five cups of cabbage juice taken throughout the day can help heal some ulcers in seven to ten days. Drink slippery elm tea. Take goldenseal root or colloidal silver to help inhibit bacterial growth. Check with your physician to find out if you have the bacteria called *helicobacter pylori* or *H. pylori*. This virus may be the cause of ulcers.

VARICOSE VEINS

Varicose veins are quite common and affect about 60 percent of Americans. They are often raised lumpy areas, dark blue or purple and appear on the backs of the legs or calves and sometimes on the insides of the legs. Varicose veins result when the veins lose their elasticity and stretch. Valves in the legs may stop working, causing blood to flow backward away from the heart. Constipation, pregnancy, and standing jobs can all contribute to varicosities because of pressure placed on the veins. To help heal varicose veins, take a warming bath with ginger four to five times per week. Dry off well and apply a cabbage poultice to the areas with varicosities. Sleep with your legs propped up. Drink three to four cups of oatstraw tea per day. Oatstraw tea is high in silicon, which builds connective tissue. Use horse chestnut cream to help strengthen veins. Take two thousand milligrams of bioflavonoids and two hundred milligrams of rutin per day. Bioflavonoids build and repair connective tissue as well. If you are constipated, see and follow directions under "Constipation." If you have a job where you have to stand on your feet all day, do your best to change jobs to one that allows more sitting. If legs become swollen and red or painful, see your doctor right away because it may indicate a blood clot.

WARTS

Warts are produced on the skin by a virus from the human papillomavirus (HPV) family. They can be passed from one person to another. Some people have very strong immune systems and do not get warts as easily as others. To heal warts, combine equal parts castor oil and oregano oil or garlic oil. Massage the mixture onto warts in a circular motion ten times, three times per day. Work to boost the immune system by eating properly, drinking purified water, exercising, and taking two propolis tablets daily. Eating garlic can also be helpful.

YEAST INFECTIONS

Yeast infections of the vaginal tract often occur when a person is under stress or consuming lots of sugar or beer. Vaginal yeast can be contracted from a sexual partner that has a yeast infection. Try taking four tablets of propolis three times per day. Use two capsules of acidophilus every two hours until well, then two capsules three times a day for one month. Use two capsules of grapefruit seed extract two times per day. Use caprylic acid as directed on the label (this comes from coconut). Take one capsule of essential fatty acids (black currant seed oil, flaxseed oil, borage oil, and pumpkin seed oil are good sources) three times per day. Drink one cup of Pau d'Arco tea per day and one cup of clove tea per day (both teas are antifungal and antibacterial).

Your diet must be fruit-free, sugar-free, and yeast-free. Avoid aged cheeses, alcohol, chocolate, honey, maple syrup, fermented foods such as pickles and vinegar, and grains containing gluten. Eat vegetables, fish, brown rice, quinoa, and millet. Eat plain yogurt that contains live yogurt cultures. Drink distilled water only.

Vaginal Douche for Yeast Infections

16 ounces distilled water
1 teaspoon ground Pau d'Arco bark
6 capsules goldenseal root powder
6 capsules acidophilus
6 drops tea tree oil or 4 drops oregano oil
2 droppers colloidal silver at 250 parts per million

Boil the distilled water and pour it over the Pau d'Arco bark. Steep the mixture for fifteen minutes, then strain it. Break open the capsules of goldenseal root powder; pour the Pau d'Arco tea over the goldenseal. Stir the mixture well, then let it cool. Add the remaining ingredients, and stir everything together. Pour the mixture into a douche bag. Stand in the shower and gently insert the tip of the douche tube, lubricated with olive oil, into the vagina. Let the contents of the bag flow in. A large part will flow back out, but some of the ingredients will remain and work to heal the yeast infection. Douche in the morning and at night for seven days.

A vaginal implant will also help heal a yeast infection. Insert a garlic clove that has been dipped in olive oil into the vagina each night before going to sleep. It will come out easily in the morning. On the third night, cut the garlic clove once with a sharp knife before inserting it. On the fourth night, cut the garlic clove twice before inserting it. Garlic cloves may be worn during the day as well with a sanitary napkin. Discontinue when the vaginal tract is healthy.

An alternate vaginal implant requires a large two-ounce syringe. Mix the implant as follows.

Vaginal Implant for Yeast Infections

- 2 ounces plain raw yogurt
- 6 capsules acidophilus
- 3 capsules goldenseal
- 1 dropper colloidal silver
- 1 dropper fresh-squeezed wheatgrass juice

Break the capsules open, and pour the contents into a bowl with the yogurt, wheatgrass juice, and liquid colloidal silver. Stir all the ingredients together. Draw some of the mixture up into a syringe. Insert the contents into the vaginal tract. Lie with your hips up on a pillow for at least one hour. This mixture can be inserted at night before bed.

Natural Supplements

The prime purpose of food supplements is to fill in the nutritional gaps
produced by faulty eating habits and by nutritionally-inferior foods.
–Dr. Paavo Airola

IN AN IDEAL WORLD where the topsoil layers were still deep and rich with nutrients, where foods were grown organically and free from pesticides, where air was clean and water was pure, we would not need to add supplements to our diets. Ideally, we would be able to get all of our vitamins and minerals from our foods. In today's world however, most fruits and vegetables have been grown on very thin layers of soil, watered with polluted water, and heavily sprayed with chemicals. Most meat has high doses of antibiotics and hormones, and much of our world's water has had toxic wastes dumped into it. Even organic foods in our health food stores are many days old and the vitamin content has been significantly reduced. In addition, many families are so rushed and hurried they don't take the time to properly prepare healthy meals or don't have access to natural organic foods. Food supplements help replace important vitamins and minerals that are sorely lacking in our diets today. They also help protect us from the poisonous elements in our foods, water, and air. Supplements can help strengthen our immune systems and strengthen our bodies so they become resistant to viruses, bacteria, and fungi. The tool kits in this chapter provide you with knowledge about vitamins, minerals, and super food supplements and the roles they play in building good health. They will help you understand symptoms you would have if these nutrients were missing and give you suggestions for foods that provide them. I am all for getting as much as we can from foods. But if eating the foods does not eliminate the health condition, these vitamins, minerals, and super food supplements can also be purchased at most health food stores. Consult a knowledgeable nutritionist or natural health practitioner for additional guidance in using any of these supplements. Remember, more of certain nutrients might be required if you fighting an illness than if you are well. (For additional in-depth information on vitamins and minerals, I recommend the book, *Encyclopedia of Nutritional Supplements* by Michael T. Murray, ND.)

Tool Kit for Buying Healthy Vitamins

Vitamins are essential for health and well-being. They work together with enzymes to release energy into our bodies. Vitamin deficiencies can cause illness. Be very careful when selecting vitamins. Many vitamins on the market today are synthetic and do not come from whole foods. These vitamins often contain fillers and food colorings that are not good for us. Natural vitamins come directly from foods. Our bodies are made to utilize elements from natural foods. Read labels and make sure the vitamins come from food sources. Some of the natural vitamins, including C and B complex, are water-soluble and others, including A, D, E, and K, are fat-soluble. The body cannot store water-soluble vitamins. They are excreted within hours of taking them in. The body can store fat-soluble vitamins within the liver and in fatty tissue. Since we can't be assured of getting all of our vitamins in our food, a good multiple vitamin can help supplement what we are missing. If you are ill or feel you need specific vitamins in addition to a good multiple, it is always best to consult with a natural health practitioner who can help you with your specific needs. Check with your doctor if you are taking a medication to make sure the supplement does not interfere.

VITAMIN A: FAT SOLUBLE

Vitamin A strengthens the immune system. It fights infections and helps prevent colds and flu. A powerful antioxidant, vitamin A fights free radicals and defends the body from cancer. It also lowers high cholesterol levels and prevents heart disease and stroke. Necessary for growing and maintaining skin tissue, vitamin A helps prevent acne and other skin disorders, keep the skin soft, and inhibit wrinkles. Vitamin A also promotes eye health and prevents night blindness.

Food Sources

Apricots, asparagus, beet greens, broccoli, butternut squash, carrots, chard, collards, dandelion greens, dulse, fish liver oils, kale, liver, mustard greens, papaya, peaches, pumpkin, spinach, sweet potatoes, turnip greens, watercress, and yellow squash.

Natural Supplement Sources

Beta-carotene, which is converted to vitamin A in the liver, and fish liver oil.

NOTE: Do not take more than 100,000 International Units (IU) of vitamin A for prolonged periods without supervision. A dosage this high could become toxic to the liver. If you have a liver disease, consult your physician before taking vitamin A. Pregnant women should not take more than 10,000 IU's of vitamin A daily as it may affect fetal development. Children should not take more than 10,000 IU's daily. Diabetics and people with hypothyroid function may have difficulty converting beta-carotene to vitamin A.

THE B VITAMINS: WATER SOLUBLE

Several different B vitamins often come in a combination called B complex. B vitamins help nourish and calm the nervous system and may relieve anxiety or depression. The B vitamins work together and should be taken together. If you need an additional amount of one of the B vitamins, take it along with a B complex.

Vitamin B1 (Thiamine)

Vitamin B1 helps keep the nervous system healthy. It metabolizes carbohydrates, assists in blood formation, improves circulation, and is necessary for good muscle tone. It also aids in the production of hydrochloric acid. Vitamin B1 prevents beriberi, a disease of the nervous system.

Food Sources

Beans, brown rice, chicken, egg yolks, liver, nuts, peas, wheat germ, and whole grains.

Natural Supplement Sources

Brewer's yeast and rice bran.

Vitamin B2 (Riboflavin)

Vitamin B2 assists in the formation of red blood cells and antibodies. It is needed for proteins, fats, and carbohydrates to metabolize. It also helps to prevent cataracts. Vitamin B2 prevents inflammation of the tongue and mouth as well as cracks at the corners of the mouth.

Food Sources
Avocados, broccoli, cheese, dandelion greens, dulse, egg yolks, fish, goat's milk, nuts, poultry, spinach, watercress, whole grains, and yogurt.

Natural Supplement Sources
Rice bran and whole grains.

Vitamin B3 (Niacin, Nicotenic Acid, and Niacinamide)
Vitamin B3 aids in good circulation, which helps prevent numbness in arms and legs and promotes good nerve and brain function. It also helps maintain healthy skin. Vitamin B3 aids in proper digestion and helps lower cholesterol. Vitamin B3 also relieves headaches and helps prevent cold sores. A deficiency of vitamin B3 causes pellagra, which has symptoms of diarrhea, dermatitis, and dementia (a decline in mental ability).

Food Sources
Carrots, beef liver, broccoli, cornmeal, dandelion greens, potatoes, and wheat germ.

Natural Supplement Sources
Brewer's yeast, rice bran, and wheat germ.

Vitamin B5 (Pantothenic Acid)
Vitamin B5 boosts stamina and helps proteins, fats, and carbohydrates release energy. It also aids in proper metabolism and digestion. It assists in the production of adrenal hormones. Vitamin B5 relieves stress, anxiety, and depression.

Food Sources
Avocados, beef, chicken, eggs, legumes, liver, mushrooms, nuts, potatoes, salmon, trout, vegetables, and yogurt.

Natural Supplement Sources
Brewer's yeast and royal jelly.

Vitamin B6 (Pyridoxine)

Vitamin B6 assists in the formation of antibodies. It helps build red blood cells and prevent anemia, and it helps prevent cholesterol deposits around the heart, arteriosclerosis, and heart disease. It also aids in keeping sodium, potassium, and phosphorus in balance. In addition, it helps protein, fat, and carbohydrate metabolize. Vitamin B6 acts as a natural diuretic for those retaining fluids, and it helps relieve nausea during pregnancy.

Food Sources

Brown rice, carrots, corn, dulse, fish, legumes, liver, peas, potatoes, sunflower seeds, and walnuts.

Natural Supplement Sources

Brewer's yeast and rice bran.

Vitamin B12 (Cyanocobalamin)

Vitamin B12 helps red blood cells develop in bone marrow and thereby prevents anemia. It helps maintain nerve sheaths and keep the nervous system healthy. It also helps the body metabolize protein, fats, and carbohydrates, and aids in digestion. Vitamin B12 helps to produce acetylcholine, which supports learning and memory.

Food Sources

Alfalfa, beef liver, dulse, eggs, halibut, herring, kelp, mackerel, nori, salmon, and yogurt.

Natural Supplement Sources

Beef liver and brewer's yeast.

BIOTIN: WATER SOLUBLE

Biotin is necessary for healthy hair and skin, and it can help prevent cradle cap in infants. Shampoos that strengthen hair and prevent hair loss often contain biotin. It is important in the production of fatty acids and the utilization of other B vitamins. It helps protein, fats, and carbohydrates metabolize and aids cell growth. Biotin is necessary for healthy nerves and bone marrow, and it can relieve muscle pain.

Food Sources
Beef liver, black-eyed peas, Brazil nuts, cod, egg yolks, halibut, hazelnuts, herring, oatmeal, and yogurt. Eating raw egg whites can deplete the body of biotin. Raw egg whites contain an indigestible protein called avidin, which interferes with the absorption of biotin.

Natural Supplement Sources
Beef liver, brewer's yeast, and soy.

CHOLINE: WATER SOLUBLE

Choline is necessary in the formation of lecithin and it helps fats and cholesterol metabolize. It also helps regulate liver and gallbladder function. Choline aids nerve impulse transmissions and proper brain function, and it is used with nervous system disorders, such as multiple sclerosis, tardive dyskenesia, and Parkinson's disease. Choline keeps the cardiovascular system healthy and prevents arteriosclerosis.

Food Sources
Beans, beef, egg yolks, goat's milk, and whole grains.

Natural Supplement Sources
Lecithin and soybeans.

FOLIC ACID (FOLACIN): WATER SOLUBLE

Folic acid ensures the formation of red blood cells and prevents anemia. It also helps with the formation of white blood cells, which strengthens immunity. It helps prevent the tongue from becoming sore or red. Folic acid feeds the brain and nervous system and it helps inhibit the formation of homocysteine, a toxic chemical that allows cholesterol to deposit around the heart.

Folic acid also supports proper cell division through the synthesis of RNA and DNA, and it is vital to the normal development of fetal nerve cells. The mother should take four hundred micrograms of folic acid prior to and throughout pregnancy to ensure proper development of fetal brain and nervous system and prevent a premature birth or anencephaly (where parts of the brain are missing).

Folic acid is best utilized if taken together with vitamin B complex, including B12, and vitamin C.

Food Sources
Asparagus, barley, black beans, brown rice, garbanzo beans, green leafy vegetables, kidney beans, lima beans, liver, nuts and seeds, oranges, parsnips, salmon, and tuna.

Natural Supplement Sources
Brewer's yeast, liver, and rice bran.

INOSITOL: WATER SOLUBLE

Inositol is important in the formation of lecithin and the proper utilization of cholesterol and fat. It is also essential for hair growth. Inositol helps prevent hardened arteries, high cholesterol, skin eruptions, depression, anxiety, and compulsive disorders.

Food Sources
Beef, blackstrap molasses, legumes, vegetables, whole grains, and yogurt.

Natural Supplement Sources
Brewer's yeast and rice bran.

PABA (PARA-AMINOBENZOIC ACID): WATER SOLUBLE

With the assistance of intestinal bacteria, PABA is converted to folic acid, which then helps the body assimilate pantothenic acid (vitamin B5). PABA is used in the formation of red blood cells. It also works as a coenzyme to break down and utilize proteins. It acts as an antioxidant and absorbs harmful ultraviolet-B radiation from the sun, thus protecting against sunburn and skin cancer. As an antioxidant, it also protects the body from cigarette smoke. In addition, PABA helps maintain healthy intestinal flora. Taking PABA can help restore to color gray hair, if the graying occurred as a result of B vitamin and PABA deficiency and stress. It may also help restore pigment to areas of white skin patches.

Food Sources
Blackstrap molasses, liver, mushrooms, spinach, and whole grains.

Natural Supplement Sources
Liver and whole grains.

VITAMIN C (ASCORBIC ACID): WATER SOLUBLE

Vitamin C strengthens the immune system by helping to produce antibodies. A powerful antioxidant, it fights free radicals that can cause damage to the cells, thus fighting infection and protecting against cancer. It assists in tissue growth and repair and helps heal wounds. Vitamin C is essential in the utilization of folic acid and the absorption of iron. It also helps the body excrete lead and other harmful heavy metals.

Vitamin C is important in maintaining healthy collagen and in forming strong connective tissue, healthy gums, and bones. It also helps prevent varicose veins, bruising, hemorrhoids, and hernias. Additionally, it assists in lowering cholesterol levels and high blood pressure. Vitamin C also helps block the release of histamines and reduce the intensity of allergic reactions. It can even help minimize the symptoms of asthma. In high doses, vitamin C can help negate the harmful effects of a black widow spider bite. The body does not manufacture vitamin C, so it must be obtained from nutritional sources. If large amounts of vitamin C are required, it is best given intravenously. Taken in large doses with aspirin, ascorbic acid can cause burning in the stomach and ulcers. Vitamin C from the sago palm tree is a mild and gentle form of vitamin C that will not burn the stomach but still should not be taken with aspirin. To learn about effective aspirin replacements, read *Beyond Aspirin* by Thomas M. Newmark and Paul Schulick.

Food Sources
Bell peppers, berries, broccoli, citrus fruits, green leafy vegetables, mangos, melons, onions, persimmons, pineapple, potatoes, strawberries, and tomatoes.

Natural Supplement Sources
Acerola cherries, rose hips, and sago palm.

VITAMIN D: FAT SOLUBLE

Vitamin D is essential for the absorbtion of calcium and phosphorus; thus it is needed for developing bones and teeth in children and for maintaining strong bones and teeth in adults. It also helps prevent osteoporosis and osteoarthritis. Vitamin D keeps the muscles strong (including the heart) and keeps the nervous system balanced. It ensures normal blood clotting, thyroid function, and healthy immune activity. Vitamin D prevents rickets in children; rickets can lead to bone deformities and osteomalacia, a condition that softens, weakens, and demineralizes the bones. Sunshine is a wonderful source of vitamin D. People who live in regions where sunshine is limited in the winter cannot produce enough vitamin D and should take a supplement. The liver and kidneys convert the vitamin D from food supplements so it can be completely utilized. People with liver or kidney disorders, who cannot take full advantage of vitamin D supplements, are more likely to develop osteoporosis.

Food Sources
Butter, dandelion greens, eggs, feta cheese, fish liver oils, halibut, liver, oatmeal, salmon, sardines, sweet potatoes, tuna, and yogurt.

Natural Supplement Sources
Cod liver oil and fish liver oil.

VITAMIN E: FAT SOLUBLE

Vitamin E neutralizes the damaging effects of free radicals, blocks the formation of carcinogens (cancer-producing compounds), and stimulates the immune system. It also protects other fat-soluble vitamins from damage by oxygen, and it protects the body's cells, including red blood cells. It helps regulate blood pressure, strengthens arterial walls, promotes normal blood clotting, and helps wounds heal without scarring. Vitamin E promotes healthy skin, hair, and nerves. In addition, it slows the aging process and helps prevent age spots from developing. It may postpone the development of cataracts, and it may slow the progression of Parkinson's disease.

Vitamin E relieves muscular cramping, including leg cramps. It also helps regulate menstrual periods, relieve symptoms that occur with PMS such as abdominal cramping, prevent fibrocystic breast disease, and reduce hot flashes in perimenopausal women. Vitamin E can help increase the sperm cell count in men.

According to Phyllis A. Balch, CNC, and James F. Balch, MD, in *A Prescription for Nutritional Healing*, ". . . studies have shown daily use of

Vitamin E to be more protective than aspirin for prevention of heart attacks, with no harmful side effects. The misuse of aspirin, in contrast, causes or contributes to an estimated 3,000 deaths in the United States each year." If you are taking blood thinners or have high blood pressure you can take vitamin E, but consult a qualified health practitioner for an appropriate dosage.

Read labels! Natural vitamin E is much more potent and better for you than a man-made form. Natural vitamin E is d-alpha-tocopheral. The label may also say d-alpha-tocopherol and mixed tocopherols of alpha, beta, gamma, and delta. Synthetic vitamin E is listed as dl-alpha-tocopherol, with an "l" after the "d." This type may not cost as much, but it also will not provide as much healing.

When combining food supplements, avoid inorganic iron, called ferrous sulphate; it will destroy vitamin E. Natural iron or organic sources of iron, such as ferrous fumerate or ferrous gluconate, does not harm it.

Food Sources
Brown rice, cold-pressed oils, green leafy vegetables, nuts, raw milk, raw wheat germ, and seeds.

Natural Supplement Sources
Soybean oil and wheat germ oil.

VITAMIN K: NOT WATER SOLUBLE

The liver uses vitamin K to make prothrombin, which is needed for clotting blood. Vitamin K also prevents internal bleeding and excessive external bleeding. It is necessary for forming and repairing bones. Vitamin K works in the intestines to help convert glucose into glycogen, which is stored in the liver and is important for keeping the liver healthy.

Vitamins K1, K2, and K3
There are three types of vitamin K. Vitamin K1 (phylloquinone) is derived from plants. Vitamin K2 (menaquinone) is made by bacteria in the intestinal tract. These two types of vitamin K are natural.

Vitamin K3 (menadione) is a synthetic form, and it can be toxic in large doses. It can cause jaundice in infants and anemia in children and adults. Taking antibiotics can inhibit the natural production of vitamin K2 by intestinal bacteria. Mineral oil attaches to vitamin K and carries it out of the body. Therefore, it is important to avoid taking mineral oil, which is a harsh laxative that can deplete your body's supply of vitamin K. Those taking blood thinners should not take vitamin K without the advice of a physician.

Food Sources of Vitamin K₁
Asparagus, brussels sprouts, cabbage, egg yolks, garbanzo beans, green leafy vegetables, green tea, lentils, liver, oatmeal, spinach, and turnip greens.

Natural Supplement Sources
Fermented soy, leafy greens.

VITAMIN P (BIOFLAVONOIDS): WATER SOLUBLE

Vitamin P helps the body absorb vitamin C, and it is often combined with vitamin C in tablet or capsule form. Bioflavonoids and vitamin C should be taken together. Vitamin P comes in several forms, including citrin, flavones, hesperetin, hesperidin, quercetin, quercetrin, and rutin. It builds and repairs connective tissue and keeps the arterial walls strong.

Rutin (taken by itself or in addition to vitamin C) and bioflavonoids can help heal the swelling and pain of hemorrhoids. It is also very effective in reducing the severity of varicose veins. Vitamin P also helps prevent hernias and relieve pain. Acting as a natural antibiotic, when taken with vitamin C it relieves the pain and swelling of herpes sores around the mouth. It may also relieve the pain and swelling of shingles. Quercetin taken with vitamin C and bromelain from pineapple can prevent the symptoms of asthma. Vitamin P improves circulation and helps lower cholesterol levels.

Food Sources
Bell peppers, blackberries, black cherries, black currants, buckwheat sprouts, grapes, plums, and the white part of all citrus fruits (just inside the peeling).

Natural Supplement Sources
Bell peppers, cherries, and rose hips.

Tool Kit for Selecting Healthy Minerals

Minerals occur naturally in the earth and are absorbed by plants and transmuted into forms we can utilize. Minerals are vital to all life. Every plant and living creature must have minerals in order to survive. In our bodies, every cell requires minerals in order to function. Minerals build strong bones, promote healthy nerve function, and help maintain proper muscle tone. Minerals support the heart muscle and cardiovascular system as well as all other bodily systems. Minerals work with vitamins and enzymes to help our bodies produce energy and heal from illness. This tool kit will teach you about the minerals, what they do for the body, and food sources they can be found in. When buying minerals, you will find they come in various forms. Liquid minerals are probably the most easily absorbed. Some minerals are chelated or bound to a protein, which enhances absorption. If you feel you need minerals, a good multimineral will often ensure that you get what you need. If you have questions about the minerals you need, consult a good natural health practitioner.

BORON, THE "MAINTAINER"

Boron in trace amounts helps maintain strong bones. It helps with the metabolism and absorption of calcium, magnesium, and phosphorus. According to James F. Balch, MD, and Phyllis A. Balch, CNC, in *Prescription for Nutritional Healing*: "A study conducted by the U.S. Department of Agriculture indicated within eight days of supplementing their daily diet with 3 milligrams of boron, a test group of post-menopausal women lost 40 percent less calcium, one-third less magnesium, and slightly less phosphorus through their urine than they had before beginning boron supplementation." One should not take more than three milligrams of boron daily.

Natural Supplement Sources
Trace minerals and boron combined with calcium supplements.

Food Sources
Apples, carrots, green leafy vegetables, nuts and seeds, pears, and whole grains.

CALCIUM, THE "KNITTER"

Calcium is a wonderful mineral that builds strong bones, teeth, and fingernails. It is also needed to mend and repair bones, muscles, ligaments, and tissues. Calcium promotes healing during illness.

Natural Supplement Sources
Calcium citrate and gluconate. Calcium from dolomite (a type of stone) or oyster shell is difficult to absorb.

Synthetic Sources
Di-cal phosphate.

Food Sources
Almonds, beet tops, broccoli, cabbage, green leafy vegetables (such as kale, mustard greens, turnip greens), raw milk and cheese, seaweeds (such as dulse and kelp), and sesame seeds.

CARBON, THE "BUILDER"

Carbon promotes growth. Together with oxygen, it brings heat to the body. Carbon is the basic element of cell birth and life. When there is too much carbon in the body, it leads to obesity.

Natural Supplement Sources
Trace minerals.

Food Sources
Almonds, avocados, butter, egg yolks, olive oil, raw cheese, and whole grains.

CHLORINE, THE "CLEANSER"

Chlorine nourishes the nerves, maintains electrolyte and fluid balance, cleanses the liver, helps with tissue construction, assists in the production of hydrochloric acid, and assists in peristalsis.

Natural Supplement Sources
Trace minerals.

Food Sources
Asparagus, avocados, cabbage, celery, chard, cucumbers, goat's milk, kale, leeks, olives, saltwater fish, turnips, and watercress.

CHROMIUM, THE "ENERGIZER"

Chromium helps balance blood sugar levels and assists in metabolizing glucose. Therapeutically, it is helpful in cases of diabetes and hypoglycemia. It helps people not to crave sweets. Chromium plays a vital role in the synthesis of fats, cholesterol, and protein. Without chromium, people become tired and fatigued.

Natural Supplement Sources
Chromium carbonate and chromium picolinate. Herbs that contain chromium are licorice root, oatstraw, and horsetail.

Food Sources
Brewer's yeast, brown rice, corn, corn oil, dried beans, eggs, mushrooms, raw cheese, and whole grains.

FLUORINE, THE "DECAY RESISTOR"

Natural fluorine, from food sources, is important to the health of our bones, teeth, and hair. It helps the teeth resist decay.

Natural Supplement Sources
Multivitamins and trace minerals.

Synthetic Sources
Mouthwash and toothpastes.

Food Sources
Avocados, brussels sprouts, cabbage, quince, raw fish, and raw goat's milk.

IODINE, THE "METABOLIZER"

Iodine is important to the thyroid gland's health. People who live near the ocean and eat lots of food from the sea do not get goiter. In mountainous regions where iodine is not readily available in the foods, we find a great deal of goiter and other thyroid disorders. Without iodine, the body is not able to metabolize nutrients well and the thyroid cannot manage blood circulation and body temperature. (See "Hyperthyroidism and Hypothyroidism" in chapter 4.)

Natural Supplement Sources
Dulse or kelp in tablets, powder, or capsules. Nova Scotia dulse, grown in the cold waters of that region, is highest in iodine.

Synthetic Sources
Potassium iodide.

Food Sources
Agar, eggplant, fish, garlic, kale, and all seaweeds.

IRON, THE "FRISKY HORSE"
Iron builds strong blood cells and keeps people from feeling tired and anemic. Iron is called the "frisky horse" mineral because it keeps us active. Iron attracts oxygen into the cells of the body. Oxygen has been called "the giver of life"; we would die without it. Harmful bacteria cannot live in the presence of oxygen. The lungs, nerves, brain, and liver are organs that particularly need iron.

Natural Supplement Sources
Bone marrow supplements, brewer's yeast, desiccated liver, ferrous fumerate, ferrous gluconate, and iron oxide.

Synthetic Sources
Ferrous sulfate and iron peptonate.

Food Sources
Black cherries, blackstrap molasses, brewer's yeast, rice bran, dulse, figs, green vegetables, kelp, lentils, liver, raisins, prunes, and walnuts.

MAGNESIUM, THE "RELAXER"
Magnesium soothes and relaxes the muscles and helps prevent muscle cramping. It calms the nervous system and promotes rest. Magnesium also relieves and prevents constipation. Magnesium helps the heart and arteries

function properly and can help prevent a heart attack. It also strengthens and builds bones and teeth. A deficiency in magnesium can cause high blood pressure.

Natural Supplement Sources
Brewer's yeast and magnesium oxide.

Synthetic Sources
Magnesium sulfate.

Food Sources
Almonds, apples, black walnuts, dulse, figs, goat's milk, green leafy vegetables (such as chard, kale, and endive), sesame seeds, sunflower seeds, turnip greens, yellow corn and cornmeal, and yellow squashes.

MANGANESE, THE "LOVER"

Manganese is important to healthy brain and nerve functioning. It helps reproduction and sex hormone production, and it is important in tissue respiration and muscle coordination. People with a hearing loss or with ringing in the ears need manganese.

Natural Supplement Sources
Manganese carbonate.

Synthetic Sources
Manganese gluconate.

Food Sources
Almonds, apricots, black walnuts, butternut squash, egg yolks, grains, green beans, peas, and spinach.

NITROGEN, THE "RESTRAINER"

Nitrogen helps to restrain oxygen that is otherwise too volatile in the body. Nitrogen builds, preserves, and protects body tissues, also giving vitality to body tissues. It is important for skin and muscle health and elasticity.

Food Sources
Almonds, black-eyed peas, butternut squash, kidney beans, legumes, and salmon. NOTE: There are no supplement or synthetic sources of nitrogen for human consumption.

PHOSPHORUS, THE "LIGHT BEARER"
We can see phosphorescent qualities in many life forms, such as the firefly that glows in the dark on summer nights, glowworms, and certain types of eels and fish. Phosphorus is the medium for the soul's expression through brain activity. Without phosphorus, we could not think or reason, study or visualize, read or comprehend. Phosphorus helps us be intuitive and sensitive. Bones are made more dense and the nerve networks strong with phosphorus. Phosphorus is responsible for cellular repair, energy production, kidney function, metabolism, and heart muscle contraction.

Natural Supplement Sources
Bonemeal and ionic trace minerals.

Food Sources
Almonds, egg yolks, fish, goat's milk and cheese, lentils, pumpkin seeds, rice bran, and sunflower seeds.

POTASSIUM, THE "GREAT ALKALIZER"
Potassium nourishes the muscles, including the heart, and helps keep them strong and functioning properly. It helps them contract and relax. Potassium is also important for blood, kidneys, nerve, and skin health.

Natural Supplement Sources
Potassium citrate.

Synthetic Sources
Calcium phosphate.

Food Sources
Almonds, apricots, bananas, beets, cantaloupe, grapes, organic ripe citrus fruits, parsley, parsnips, pears, potato peeling broth, potato peelings, sunflower seeds, tomatoes, and turnips.

SILICON, THE "MAGNET"

Silicon builds and repairs skin, teeth, hair, fingernails, and bones. It also builds connective tissue. It strengthens blood vessels and helps prevent bruising, varicose veins, hemorrhoids, and hernias. Silicon nourishes the brain and nervous system as well. It is called the "magnet" because a person with sufficient silicon in their bodies will have beautiful teeth; strong, shiny hair; good skin; and beautiful fingernails. Their brains and nerves are strong and they usually have good personalities. Because of their beauty, strength, and happy dispositions, others are drawn to them.

Natural Supplement Sources
Silica capsules. Horse chestnut, horsetail, oatstraw, and shavegrass in liquids or capsules. Rice bran syrup. Horse chestnut cream used topically on varicose veins.

Food Sources
Alfalfa tea, flaxseeds, oats, oatstraw tea, onions, parsnips, red bell peppers, rice bran, rice polishings, and sunflower seeds.

SODIUM, THE "FOUNTAIN OF YOUTH"

Natural sodium (not table salt) nourishes the lymph system and helps hold fluids in areas where they are needed, such as around the eyes, in the sinus cavities, mouth, and lungs, and around the joints. Sodium helps us stay limber and pliable. Babies have a lot of sodium in their bodies and are very soft. Sodium holds calcium in solution where it is needed in the tissues and bones, instead of forming crystals in the joints and stones in the kidneys and gallbladder. It normalizes glandular secretions and maintains a proper balance in blood pH as well as a balance of water in the cells. An adequate amount of sodium may help prevent cataracts as well.

Natural Supplement Sources
Dulse tablets and goat's whey capsules.

Synthetic Sources
Sodium chloride.

Food Sources
Beet tops, celery, celery juice, green leafy vegetables, goat's whey, okra, parsley, seaweeds, strawberries, and turnips.

SULFUR, THE "HEATER"
Sulfur warms the body. It energizes each cell, enabling it to eliminate toxic substances. Because it drives toxins from tissues, it can help to heal skin disorders, such as psoriasis, eczema, and rosacea. Such protection against toxic substances, radiation, and pollution slows down the aging process. Sulfur also assists in tissue formation and repairs and restores collagen elasticity. It helps relieve the pain of arthritis, bursitis, and gout. Sulfur disinfects the blood and helps the body resist bacteria.

Natural Supplement Sources
Trace minerals, multimineral supplements, and ointments. Methylsulfonylmethane (MSM) is highly bioavailable and can be found in capsules, powder, lotions, creams, and facial cleansers.

Food Sources
Brussels sprouts, cabbage, celery, dried beans, eggs, fish, garlic, kale, onions, and turnips.

ZINC, THE "REGULATOR"
Zinc ensures that the reproductive organs and prostate gland function well. It helps with collagen formation, tissue repair, and immune function. Zinc helps maintain our ability to smell and taste. It also regulates the production of oil from the oil glands and therefore is beneficial in treating skin disorders, such as oily skin and acne. Without zinc, our fingernails become thin, get ridges in them, and crack and peel. Do not take more than fifty to one hundred milligrams of zinc daily.

Natural Supplement Sources
Zinc oxide.

Synthetic Sources
Zinc sulfate.

Food Sources
Brewer's yeast, egg yolks, green leafy vegetables, lecithin, legumes, pumpkin seeds, seafood, soaked almonds and sunflower seeds, and whole grains.

Tool Kit for Choosing Super Food Supplements

Super food supplements include a wide variety of foods or nutrients that provide super nourishment to the body and/or wonderful health benefits. Many of the super food supplements can be used in place of food when one is traveling or in case of emergency when food is scarce. For example, if people are not eating salads, alfalfa tablets or chlorella can give them the fiber and nutrients they are missing by not getting salad. Bee pollen is another great example of a super food supplement because it contains 40 percent protein and all the essential components of life. It helps correct allergies, strengthen the body, and provide energy. This tool kit will provide you with information about some of the best super food supplements available.

ALFALFA

Alfalfa is a super green food rich in vitamins, minerals, and chlorophyll. The roots of the alfalfa plant reach far into the earth to gather nourishment, sometimes as far as 120 feet! Alfalfa can be taken in liquid, tablet, or capsule form. As a liquid, it is great for people on a cleanse or fast, who are not eating solid foods. As a tablet, it helps tremendously with bowel cleansing. The fiber in the tablets helps scrub the colon wall clean. Crack alfalfa tablets with your teeth before swallowing to aid digestion. Alfalfa also helps promote good peristalsis in the bowel, because it provides the fibrous bulk the bowel needs for squeezing and pushing. It gives the bowels a great exercise workout.

Alfalfa helps cleanse and build the blood and liver and improve digestion, and it may help prevent cancer and liver disease. Alfalfa can help heal and relieve arthritis, gout, hemorrhoids, diverticulitis, intestinal ulcers, constipation, bad breath or body odor (including smelly feet), athlete's foot, and bleeding gums. It can balance blood sugar, making it beneficial for both hypoglycemics and diabetics. It even helps people who are dieting feel fuller longer and resist sweets.

ALOE VERA JUICE AND GEL

Aloe vera can be taken orally as a juice or gel, and it soothes the entire digestive tract. Aloe vera is a natural anti-inflammatory and helps tremendously with cases of gastritis, heartburn, acid reflux, colitis, diverticulitis, ulcers, and irritable bowel syndrome.

Irritable bowel syndrome causes people to swing from diarrhea to constipation. For relief, grind flaxseeds, soak them in aloe juice, and drink the juice twice a day. Flaxseeds are mucilaginous and very beneficial for the colon. This aloe-flaxseed combination helps relieve both constipation and diarrhea.

Aloe vera helps fight infection in the body. Aloe vera gel is reputed for its ability to heal burns and relieve dry skin. It is wonderful for acne, cuts, insect bites, skin ulcers, eczema, psoriasis, dandruff, cradle cap, and poison oak or poison ivy. Aloe vera soothes and softens the skin and can be used as a facial mask. Look for aloe vera in lotions, salves, ointments, and creams.

There are approximately two hundred species of aloe. If you like growing plants, you might enjoy growing your own aloe vera plant. When it is large enough, you may break or cut a leaf, and squeeze out the gel to treat a burn, insect bite, or wound. Properly cared for, an aloe vera plant can provide years of service. Enjoy!

BARLEY GRASS

Barley grass is available in powder or capsule form. As a powder, it can be stirred in distilled water to provide a nutritious low-calorie drink. It is high in chlorophyll, vitamin C, protein, enzymes, and minerals, including calcium and iron. It is great for vegetarians because it also has some vitamin B12. (B12 is predominantly found in animal products.) Barley grass nourishes the entire body. It is also an anti-inflammatory, which makes it beneficial for any inflammation of the gastrointestinal tract.

BEE POLLEN

Bee pollen is a wonderful food for humans, rich in protein, vitamins, and minerals. Bee pollen is different from the pollen that many people are allergic to. Pollens that cause allergies are called anemophiles; they are very light and easily blown through the air. Bee pollen is called entomophiles, which means "friends of the insects," and it is heavy and sticky. This pollen is collected from the legs of the bees by a special device placed near the opening of the beehives. Allergies caused by bee pollen are rare, and local bee pollen can help alleviate allergies to airborne pollens. Take it six weeks prior to allergy season, starting with small amounts—one granule the first day, two the second day, and three the third day, until you are taking one-half teaspoon one to two times per day. Mankind has consumed bee pollen for centuries. It was praised in the Bible, used in ancient Chinese medicine, and prescribed by traditional doctors for its healing properties. Bee pollen contains all the known nutrients necessary for survival and has been used consistently to build energy levels. Athletes have used it since the earliest Olympic games in Greece. Bee pollen builds the blood and improves endurance and vitality, has antibiotic properties, and helps prevent colds and flu. It also has been used successfully to reduce cravings and addictions to sugar, caffeine, nicotine, and alcohol. (See resources for where to find good bee pollen.)

Royden Brown writes extensively in *The World's Only Perfect Food* about the wonderful value of consuming bee pollen. In addition to its other uses, he notes that bee pollen can help balance hormones in both men and women and restore potency. He also explains the tremendous value of using bee pollen to prevent illness, build the immune system, and promote longevity. And according to Steven R. Schechter, ND, in *Fighting Radiation and Chemical Pollutants with Foods, Herbs and Vitamins*, a study in Sarajevo, Yugoslavia, reports findings that bee pollen successfully corrected radiation sickness.

BEE PROPOLIS

Bee propolis is a resinous substance that bees collect from the bark of trees and leaf buds. They mix it with beeswax and pollen to form a sealer that protects the hive from harmful bacteria and viruses.

Bee propolis can be taken internally in a liquid or tablet form. It is high in vitamin A (carotene), vitamin C, bioflavonoids, vitamin E, and some of the B vitamins. It also contains a large number of minerals. It is antibacterial, antiviral, and protects us from radiation. Bee propolis acts as a powerful antibiotic and immobilizes bacteria and viruses. It helps fight colds, flu, tonsillitis, and infections, including those in the mouth and throat. Propolis is also very effective when used externally in salves and ointments.

Its antibacterial properties fight infection in cuts and other wounds. Propolis can be taken on a regular basis with no side effects and be consistently effective because bacteria and viruses cannot build a tolerance to it. This differs from penicillin and other antibiotic drugs, which germs grow resistant to over time.

BEET TABLETS AND BEET POWDER

Beets are deep red root vegetables that are rich in vitamins and minerals, especially iron. Beet juice, according to German research, can help heal anemia. Beets can also cleanse the liver, gallbladder, and kidneys. They can help reduce inflammation in the nervous system and promote good peristaltic action in the bowel. According to Steven R. Schecter, ND, in *Fighting Radiation and Chemical Pollutants with Foods, Herbs and Vitamins*, "Beets have been shown to rebuild hemoglobin of the blood after exposure to radiation. Rats fed a diet of 20 percent beet pulp were able to prevent cesium-137 absorption 97 to 100 percent more effectively than rats exposed to the same radiation but given no beets."

Beets and raw organic beet juice are available in powdered form as well as tablet form for those who don't like beets, haven't the time to juice them or prepare them, or simply want to supplement their nutritional program.

BETA-1,3-D-GLUCAN

This supplement is made from the cell walls of yeast, the type used for baking. It does not, however, contain any yeast in supplement form. Beta-1,3-D-glucan works to boost the immune system by stimulating destroyer cells, or macrophages, to devour and destroy bacteria, viruses, and fungi. It has even been used to kill tumoral cells.

BIFIDOBACTERIUM BIFIDUM (BIFIDUS)

Probiotics are friendly bacteria in the digestive tract that build a healthy intestinal flora and improve digestion. One type of probiotic is called bifidobacterium bifidum or bifidus. Bifidobacterium bifidum fight harmful bacteria in the gut as well as yeast infections, including those of the vaginal tract. These good bacteria promote healthy intestinal movement and help relieve constipation and gas. They provide a conducive environment in the intestines for the manufacture of B vitamins and vitamin K.

Bifidobacterium bifidum should be taken after a round of antibiotics to replace the healthy bacteria in the bowel. Antibiotics kill harmful bacteria, but they also destroy friendly bacteria. If these friendly bacteria are not replaced, yeast infections can grow rapidly and harmful bacteria can grow strong.

Ammonia is often the by-product of destructive bacteria and faulty digestion. Tears and holes can develop in the intestinal walls, resulting in leaky gut syndrome. The blood will carry toxins from the bowel to the liver, causing tremendous strain on the liver. Undigested food can cause the body to produce too much histamine, and allergies can result. Unhealthy intestinal flora can cause exhaustion, headaches, and nausea. By replenishing bifidobacterium bifidum, we can prevent or heal a lot of these problems and keep our digestive tract healthy and working smoothly.

BLACK CHERRY CONCENTRATE

Black cherry concentrate is a delicious syrup made from the finest black cherries. It is rich in vitamins and minerals and is a wonderful source of natural iron. You can add water to make a great juice. It can be used occasionally over yogurt as a nutritious dessert. It is even great on pancakes made from sprouted whole grains, and much better for you than a lot of commercial syrups made from sugar and water. Children love it! Incorporated into your nutritional plan, black cherry concentrate can help prevent anemia, heal gout, and dissolve kidney stones and gallstones.

BLUE-GREEN ALGAE

Blue-green algae is a green freshwater algae grown in the great Klamath Lake in Oregon. It can be acquired in powder, capsule, or tablet form. Blue-green algae is filled with chlorophyll, which cleans the blood and liver, as well as with protein, vitamins, and minerals. It is a whole food that boosts energy levels because it is quickly and easily absorbed. For this reason, blue-green algae helps balance blood sugar levels and stop cravings for sweets. It nourishes the brain and nervous system and promotes clear thinking.

CHLORELLA

Chlorella is a single-celled alga that is grown in freshwater. One of the best sources of chlorella is grown and harvested in Japan. This nutritious green algae is over two and a half million years old, which makes it one of the most stable sources of food on the planet. Chlorella can be obtained in liquid, tablet, capsule, or powder form. When purchasing chlorella, make sure the label says that the cell wall has been pulverized. This ensures proper digestion and absorption. In fact, one of the best ways to know the chlorella cell wall has been sufficiently pulverized is to look for the DYNO-Mill name. "DYNO-Mill" refers to the machine that pulverizes the cell walls, making the chlorella over 80 percent absorbable. Most chlorella has had the cell wall broken with intense heat or chemical treatments, and is only 40 percent absorbable or less.

Chlorella is one of the most nutritious plant foods and contains the highest amount of chlorophyll in the known plant world, making it a great blood cleanser. About 58 percent of chlorella is protein, so it is especially nourishing for vegetarians.

Chlorella contains one of the highest contents of RNA and DNA of any known food substance. The RNA and DNA in chlorella provide materials for cellular repair and can protect against the effects of ultraviolet radiation, contribute to rapid healing, and promote longevity. Chlorella is rich in beta-carotene and contains all the B vitamins, including more B12 than liver; vitamins C and E; and rare trace minerals. In addition, one of the most important aspects is the presence of a substance called chlorella growth factor (CGF), which is often extracted and sold as a separate product. Experiments have shown that CGF increases the rate of tissue healing. Chlorella can help reduce the cellular damage that accompanies chemotherapy and radiation. Chlorella tablets taken with flaxseed oil is a wonderful stool softener and can relieve constipation. (See resources for where to find good chlorella.)

CHLOROPHYLL

Chlorophyll is the green juice of plants that is created during photosynthesis, their interaction with sunshine. Chlorophyll is a rich source of absorbable iron, which helps attract oxygen to cells and builds hemoglobin. It is high in potassium, which supports the muscles and heart; magnesium, which helps tone and relax the muscles; calcium, which helps build teeth and bones; and many other minerals and trace minerals. Chlorophyll is also rich in vitamins, including vitamins A and C, making it wonderful for the immune system, and some vitamin D, which helps in the absorption of calcium. Chlorophyll also contains vitamin K, which assists in normal blood clotting.

Chlorophyll benefits the body in many ways. It builds the blood, neutralizes acids, cleans and deodorizes the bowels, purifies the liver and blood, helps prevent bad breath and body odor, helps relieve sinus drainage, soothes a sore throat, reduces inflammation, soothes ulcers, regulates menstruation, and improves milk production.

Chlorophyll can be obtained in liquid form and added to water. It can be obtained from the raw juice of wheatgrass or green leafy vegetables. You can also buy green powdered drinks, such as raw powdered wheatgrass, kamut, barley grass, chlorella, and blue-green algae.

COENZYME Q10

Coenzyme Q10 is responsible for helping the body's cells produce adenasine triphosphate (ATP), an important source of energy. When people are deficient in coenzyme Q10, they can become fatigued. The muscles may ache or feel tired. Cardiovascular disease can develop, because the heart will lack the energy necessary to perform its vital functions. Coenzyme Q10 also plays a role in metabolizing fats and carbohydrates.

COLLOIDAL SILVER

Colloidal silver is a clear golden liquid that contains the purified trace mineral silver in a water-based solution. Medical doctors in America used it to treat a variety of diseases from the late 1800s to 1938, before man-made antibiotics became available. Settlers in the Old West used to keep their milk from spoiling by putting a silver dollar in it.

Colloidal silver is a powerful germicidal agent. Silver acts by crippling the oxygen-metabolizing enzyme in single-celled organisms (germs and viruses). The organisms are suffocated in a matter of minutes, and they are carried out of the body through the elimination channels.

An article titled "Silver, Our Mightiest Germ Fighter" (Science Digest, 1978), reported that silver kills over 650 disease-causing organisms.

Colloidal silver is nontoxic to mammals and plants, but a powerful destroyer of bacteria, viruses, and fungi. Topically, it fights fungal infections such as athlete's foot. It works wonders on acne, boils, eczema, herpes, ringworm, staph infections, warts, and impetigo.

Colloidal silver can be used in vaginal douches to clear up yeast infections. It works well when used as eyedrops, nose drops, and throat gargle. It can be used to heal gum infections or clear up bad breath. It helps get rid of dandruff, cradle cap in infants, and bedsores in the disabled. Colloidal silver also can be mixed with distilled water in a spray bottle and sprayed through the home or office to kill airborne viruses and bacteria. It can be added to bottled water when traveling.

Internally, colloidal silver that has been formulated correctly is safe for adults as well as children. It helps heal colds and flu, pneumonia, strep throat, bladder infections, and many other internal infections. (See resources for where to find good colloidal silver.)

COLOSTRUM

Colostrum is the nourishing fluid that is secreted by the milk glands of all mammal mothers for the first few days after birth, before the milk begins to flow. This is nature's way of providing powerful immune factors, friendly bacteria, and high levels of protein to ensure good health in the newborn. The immune factors protect the body against infection and the friendly bacteria provide a healthy intestinal flora.

Colostrum (from bovine sources) can be purchased in capsule, tablet, and powder form, and both children and adults may take it. It helps build and strengthen the immune system and is especially helpful for those who were never nursed by their mothers. It may help alleviate allergies, strengthen frail children and adults, and relieve chronic fatigue, constipation, environmental illness, and fibromyalgia. Colostrum is great for dieters. It nourishes the body, reduces hunger, and helps burn fat and build lean muscle.

DULSE

Dulse is a seaweed that is sold in dried form, powder, tablets, and capsules. It is high in natural iodine and a multitude of vitamins and minerals, including calcium. Dulse from the cold ocean water of Nova Scotia is one of the best sources available. It can be very effective in treating obesity because it greatly improves metabolism. Dulse is also good for the nervous system, brain, and spinal cord. It is beneficial in restoring hair after hair loss and strengthening the nails. Dulse and all the edible seaweeds—including kelp, hijiki, arame, and kanbu—are high in iodine. They nourish the thyroid gland and protect from the effects of radiation. They also bind with harmful heavy metals and remove them from the body or neutralize them. Dulse and kelp in powdered form can be used in a salt shaker on the table in place of salt. Both are nutritious, add a delicious salty flavor to foods, and are much more nutritious than table salt.

ESSENTIAL FATTY ACIDS (EFAs)

Essential fatty acids have also been called vitamin F. Though our bodies cannot produce them, they are vital to good health. None of our cells can survive without fatty acids, and our bodies need them to produce new cells. We also need them to produce prostaglandins, which are similar to hormones, and to help regulate important bodily functions. EFAs keep our skin soft and our hair shiny. They protect nerve sheaths and the heart and help lower cholesterol and blood pressure. They also help keep the joints limber and prevent arthritis.

There are two categories of essential fatty acids. The omega-3 EFAs are found in fresh ocean fish, such as salmon, herring, sardines, and mackerel, as well as fish oil, flaxseed oil, and walnut oil. Omega-6 EFAs are in beans, borage oil, Brazil nuts, grape seed oil, pecans, pumpkin seeds, primrose oil, raw almonds, sesame oil, sesame seeds, and sunflower seeds.

FIBER

If you have high cholesterol, fiber can help lower it. For those with blood sugar imbalances, fiber can stabilize the blood sugar. Fiber helps keep the intestinal tract working well and promotes good peristalsis and regular bowel movements. Fiber also helps prevent and heal hemorrhoids. It relieves constipation as well as diarrhea and even helps prevent colon cancer. Most Americans are not getting nearly enough fiber. Some good sources of fiber are beans, fruits, nuts, seeds, vegetables, and whole grains. Oat bran and rice bran are options for people who are allergic to wheat. Oat bran and rice bran can be added to cereals and baked in muffins.

Another source of fiber is pectin. It is found in apples, cabbage, carrots, and okra. Apple pectin can be purchased in powdered form and stirred in water to drink. It cleans the colon, lowers cholesterol, and helps balance blood sugar.

Psyllium seed is a good source of fiber that is great for cleansing the bowel. The best way to take it is mixed in water or juice. Some people have such poor peristalsis, and they have difficulty pushing this through the bowel. The psyllium may swell in the colon and cause the abdomen to extend. If this happens, drink more water. If it doesn't work for you, use flaxseed meal, apple pectin, alfalfa tablets, or chlorella to keep the colon clean. Psyllium works well when you are cleansing with colemas, which are discussed in chapter 6.

FLAXSEEDS

Flaxseeds are high in fiber, very nutritious, and have a nutty flavor. They are digested best when they have been ground. A small coffee grinder is ideal for this job. Ground flaxseeds help soften the stool and relieve constipation. They can be sprinkled on salads, cereal, soups, and yogurt, and taken in vegetable juice. They contain omega-3 essential fatty acids, protein, B vitamins, magnesium, zinc, and potassium.

Try grinding flaxseeds together with almonds, sunflower seeds, pumpkin seeds, and walnuts, and sprinkle this mixture over a bowl of hot millet or quinoa for breakfast. It tastes delicious and gives you additional nourishment throughout the morning. Try it!

FLAXSEED OIL

Flaxseed oil should be taken only if it is organic and cold-pressed. It is a rich source of omega-3 EFAs and can help reduce inflammation in the body, keep the arteries limber, and lower cholesterol and triglyceride levels. People with symptoms from arthritis, multiple sclerosis, Parkinson's disease, and fibrositis improve after taking flaxseed oil.

Flaxseed oil does not have the fiber and nutrients contained in flaxseeds, and it will not relieve constipation as well. However, you would have to eat a lot of the seeds to get the same omega-3 benefits found in one tablespoon of flaxseed oil. I recommend using both.

GARLIC

Garlic is a wonderful super food that can save a life. It helps lower choles-terol and blood pressure, and it prevents abnormal blood clotting and pro-tects the heart. Garlic contains allicin, which is a powerful antibiotic. There are also many sulfur compounds in garlic, which give it wonderful healing properties. Taken internally, garlic can stimulate the immune system and help heal colds, flu, bronchitis, and pneumonia. It also has a cleansing effect on the colon. It even helps to prevent and fight cancer. According to James F. Scheer, Lynn Allison, and Charlie Fox, in *The Garlic Cure*, "Sloan-Kettering cancer authorities, doctors John F. Pinto and Richard S. Rivlin, write that at least 20 ingredients in garlic prevent cancer or help to cope with it in as many as three ways: (1) block tumors from developing from precursor cells, (2) prevent cancer from spreading to vulnerable target cells, and (3) delay or reverse malignancy." One of the best ways to take garlic is raw, chopped in salads or with vegetables. It can also be added to olive oil and used as a salad dressing. It can be juiced with apples. Garlic oil can be taken in capsule form to protect the heart, fight bacteria and viruses, and kill parasites and candida. Garlic oil can be used externally as an antibiotic on cuts, wounds, fungal infections, and cold sores. For ear infections, rub it inside the ear. If you don't like the taste of garlic, or to freshen the breath after eating garlic, gargle with chlorophyll or baking soda and water, or chew some fresh mint leaves or fennel seeds. Bathing in baking soda baths staves off bad breath from the garlic.

GLUCOSAMINE SULFATE

Glucosamine is produced naturally in our bodies and helps build connec-tive tissue, tendons, ligaments, bones, skin, and nails. It cushions the joints and helps keep them functioning smoothly. It helps prevent and heal osteoarthritis and build joint cartilage.

Glucosamine sulfate can be taken in supplement form to reduce the pain of and help heal arthritis, bursitis, and osteoporosis. It is often found combined with chondroitin sulfate, which also helps build cartilage.

GOAT'S MILK WHEY OR MINERAL WHEY

Whey is the translucent liquid that separates from milk solids during the process of making cheese. High in minerals, goat's whey drink is prized in Europe and the Middle East as a youth elixir that promotes health and long life.

Goat's milk whey is a golden-brown powder, rich in minerals, that has been dehydrated and is free from chemical additives. A tablespoonful stirred in hot water is delicious, tasting like a slightly salty broth. It is an ideal way to correct mineral deficiencies and the multitude of health problems that occur because of them. Goat's milk whey or mineral whey can be purchased in most health food stores.

Mineral whey is high in organic potassium, calcium, chloride, phosphorous, sodium, magnesium, zinc, and iron. It also has some manganese, chromium, silicon, and selenium. In addition, it contains many of the important trace minerals that are vital to good health. Electrolytes are plentiful in mineral whey, and they make up the electrically charged ions that help regulate acid-alkaline balance, water balance, muscle contraction, nerve impulse conduction, osmotic pressure, and the transport of nutrients into and out of the cells.

High in sodium and potassium, mineral whey can prevent or help heal conditions such as chronic indigestion, constipation, intestinal irritation, colitis, and ulcers when mineral deficiencies, acidity, and stress are the causes.

Mineral whey also replaces the sodium content that helps hold calcium in solution. This can help prevent and heal arthritis, osteoarthritis, and osteoporosis by restoring minerals to the lymph fluid, joints, and bone. Capra Mineral Whey, with its high content of potassium and sodium, can reduce muscular pain and fatigue, and help the heart beat with a normal healthy rhythm. Whey provides the nutrients necessary to keep a balanced pH. In addition to all these wonderful health benefits, mineral whey is also being used successfully to detoxify heavy metals from the body (see resources). See chapter 1 for a delicious warming mineral whey drink.

GRAPE SEED OIL

Grape seed oil is one of the richest sources of omega-6 EFAs and is the only oil with the exception of olive oil that can be heated without producing free radicals. It is delicious on salads and in cooked dishes such as stir-fried vegetables. Grape seed oil can be added to night creams and hand lotions to keep the skin soft, young, and healthy. Purchase organic grape seed oil, as grapes are one of the most chemically sprayed crops.

GYMNEMA SYLVESTRE

Gymnema sylvestre is a plant that grows in India and has been used for medicinal purposes for hundreds of years. It has been used in Ayurvedic medicine as a natural diuretic and for the relief of upset stomach. Hindus use the powdered root on snakebites while having the patient drink a decoction from it.

One of the most wonderful benefits of gymnema sylvestre is that it has blood sugar-lowering actions. Extracts from the leaves are being used successfully as a remedy for diabetes mellitus. Excessive secretion of glucose in the urine has been greatly reduced in diabetics using this botanical, without side effects. In addition, gymnema sylvestre has been shown to increase beta cells that naturally produce insulin in the islets of Langerhans within the pancreas. This activity decreases the body's requirement for additional insulin treatments. Thus gymnema sylvestre has proven to be very promising in treating and healing of type 1 and type 2 diabetes. However, it is not a panacea. Diabetics should follow a healthy nutritional plan and never lower their insulin dosages before consulting with their doctor.

LACTOBACILLUS ACIDOPHILUS

Lactobacillus acidophilus is a friendly bacteria that helps establish a healthy flora in the colon. Taking antibiotics will kill these friendly bacteria and often cause yeast infections to develop. Lactobacillus acidophilus works to prevent the overgrowth of candida, fights fungus, inhibits pathogenic organisms, improves digestion and absorption of nutrients, helps reduce cholesterol, and prevents leaky gut syndrome. It is also involved with the digestion of proteins and the production of B vitamins and certain enzymes in the intestinal tract.

Lactobacillus acidophilus can be purchased in powder, tablets, or capsules. It is often derived from cow's milk, but there are nondairy formulas available for people allergic to dairy products. It is best to take it when the stomach is empty—first thing in the morning, between meals, and before bed. If you are taking an antibiotic, you can and should take acidophilus, but at different times during the day than when you take the antibiotic.

LECITHIN

Lecithin is a lipid, or good fat, that is essential to the entire body, ensuring proper cellar functioning in the brain and nervous system. It makes up the protective sheaths of the brain and nervous system. Lecithin is an emulsifier that helps dissolve plaque in the arteries and lower cholesterol. It helps keep the arteries from hardening, and it can prevent heart disease. Lecithin helps repair damage to the liver and keeps it working well.

Lecithin often comes from soybean sprouts or eggs and contains choline (a B vitamin), inositol, and linoleic acid, which is an omega-6 EFA. Other sources of lecithin are legumes, grains, and brewer's yeast.

METHYLSULFONYLMETHANE (MSM)

MSM is organic sulfur that is found in broccoli, brussels sprouts, cabbage, cauliflower, fish, raw cow's milk, and raw goat's milk. MSM is necessary for good health because it helps detoxify cells. It helps the body heal itself from injury, repair cellular damage, reduce inflammation, relieve pain such as that associated with arthritis or headaches, improve allergic symptoms, and strengthen the immune system. MSM also acts to heal gastrointestinal disorders and lung congestion. MSM is an important nutrient for the skin, hair, and nails.

OLIVE LEAF EXTRACT

Studies have proven olive leaf extract to be extremely effective against viruses, bacteria, and fungal infections. Taken orally, this herbal extract can help heal sore throats, colds, flu, bronchial infections, sinus infections, and intestinal viruses. It can even help protect against viruses such as herpes and HIV (human immunodeficiency virus).

OREGANO OIL

Oregano oil taken from wild-crafted oregano (oregano grown in the wild) is a powerful antiseptic and fights bacteria, viruses, and fungi. It contains phenols, which are natural chemicals that act as strong antiseptics that destroy harmful germs. Rubbed on the skin, oregano oil can heal cold sores and destroy fungal infections, including ringworm and athlete's foot. It can be rubbed on the gums to heal gum disease. Oregano oil has even helped heal warts, which are caused by a virus, and may even diminish moles. Oregano oil can be taken internally as well to knock out infections, viruses, and even food poisoning. For more information on this wonderful natural medicine, read *The Cure Is in the Cupboard: How to Use Oregano for Better Health* by Dr. Cass Ingram.

POLICOSANOL

Policosanol is a natural food substance taken from the sugar cane plant that dramatically reduces elevated levels of cholesterol. Though it is from the same plant that sugar comes from, policosanol does not affect blood sugar levels. Studies have shown that it lowers cholesterol without the harmful side effects caused by drugs. In addition to reducing the LDLs (low-density lipoproteins), or bad fats, in the body, policasonal helps raise HDLs (high-density lipoproteins), or good fats, in the body. According to Raj Pal, PhD, RNC, author of *Hardening of the Arteries: Intravenous (I.V.) Chelation/ Antioxidant Approach*, "Policosanol inhibits the formation of lesions in arteries, reduces inflammation-promoting thromboxane, and inhibits platelet aggregation (a cause of arterial blood clotting) and doesn't interfere with sex life."

If you would like to try policosanol but are already taking cholesterol-lowering medications, consult with your physician before discontinuing any prescription drug.

RICE BRAN AND RICE BRAN SYRUP

Rice bran syrup is concentrated from the juice of the bran, or outer husk, of brown rice. This is the nutritious part of the rice that is discarded from refined white rice. It is high in the B vitamins that keep the nervous system healthy and minerals, including silicon, which keep the hair, skin, joints, bones, and nails healthy. Rice bran syrup is high in niacin (vitamin B3), which promotes circulation. If taken on an empty stomach, a flush will come to the cheeks. Take a spoonful after a meal to avoid the flush. It can be sprinkled on cereal or baked in breads. Rice bran is sweet so it will curb the desire for a dessert.

ROYAL JELLY

Royal jelly is the food that worker bees give to the queen bee to help her grow twice as large and live six times as long as all the other bees. It gives her the nourishment she needs to lay eggs and procreate. This magnificent sweet, creamy food is produced in the glands of the worker bees. It contains enzymes to aid in digestion and absorption, and eighteen amino acids, making it a good source of protein. It also contains vitamin A; all the B vitamins; vitamins C, D, and E; minerals; and hormones. Royal jelly has antibacterial components as well. It nourishes the body and helps fight bacteria and free radicals, thus strengthening the immune system. It balances hormones and promotes longevity.

Royden Brown, one of the world's leading experts on bees and bee products, said we should take royal jelly that is no more than twenty-four hours old. In *The World's Only Perfect Food*, he explains that royal jelly should be freeze-dried immediately to maintain its potency. Take twenty-four-hour royal jelly to maintain youth and energy.

S-ADENOSYL-L-METHIONINE (SAM-E)

SAM-e is a wonderful compound that contains sulfur. It acts as a powerful antioxidant, helps raise serotonin levels in the brain, and detoxifies cellular membranes. It has been used successfully in Europe to treat fibromyalgia, migraine headaches, osteoarthritis, liver disorders, and neurological problems. It also has clinical applications in depression, anxiety disorders, and ADHD. SAM-e assists the body with metabolizing neurotransmitter phospholipids such as phosphatidylcholine and phosphatidylserine. SAM-e also helps increase levels of other neurotransmitters, such as serotonin, norepinephrine, and dopamine. These neurotransmitters help increase brain function and prevent or relieve depression.

SAM-e also plays a key role in producing lipotropic compounds in the liver. These ensure the utilization of fats and help eliminate toxins. Thus, it has been very beneficial in promoting liver health. Liver dysfunction can cause fatigue, insomnia, weight gain, poor digestion, allergies, PMS, and hormonal imbalance. SAM-e helps increase the flow of bile in the liver that is needed to digest fat. It has even been shown to be useful in serious liver disorders such as cirrhosis.

SAM-e is produced naturally in the body and is manufactured from the amino acid methionine. When there is an illness or the absence of methionine, B12, or folic acid, the synthesis of SAM-e can be compromised.

SPIRULINA

Spirulina is a green algae that grows in water in areas where there is a lot of sunshine. Spirulina is an excellent food that contains as much as 70 percent protein; minerals including iron; vitamins including B12, RNA and DNA; and essential fatty acids. Spirulina is also high in chlorophyll. It is a powerful nutritional supplement and has been used successfully by dieters to lose weight and by hypoglycemics to balance blood sugar. Spirulina is a great cleanser for the kidneys. It helps remove heavy metals, drugs, and radiation. Spirulina can be taken in capsule form, but it makes a nice green drink when stirred in water.

VITA BIOSA

Vita Biosa is an herbal drink produced in Denmark under the control of the Danish Food and Health Ministry. It was developed by Erik Nielsen, a Danish organic farmer who was inspired by the research of Japanese professor Dr. T. Higa and German herbalist Friedrich Weinkath. Vita Biosa is composed of a mixture of herbs and plants that have been fermented by lactic acid cultures. These cultures are made from friendly bacteria known as effective microorganisms (EMs), which are normally present in well-functioning healthy bowels. The herbs in Vita Biosa consist of angelica, anise, basil, chamomile, chervil, dill, elder, fennel, fenugreek, ginger, juniper, licorice root, nettle, oregano, parsley, peppermint, rosemary, sage, and thyme. The herbs supply the body with beneficial antioxidants, which counteract the development of free radicals. They are also quite beneficial to the digestive tract, helping to improve digestion.

The Vita Biosa's pH is 3.5. This low pH prevents the development of harmful bacteria both in the product and in the body. The lactic acid in the drink works together in the alimentary tract with other friendly microorganisms to abolish harmful bacteria, fungi, viruses, parasites, and yeast infections. Vita Biosa acts directly upon the mucus membranes of the intestines, helping to heal and repair leaky gut syndrome and to develop a powerful defense so harmful bacteria are killed before they can leak out of the gut and cause damage in the body and bloodstream. The effective microorganisms in Vita Biosa work amazingly well to heal Crohn's disease, ulcerative colitis, food intolerances, constipation, diarrhea, and *Candida albicans* (see resources for where to buy good Vita Biosa).

WHEATGRASS JUICE

Wheatgrass juice is a bittersweet rich green juice that has been extracted from green grass grown from grains of wheat. It was made popular by Dr. Ann Wigmore, who founded the Hippocrates Institute in Boston to educate people about healing through good nutrition. Wheatgrass juice is high in chlorophyll, iron, vitamins, and minerals. Taken internally, it fights free radicals in the body and slows the aging process. Wheatgrass juice has helped heal cancerous growths. People drinking the juice report feeling greater energy and vitality. For best results, drink the juice on an empty stomach. Wheatgrass juice can be used externally as an eyewash, a throat gargle, eardrops, a vaginal douche, and a rectal implant. It can be used in the mouth to heal gum infections. Wheatgrass juice promotes healing when placed on cuts, burns, and wounds.

WHEY

See "Goat's Milk Whey."

YEAST, BREWER'S YEAST, AND TORULA YEAST

Brewer's yeast and torula yeast are nutritional yeasts, different from the yeast used for baking. Brewer's yeast is grown on the herb called hops and torula yeast is grown on wood bark or blackstrap molasses. Nutritional yeast is high in protein, B vitamins (except for B12), and vitamins and minerals, including phosphorus. It is beneficial to people with hypoglycemia because it helps with sugar metabolism. High in niacin (vitamin B3), it helps improve circulation. The cheeks may become flushed after eating nutritional yeast because more blood is flowing to the head and brain. This is good because the blood is carrying nutrients to the brain, eyes, ears, nose, and throat, and carrying away toxins. Nutritional yeast can be sprinkled on salads or taken in water or vegetable juice.

chapter 6 ꙮ

Cleansing the Body
from Within

*The body heals from within out, from the head down
and in reverse order of how the illness began.*
–Hering's Law of Cure

THE SECRET TO VIBRANT HEALTH, youth, and vitality is in cleansing the body and mind and then adopting a lifestyle that includes clear thoughts, natural foods, pure water, fresh air, sunshine, and exercise. Learning to cleanse the body and the mind is an essential part of healing. When the body is burdened with toxic waste material, it will be tired and have low immune function. When the body is clean, it can absorb the essential nutrients it needs to heal, repair, and maintain good health.

Whole Body Cleansing through
Bowel Management

Throughout the ages, people from all walks of life have cleansed their bodies of morbid waste. Whole body cleansing through bowel management has saved some people from severe illnesses that could not be healed through any other means. Unfortunately, in today's modern society, many people are unaware of the healing miracles that can come from cleansing the body internally. Dr. Bernard Jensen, Dr. Max Gerson, Victor E. Irons, Dr. Norman Walker, Dr. Herbert Tilden, Dr. Paul Bragg, Dr. John Harvey Kellogg, and many other pioneers in the field of tissue cleansing have recorded remarkable case studies in which patients with terminal diseases were able to get well after cleansing the colon (part of the bowels). Dr. Jensen's book, *Tissue Cleansing through Bowel Management*, has guided thousands of people through cleanses and brought remarkable healing results. In addition, Dr. Gerson's book, *A Cancer Therapy*, presents numerous case studies of chronically ill patients who completely regained their health through good nutrition and cleansing. His daughter, Charlotte Gerson, continues to carry on his work with great success. Other modern-day doctors, including Dr. Rich Anderson, Dr. Jeffrey Bland, and Dr. Hugo Rodier, recommend various forms of cleansing in their practices.

Faulty digestion can keep food from being properly processed and sent out of the body. Undigested food remains in the body and creates fermentation, putrefaction, and free radicals, which cause us to age before our time. In addition, parasites feed on undigested waste materials as well as starch and sugar. It is not uncommon for people to have a tapeworm, hookworm, or liver flukes! No wonder people are fatigued and can't think clearly. Their bodies are toxic. All the blood flows through the colon by osmosis and will either pick up nutrients that nourish the body or toxins that can cause exhaustion and disease. Cleansing the colon can greatly improve the quality of the blood that circulates throughout the body, eventually cleansing all the tissues.

What is whole body cleansing? Whole body cleansing is a ten-day program during which you eat whole natural organic foods (mostly vegetables) that have been prepared to be as soft as possible or made into a soup for easy digestion. During the cleanse, you drink purified water, herbal teas, broths, and raw vegetable juices.

Each day, you spend time lying on your back in a comfortable position, on a special colon-cleansing board. The board is fixed above a toilet with a five-gallon bucket of water stationed close by and just above the board. The water contains healing herbs and flows from the bucket through a tube and into your colon via a soft tip held in the rectum. This is a very gentle process because the water is moved by gravity rather than pressure and does not require you to move off the board. You may listen to soft music and completely relax while the water flows in and then back out into the toilet. Cleansing the colon allows the body to release old fecal matter, which has often been held for years! Pennies that one swallowed as a child have been evacuated. Popcorn husks that were eaten weeks earlier, as well as parasites of all sorts, both living and dead, have been expelled into the toilet. People usually feel tremendous relief, especially if they are, and have been, chronically constipated.

TOXIC WASTE IN THE BOWEL

Toxins accumulate in the body for various reasons. Many of my clients have reported having only one small bowel movement a week! When we eat three meals a day, the bowel should move three times a day. Colons can become impacted with old rubbery fecal matter. During a cleanse, this matter—which can look like pieces of an old black tire—will be visible in the toilet. Dr. Rich Anderson, in *Cleanse and Purify Thyself, Book Two*, calls this old rubbery material "mucoid plaque" and describes it this way:

> *Mucoid plaque appears to develop in the presence of acids, wherein the mucus is secreted and coagulates. It can then compound with other elements, forming an increasingly firm substance. For those who have followed the standard American lifestyle and diet, which are acid producing, it is common for mucoid plaque to form over the glycocalyx (normal thin layer covering the microvilli in the intestines where nutrients are absorbed) of the small intestine, as well as in the stomach and large intestine. In most cases the layer (or layers) has become intermingled with a variety of damaging toxic constituents. These may include drugs, noxious fecal compounds, heavy metals, pesticides and more depending on what the person eats . . . mucoid plaque contributes toward a high percentage of pathological problems, as well as premature death.*

Dr. Anderson goes on about mucoid plaque to say:

> *This profile weakens intestinal function, causes interference of nerve meridians, and development of bowel disease. . . . Clinical studies have shown that intestinal mucins are frequently altered in such a way as to trigger the evolution of epithelial cells into cancer cells. . . . Gastric carcinomas have also been shown to develop from intestinal metaplasia that has mutated from mucoid plaque.*

Most of the foods and water people ingest today are laden with chemicals, and not all of them are eliminated. In their article "Detoxing from Toxins," Jeffrey Anderson, MD, and Jerry Stine stated that:

> *. . . [There are] contaminants that are ingested not by design, but primarily because of contaminated food and water. This category includes food additives, pesticides, agricultural contaminants in meats and*

dairy products, and heavy metals in fish. Water may contain chemicals and their by-products, pesticides, and heavy metals as well.

In addition, when people live in polluted cities, or if they smoke, the lungs become laden with tar and soot. The blood eventually carries some of this into the liver and intestinal tract.

LEAKY GUT SYNDROME

A lot has been written about the leaky gut syndrome, or hyperpermeability. It is a common condition that occurs when there is inflammation and holes or openings in the lining of the gut. Toxic by-products from foods and a proliferation of harmful bacteria leak through the lining of the gut and are carried to the liver and throughout the body. These toxins affect different areas in different people. They may cause food sensitivities, allergies, skin disorders, headaches, fatigue, irritable bowel syndrome, diarrhea, brain fog, lowered immune function, chemical sensitivities, and painful inflammation of the joints.

There are many causes of hyperpermeability, including malnutrition, long-time use of processed foods, not enough friendly bacteria in the intestinal tract, allergies, parasites, certain medications, ulcerative colitis, Crohn's disease, celiac disease, and cancer. If leaky gut persists, the liver will become overloaded with toxins, and the immune system will become severely compromised. Hugo Rodier, MD, in *10 Most Common Diseases*, tells about a landmark study reported in *Immunology Today* (1994: 15: 504), which stated that "the immune system (remember 60 percent of it is found in the G.I. tract), the nervous system, and the hormonal system are virtually inseparable!"

Through colon cleansing, we can cleanse our intestinal tract of toxic by-products that can create holes and leak through the gut. This allows the walls of the intestines to mend and repair, thus healing the symptoms caused by the leaky gut. We replace the friendly bacteria during cleansing to stand guard and protect our intestinal tract from any new invaders.

THE HEALING BENEFITS OF
WHOLE BODY CLEANSING

If you are plagued with leaky gut syndrome, arthritis, skin afflictions, low-ered immune function, liver toxicity, parasites, Crohn's disease, ulcers, coli-tis, chronic fatigue, allergies or excessive mucus, and many other disorders, cleansing the colon and subsequently all the bodily tissues can help immensely. During a ten-day period, a special mucus cleanse is followed for three days, a kidney and bladder cleanse for two days, and a liver cleanse for one day. When the colon is clean and reinforced with healthy flora, the three other elimination channels—lungs, kidneys, and skin—will cleanse themselves naturally. Lung congestion, kidney infections, and skin afflic-tions such as psoriasis, acne, and dandruff heal beautifully following a cleanse.

When the body's cells and tissues have been cleansed they can function much more efficiently and energy will return to a tired body. The blood will be rich with nutrients when it leaves the intestinal tract and can deliver life-giving food to each organ. The intestinal tract will be strong and effective, and able to contribute as a large part of the immune system. It is vital to eat healthy foods after cleansing so the cells don't become bogged down with toxic overload again. A clean, healthy body receiving the proper nutri-ents from natural whole foods, pure water, fresh air, sunshine, and exercise will feel vibrant and wonderfully alive!

Cleansing Excess Mucus

Millions of people in our world today suffer from excess phlegm in the back of their throats, sinus congestion, sinus infections, stuffy noses, allergies, watery eyes, lung congestion, asthma, and bronchitis. Clients have told me they cannot lie down at night because so much phlegm drains from their sinuses into their throats that they have to sleep sitting up. Many of our children suffer from runny noses and sinus congestion. More and more children suffer from ear infections, wearing polyethylene tubes in their ears to drain excess fluid from the inner ear through the eustachian tubes. Some children and adults have excess mucus in their stools. They often suffer from constipation, bloating after a meal, digestive disorders, gas, and burping. To remedy all these problems, people are taking decongestants, expectorants, antihistamines, cough suppressants, pain relievers, laxatives, antacids, and antibiotics. In the United States alone, 250,000,000 aspirins are swallowed each day! Unfortunately, medications treat the symptoms and may suppress the mucus or phlegm for a time, but if the cause is not discovered and treated, the problem will persist.

The sad thing is that most people haven't a clue as to what is causing the excess mucus production in their bodies. Since the discovery of antibiotics, Americans have relinquished responsibility for their health to quick fixes. However, bacteria are growing stronger because of the excessive use of antibiotics. There are many antibiotic-resistant bacteria today. In addition, antibiotics kill beneficial as well as harmful bacteria. Other medications have long lists of side effects that people may have to endure as well. It is time we take a long look at how we are living our lives if we want to stay well and healthy. It is time to discover the cause of our problems in order to be able to heal them.

WHAT IS MUCUS AND WHAT CAUSES IT?

First let us understand what mucus really is and what it does in our bodies. According to *The American Medical Association Encyclopedia of Medicine*:

Mucus is the thick, slimy fluid secreted by mucous membranes. Mucus moistens, lubricates and protects those parts of the body lined by mucous membrane, such as the alimentary and digestive tracts. Mucus prevents stomach acid from damaging the stomach wall and prevents enzymes from digesting the intestine, it eases swallowing and lubricates food as it passes through the alimentary tract, it moistens inhaled air and traps smoke and other foreign particles in the airways (to keep them out of the lungs), and it facilitates sexual intercourse.

So mucus in and of itself is helpful and plays an important role in good health. There are several causes for excess mucus. When the body becomes too acidic, the mucous membranes produce mucus to protect the tissues. The body tissues become overacidic when there is undue stress; lack of sleep; not enough purified water; a lack of fresh air, sunshine, and exercise; and consumption of foods that form high levels of acid. Most people need to eat more of the alkaline-forming foods, which are fresh fruits and vegetables, and fewer of the acid-forming foods, which are dairy products and meats. Processed foods that are high in starch, soda pop, all sweets, and alcohol are acid-forming.

The body may also produce mucus to protect membranes inflamed by allergies to food, which produce gas and swelling in the gut. A large percentage of the American diet is composed of starches, dairy products, meat, salty foods, fried foods, sweets, and soda pop. Most packaged foods contain hidden sugars and starches. Americans have consumed so much wheat that many people have formed allergies to gluten (the gluey part of wheat). Pasteurized cow's milk contains lots of fillers and no living enzymes to facilitate digestion. Many people have developed allergies to milk or simply cannot digest it.

Good health depends upon proper digestion and absorption of nutrients. The small intestine is lined with villi, or fingerlike projections, that increase the surface of absorption area in the small intestine up to a thousand fold. This area of absorption can be dangerously compromised by any condition that irritates the lining of the small intestine. Specialized immune cells called immunocytes line the small intestine. These immunocytes secrete IgA, a crucial component of the mucus lining that makes up our first line of defense. Inflammation destroys these important immune cells, opening the door to intestinal infections, bacteria, viruses, yeast, fungal organisms, and parasites.

RIDDING THE BODY OF EXCESS MUCUS

If you are suffering from excess mucus, phlegm, sinus congestion, lung congestion, allergies, gas, bloating, or mucus in the stool, it would be wise to adopt a more wholesome diet that is high in vegetables and lower in acid-forming foods. Avoid processed foods, foods high in gluten, salt, sugar, pasteurized milk products, fried foods, caffeinated drinks, alcohol, and sodas. Rest, fresh air, sunshine, and exercise will reduce inflammation and overacidity.

Cleansing the colon is also beneficial. Three days of the ten-day colon and tissue cleanse includes a specific mucus cleanse. This mucus cleanse incorporates alkalinizing foods such as vegetable broths high in potassium as well as herbs—such as ginger, garlic, and cayenne—to help expel mucus. It also includes drinking raw vegetable juices of celery, parsley, carrot, beet, and ginger to purify the lymph fluids, blood, and liver. There are wonderful herbal teas that rid the body of mucus as well, such as mullein, anise, wild cherry bark, yerba santa, and coltsfoot. A warm saltwater nasal douche can be made by adding a half-teaspoon of Celtic sea salt to one cup of lukewarm water. Scoop the water into the cupped palm of your hand and sniff some into each nasal cavity or take it into the sinuses through a dropper.

THE TURNIP DIET

The turnip diet is excellent for asthma, bronchial trouble, and all other catarrhal conditions. White turnips are higher in vitamin A than carrots and have a wonderful cleansing effect on mucus. In the turnip diet, use the juice, the greens, or the turnip itself—raw, cooked, or in soup form. Vary the diet by eating turnips in different ways along with a regular healthy diet or by having turnip combinations alone. Apple juice and pineapple juice can be added to raw turnip juice to make it more palatable. Grind raw turnips and serve them in a salad. The turnip diet can be taken for one to two days.

Cleansing the Kidneys and Bladder

Cleansing the kidneys and bladder will reduce the likelihood of kidney and bladder infections. Well-functioning kidneys help regulate the acid and alkaline balance that is crucial to health. They also help regulate blood pressure, and they are a major elimination channel. When the kidneys are toxic, the skin must pick up some of their elimination responsibilities. Acne, dandruff, psoriasis, and eczema often clear up when the kidneys are cleansed.

Another reason to cleanse is to prevent kidney stones. If you have ever passed a kidney stone, you know the severe agony they can cause! People with stones are often advised to have them removed surgically or by laser expulsion.

WHAT CAUSES KIDNEY STONES?

The kidneys filter minerals from the blood, including uric acid, calcium, phosphorus, magnesium, and sodium. Most kidney stones are composed of calcium, while some are composed of uric acid or magnesium and phosphorus. Over time, when the kidneys have too much of these substances to filter, the minerals settle and turn to stones. Heavy minerals can even harden the arteries, which enter the kidneys directly from the aorta, the main artery leading directly from the heart. This arteriosclerosis (arteries hardened by calcification) will cause the blood pressure to rise.

It is difficult for the kidneys to filter water that is heavily laden with inorganic minerals. People who live in areas where the water is high in limestone will notice a chalky white ring in their bathtubs and teapots. If the water is filled with iron, a rust-colored ring will appear. Heavy minerals in water clog up appliances. We do not need these indigestible hard materials in our bodies!

Excessive calcium is generally a result of poor nutritional habits. When people consume large amounts of pasteurized cow's milk and cheese that are devoid of enzymes to help digest it, the minerals are sent through the kidneys and spilled out in the urine. Similarly, a body overburdened with processing heavy loads of protein is unable to utilize calcium. Calcium is vital for health and prevents bone deterioration, but we need to absorb it rather than spilling it out into the toilet!

WAYS TO ABSORB CALCIUM AND AVOID GETTING STONES

Natural sodium helps hold calcium in the bone where it belongs. Vegetables and vegetable juices are high in absorbable organic sodium and calcium. Juices from green leafy vegetables and carrots contain just as much calcium as milk. Other great sources of calcium that do not cause kidney stones are chlorella, blue green-algae, spirulina, and sea vegetables such as dulse, kelp, nori, and hijiki.

A PERSONAL STORY

When I was six years old and in first grade, I woke up one snowy winter morning, went to the bathroom, and noticed blood in my urine. I didn't mention it to my mother and went to school that day. The next morning I woke up with a fever of 104°F. At that point, my mother and father rushed me to the doctor, who said I should go to the hospital right away. After many blood tests, urine tests, and X-rays, the doctors told my parents I had glumerulonephritis.

The glumeruli are filtering units within the nephrons of each kidney. These filtering units filter blood plasma. Blood is sent back into the body, and wastes such as bacteria, parasites, and even blood are carried out of the body in the urine. These glumeruli and nephrons can become inflamed and infected by infections such as streptococcal throat infections. (I often had a sore throat as a child.) When the glumeruli become damaged by inflammation, they will allow red blood cells to escape into the urine.

The doctors prescribed lots of antibiotics for me and complete bed rest. I ended up having to take antibiotics and stay in bed until the following summer! I had to go to the hospital and have blood drawn from my arm for examination every two weeks.

As I grew up, I still had sore throats every winter. It was not until I practiced colon cleansing in my early twenties that I stopped having sore throats. I do not recommend kidney cleanses until one cleanses the colon for at least three days.

Cleansing the Liver and Gallbladder

There are many ways to cleanse the liver and gallbladder. However, the bowel should be cleansed first, so the liver has a place to dump its toxins. If the bowel is toxic and you start cleansing the liver, the body will suffer from toxic overload. This can cause headaches, nausea, and even vomiting as the body tries to find a way to get rid of liver toxins. When the bowel is clean, it can efficiently carry toxins from the liver out of the body through the rectum. Dr. Jeffrey Bland states in *Optimal Digestion: New Strategies for Achieving Digestive Health*:

> *The overgrowth of bacteria or yeast in the GI tract may create toxic overload that can stress detoxification. When overgrowth occurs, the liver may be less able to detoxify other incoming substances that would normally go unnoticed. The buildup of these toxins in the body can result in general toxicity or in specific illness. For example, research has found that an overgrowth of E. coli bacteria is frequently present in the stool of patients with food sensitivities or Crohn's disease. The toxic by-products of bacteria and yeast are passed on to the liver for processing.*

STRENGTHENING AND CLEANSING FOODS AND HERBS

To strengthen and cleanse the liver, eat foods that are high in iron such as the bitter greens, including mustard greens, kale, turnip greens, collards, beet tops, endive lettuce, parsley, arugula, cilantro, and broccoli rabe. Other foods that are high in iron and nourishing for the liver are beets, prunes, figs, and raisins.

Several herbs help the liver tremendously. Milk thistle is a bitter tonic that is high in silymarin, a constituent that helps protect the liver against some of the most virulent liver toxins. Milk thistle helps heal hepatitis A and B and cirrhosis of the liver. Milk thistle also has been proven to lower fatty deposits in the livers of animals. Oregon grape root stimulates the flow of bile through the liver and gallbladder. Burdock is high in minerals and helps the liver by cleansing and filtering the blood. Yellow dock root is high in iron. It helps decongest the liver and fight most inflammatory liver and gallbladder ailments. Wormwood is very effective against hepatitis and jaundice and also kills parasites. Celandine has been used to decongest the liver, treat hepatitis and jaundice, and dissolve gallstones. Dandelion root tea has cured some of the worst cases of hepatitis. Turmeric helps the liver process estrogen and balance hormones, so it is very useful for people suffering from premenstrual symptoms.

Twenty-four-Hour Liver, Gallbladder, and Kidney Cleanse

This twenty-four-hour cleanse can safely dissolve stones from the liver, gallbladder, and kidneys. Here is the program to follow.

6:00 A.M. Drink one quart of distilled water.

7:00 A.M. Drink as much unfiltered, organic apple juice as desired. Freshly juiced apple juice is best, but if this is not possible, buy organic apple juice from a health food store. Apple juice and apple cider vinegar dissolve stones.

After 7:30 A.M. Take a morning enema or colema with five gallons of water.

12:00 noon. Drink no more fluids for the rest of the day except distilled water.

Shortly after noon. Take a second enema or colema with five gallons of water.

5:00 P.M. Dissolve two tablespoons of Epsom salts in one quart of distilled water and drink the mixture.

9:00 P.M. Mix four ounces of fresh lemon juice with four ounces of virgin olive oil and drink the mixture.

Lie on your right side to sleep, and prop pillows behind your back to help maintain this position throughout the night. In the morning, kidney stones will pass through bowel elimination. They should be soft and gelatinous and will harden again after they come out in the stool.

The Ten-Day Whole Body Cleanse

I have traveled far and wide studying different cleansing techniques and have worked with and participated in many wonderful cleansing programs. I worked with Dr. Jensen at his beautiful Hidden Valley Health Ranch in Escondido, California, for five years. While I was there, we held many tissue-cleansing classes. People came to the ranch from all over the world and studied the principles of tissue cleansing while cleansing their own bodies. I witnessed miracles occur in these people's health as their bodies were cleansed and healed.

The whole body cleanse that I offer in this book incorporates the best techniques and nutrients I have seen proven time and again to heal and repair the body. This whole body cleanse purifies all the elimination channels, which include the bowel, kidneys, lungs, and skin. It cleanses major organs and glands, such as the thyroid, adrenal gland, male and female reproductive systems, liver, gallbladder, spleen, pancreas, brain, and eyes. It also cleanses the sinuses and lymph fluid as well as all the other tissues, glands, and cells.

PREPARING FOR THE WHOLE BODY TISSUE CLEANSE

Approximately one week to one month before beginning a cleanse, eat only the foods recommended in the Tool Kit for Making Healthy Food Choices, and make all your drink only slections from the Tool Kit for Choosing Healthy Popular Beverages. Eat whole foods and drink natural drinks before a cleanse. This healthy nutritional program will begin the process of cleansing your body. Eating healthy foods beforehand will also prevent many of the symptoms that can accompany cleansing, such as headaches and nausea. These symptoms often occur when people are detoxing from caffeine, nicotine, sugar, processed foods, and alcohol.

WHO SHOULD CLEANSE?

This cleanse is rejuvenating for everyone. If you are elderly or at all weak, you should definitely have assistance. Children over the age of eight can do a partial cleanse with their parents or a qualified adult to assist. A syringe of warm water with chlorophyll, catnip tea, and white willow bark can be given rectally to babies and children experiencing fever, colds, flu, or constipation. Consult a qualified health practitioner in your area.

Children between the ages of eight and twelve may participate for one day of drinking raw vegetable juices and eating soups. They should cut the supplement recommendations to one third. For example, if an adult is taking nine chlorella tablets, three times per day, a child could take three tablets three times per day. Children can also go on a cleansing board using one gallon of warm water that day with herbal teas and supplements added, enough for one gallon of water. Teenagers from twelve to sixteen may participate for three days of raw vegetable juices, soups, and broths. They can go on a cleansing board and use one to three gallons of water each day for three days.

If you are seriously ill, this cleanse could be very beneficial for you. However, you will definitely need help. Friends or family may help to prepare the soups, juices, broths, cleansing boards, and buckets of water, with nutrients and implants. Their love and emotional support are valuable at this time. Remember, above all else, love heals.

If someone you love is ill, help them. Give them support and encouragement. It could save their lives!

WHAT TO EXPECT WHILE CLEANSING

While you are cleansing, you may feel a bit more tired than you usually do. If you do, make sure to get more rest. Others have reported feeling more energy. Some people have broken out with rashes on the skin but it goes away within a few days. This is the skin's way of helping the body release toxins. You may have a slight fever during the cleanse while the body is burning off impurities. If this happens, rest, drink plenty of water, and place damp cooling cloths on the head. You may release lots of mucus during the cleanse. One man reported that he ached in his joints for a few days and then all aching was gone. You may feel some nausea at times, especially during the liver cleanse. Some people have actually vomited. This doesn't happen often but is a natural occurrence. Be aware that you are actually on nature's operating table and need to slow down during this time and allow the toxins to exit the body. Your body will do this gradually and in a very intelligent, orderly manner. If symptoms become intense, if there is blood in the stool or urine, if the fever is more than 101°F for more than a day or two, consult a competent natural health practitioner or medical doctor. On the positive side, many people have very beautiful experiences during the cleanse. They feel "lighter" and more peaceful. Try to relax as often as possible, be in nature when you can, watch some funny movies, and take extra care of yourself during this time.

WHERE TO CLEANSE?

This cleanse can be accomplished in the comfort of your own home. You will need a bathroom large enough to fit a cleansing board that is forty one inches long and twenty one inches wide over your toilet and extend approximately four feet straight out in front of the toilet. You will also need room to elevate a five-gallon bucket about three feet above the board; this will allow gravity to draw water from the bucket through a hose to the rectum. Buckets are often placed on bathroom counters above the toilet and this works quite nicely. Another way to raise the bucket is to place it on top of a sturdy, wide stepladder.

You will need a kitchen where you can prepare herbal teas, raw vegetable juices, soups, and broths. Rest is crucial to cleansing. Ideally, you should have a room where you can go for silence and meditatation, reading, or writing. You will need a comfortable bed with cotton sheets.

Exercise is important during the cleanse, so you will need space to do yoga, stretch, or jump gently on a mini-trampoline. Fresh air and sunshine are important, so you will need a place to go for a walk in the morning or later in the afternoon. It's better to avoid intense sun from 11:00 A.M. to 4:00 P.M. in most areas.

SUPPLIES FOR THE CLEANSE

During this cleanse, you will be washing your colon clean with approximately twenty gallons of water per day using a comprehensive colon cleansing board, a five-gallon bucket, tubing, and tips. Water will be inserted through the tip into the rectum as you lie on the board in a relaxed position. Though this may sound frightening, it is actually soothing and relaxing. The tip that you use will be lubricated with a natural plant-based lubrication, such as olive oil or K-Y jelly. Here are the supplies you will need to do a complete ten-day whole body cleanse:

· A comprehensive colon cleansing board (forty-one inches long and twenty-one-and-a-half inches wide) with tubes and clamps (see resources for where to find boards)
· One five-gallon bucket that you will fill two to four times
· Clear pliable plastic tube (comes with the board) that is about a third of an inch wide and four and a half feet long. This tube attaches to the bucket at one end and the opening in the cleanse board that fits above the toilet. It can be cut to fit the length you need for your particular bathroom.
· Pliable plastic tips are about ten inches long with four tiny holes in the end—two on each side to disperse the water gently and evenly. You will get two or three tips with your board, but you will use only one with each cleanse. Extra tips are supplied in case you lose one. The tip fits on the end of the tube and extends through a hole in the opening of the board that fits over the toilet. An extra two-inch piece of plastic attaches the tip to the tube and fits snugly into the hole in the board to prevent it from slipping when the tip is inserted into the rectum.
· A syringe or apparatus that connects into the tubing to do implants
· A colander to place in the toilet to catch fecal material if you'd like to view the material coming from the colon
· A two-foot-square table or chair measuring from one half to one inch higher than your toilet (with the seat up) to support the cleansing board (the slight angle allows all fecal material and water to flow into the toilet easily)
· Two quarts of extra virgin olive oil to lubricate tip (will also be used throughout cleanse) or K-Y jelly to lubricate tip
· Purified water or a water filter to filter the water from your shower that goes into the bucket
· Thin rubber gloves to wear while cleaning up
· A quart-size spray bottle with two tablespoons 35 percent food-grade hydrogen peroxide or one pint regular hydrogen peroxide and the rest

distilled water to disinfect and clean everything. Soak the tip in this solution and pour it through all the tubes each day after cleansing.

· A bottle of biodegradable natural liquid soap for cleaning
· Whole body cleanse solution additives (see the list under "Whole Body Cleanse Solution Additives")
· Ingredients for the implant (see the list under "The Implant")
· Plenty of distilled water for teas
· One ten ounce jar of psyllium seeds and husks, which equals sixty teaspoons. You will use thirty teaspoons during entire cleanse (or five ounces), and the rest for maintenance. Or puchase sixteen ounces of whole flaxseeds and grind three teaspoons each day of the cleanse. Use remainder for maintenance.
· One thirty-two ounce bottle bentonite clay liquid, which equals sixty-four tablespoons. You will use thirty tablespoons during entire cleanse and the rest for maintenance.
· A pint jar with a lid
· Herbal teas as recommended
· Supplements (see list)
· Foods as recommended. All vegetables and fruits should be washed in a food-grade hydrogen peroxide solution with one teaspoon to one quart of water to remove bacteria and parasite eggs. If food-grade hydrogen peroxide is not available, soak your vegetables in a solution of raw apple cider vinegar and water. Use one tablespoon of vinegar to one quart of water. Health food stores also carry vegetable-cleaning solutions.
· Warm olive oil to massage the abdomen in case of cramps. You will need about a quarter cup for each abdominal massage.
· An oral mercury or digital thermometer to record daily temperatures
· A reliable set of scales to weigh yourself daily
· An automatic electric blood pressure monitor (available at pharmacies). Checking the blood pressure daily on the cleanse is important, especially if you have high blood pressure or very low blood pressure.

Supplements

· 1 bottle beet tablets (250)
· 1 bottle dulse tablets (100 tablets)
· 1 bottle 50 milligrams niacin tablets (100 tablets)
· 1 bottle plant enzymes (100 capsules)

- 1 bottle flaxseed oil (8 ounces) or 1 bottle essential oils with flax and borage (100) or 1 bottle wheat germ oil capsules (100)
- 1 bottle Calphonite (liquid calcium, magnesium, potassium) (15 ounces)
- 1 bottle mineral lyte homeopathic trace minerals (16 ounces)
- 1 jar mineral whey (12 ounces)
- 1 bottle Jensen's vegetable seasoning (2 to 6 ounces)

Liver Cleanse Supplies

- 1 bottle L-ornithine (30 to 60 capsules) or 1 bottle passion flower, valerian combination (60 tablets) (may use if having difficulty sleeping throughout the entire cleanse)
- 1 organic grapefruit, red or white, or 4 organic lemons
- Olive oil (you already have enough)
- 1 pint Epsom salts
- Raw organic honey

WHOLE BODY CLEANSE SOLUTION ADDITIVES

You or your practitioner will add various nutrients to the buckets of water, which may include the following.

Aloe Vera Juice

Aloe vera juice is mucilaginous. It is also high in minerals that soothe and nourish the colon.

Antiparasite Herbs

Antiparasite herbs, such as wormwood, black walnut, and clove combined in tincture or capsules will fight parasites.

Bentonite Clay

Bentonite clay is taken from the earth and purified for cleansing purposes. It has a drawing effect and helps pull toxins out of the colon.

Catnip Tea

Catnip can be added to the water when a person is having cramps. Catnip tea helps relieve cramps and relax the abdominal muscles. It can heal colic in babies as well.

Celery Juice

Celery juice is high in natural sodium. The fluid in the colon is naturally high in organic sodium, which keeps it limber and pliable. Celery juice will replace natural fluids flushed from the colon. The blood will also carry the sodium to your joints, keeping them limber and free from arthritis.

Eugalan Topfer Forte

Eugalan Topfer Forte is powdered form of lactobacillus bifidus that nourish and feed the bowel, and help to fight harmful bacteria.

Flaxseed Tea

Flaxseed is an emollient tea that is very soothing to the intestinal walls and helps rid the colon of old fecal matter.

Garlic Juice

Garlic juice fights parasites and harmful bacteria in the colon. It also helps promote peristalsis and assists the liver in releasing its load of waste products into the intestinal tract for elimination.

THE IMPLANT

After you have completed your cleanse each day, and soon after you get off of the cleansing board, you will insert, or "implant," a solution with various nutrients and probiotics—such as lactobacillus acidophilus, and Vita Biosa, with effective microorganisms—back into your colon. This is crucial to the success of the cleanse. The blood then picks up these nutrients from the colon and carries them to all parts of the body. Specific nutrients may be added for each person individually to assist him or her in healing particular conditions. The implant consists of the following ingredients.

Aloe Vera Juice

Juice from the aloe vera plant is emollient and contains lots of vitamins and minerals. Aloe vera juice is very soothing to the colon.

Antiparasite Herbs

A combination of cloves, wormwood, black walnut, and garlic is included in the implant to fight and kill parasites. Each of these herbs contains powerful properties that eliminate harmful bacteria and parasites acquired from eating rare meats, poorly washed fruits and vegetables, or lots of sugar, which feeds the parasites.

Enzymes

Enzymes aid digestion. They help break down the other nutrients in the implant. Enzymes assist in digesting and eliminating bacteria and parasites.

Lactobacillus Acidophilus

Lactobacillus acidophilus is a friendly bacteria that normally lives in the colon. During a cleanse, some of the acidophilus may be washed out. The implant replenishes it. Acidophilus helps fight harmful bacteria in the gut and is a major part of the immune system.

Greens

Greens cleanse, nourish, and build the blood that flows through the intestinal tract. Use wheatgrass juice, chlorophyll, or green powder, such as barley green, spirulina, or blue-green algae.

Grapefruit Seed Extract

Extract from grapefruit seeds acts as a natural antibiotic in fighting harmful bacteria.

Vita Biosa

Vita Biosa provides additional friendly microorganisms that fight bacteria, fungi, and viruses.

Implant Solution

- 2 capsules lactobacillus acidophilus (broken open) or 1 teaspoon Vita Biosa or Eugalan Topfer
- 1 to 2 ounces chlorophyll or wheatgrass juice or 1 teaspoon barley green powder and 1 to 2 ounces distilled water
- 1 dropperful antiparasite herbs, including wormwood, cloves, and black walnut
- 1 to 2 ounces aloe vera juice
- 5 drops grapefruit seed extract
- 1 capsule plant enzymes

Combine all the ingredients. Use no more than two to four ounces for the implant. Use a syringe or a tube hooked directly from a special holding cup connected to the cleansing board to place the implant into the rectum. A syringe will usually hold two ounces and the holding cup, four ounces. Hold the implant within you as long as possible. You may be able to hold it through the day or night without expelling it. If you can't hold it very long at first, don't worry. Whatever goes in will be beneficial.

ELECTROLYTES

When you come off the cleansing board, you will need to drink eight ounces of water containing one teaspoon trace minerals in homeopathic form, often called mineral lyte or trace lyte (see resources). These electrolytes will keep you from feeling light-headed or dizzy. They restore vitality to the body and balance pH. Drink another glass of this electrolyte mixture later in the day. If you have a particular problem with acidity or light-headedness, drink this mixture four to five times during the day.

BEVERAGES DURING THE CLEANSE

During your cleanse, you will often drink a mixture of psyllium and bentonite clay. Psyllium is a fiber that swells and is slippery. It helps to gently "scrub" the colon clean. It gets into the pocketed areas of the colon and cleans out old impacted matter. Bentonite clay absorbs toxins, heavy metals, and poisons from the bowel and carries them out of the body.

Psyllium and Bentonite Drink

  1 tablespoon bentonite clay
  1 rounded teaspoon psyllium husks and seeds or ground flaxseeds
  8 ounces water
  2 ounces organic apple juice

Mix the ingredients in a jar with a lid. Shake it well, then drink as recommended in the various stages of the cleanse.

Drink lots of fluids between meals when undergoing a cleanse. It is best not to drink during a meal because liquids can keep the body from digesting foods properly. If you feel you must drink during a meal, just sip a small amount of water. Just as your foods should not be too hot or too cold, neither should your beverages. Drink eight glasses of purified water each day. If you have arthritis, kidney stones, or gallstones, drink distilled water. In addition, you may enjoy some herbal teas or vegetable juices.

Herbal Teas

As we have learned earlier in this book, herbal teas have many healing properties. The following herbal teas are selected specifically for this cleanse because of their individual abilities to cleanse or strengthen the body.

Some of the best herbal teas to assist your cleansing process are listed here. Consult the Tool Kit for Choosing Therapeutic Herbal Teas for advice on a particular tea.

Fenugreek Tea

Fenugreek tea has a bittersweet taste. It helps cleanse the liver and also plays a tremendous role in releasing mucus buildup from the tissues. Parasites can dwell in excess mucus, so this tea is wonderful during a cleanse.

Fennel Tea

Fennel makes a delicious tea that cleanses the liver.

Flaxseed Tea

Flaxseed tea helps promote natural peristalsis while lubricating and soothing the colon. It helps to soften old fecal matter along the colon wall so it can be released.

Oatstraw Tea

Oatstraw tea is high in silicon, which builds connective tissue, skin, hair, and fingernails. This tea is very healing to the nervous system.

Red Clover Tea

If you feel tired every day, your blood may be toxic. Red clover tea cleanses the blood. Also, during a cleanse the blood may become toxic because all the organs are releasing their toxins into the blood to be carried out through the elimination channels.

Vegetable Juices

Vegetable juices are very nourishing and help strengthen the cells to release the toxicity necessary for cleansing. Each vegetable juice has specific healing properties.

Beet Juice

Beet juice is excellent for cleansing the liver and gallbladder. If the liver and gallbladder are too toxic, begin with small amounts and slowly increase over time to avoid becoming nauseous.

Carrot Juice

Carrot juice is high in beta-carotene, which is a tremendous immune-system booster and helps prevent cancerous types of growth. Carrot juice cleanses and detoxifies the liver. Eight ounces of carrot juice has the same amount of calcium as eight ounces of milk and is much easier to assimilate and utilize.

Celery Juice

Celery juice is high in chlorophyll, which cleanses and nourishes the blood, and sodium, which keeps the joints limber. Sodium also helps hold calcium in the bone so that it does not leach out and create crystals in the joints.

Ginger Juice

A little ginger added to your juice will improve circulation. If you have cold hands and feet, ginger juice is a good choice for you. Remember, a little ginger goes a long way!

Parsley Juice

Very high in chlorophyll and minerals, parsley juice is a tremendous blood, liver, kidney, and bladder cleanser.

Fruit Juices

The only fruit juices recommended on this program are the diluted apple juice used to take the bentonite clay and psyllium and the diluted lemon juice described next. The apple juice should be freshly juiced from organic apples, if possible. If this is not possible, buy organic apple juice from a health food store. Organic apple juice helps dissolve kidney stones and gallstones. Pasteurized apple juice or juice from nonorganic apples will simply feed the bacteria and parasites you are trying to get rid of!

Lemon Juice Drink

> 1 lemon
> 8 ounces distilled water
> $1/8$ teaspoon cayenne pepper
> $1/2$ teaspoon maple syrup (optional)

Squeeze the juice of an entire lemon into eight ounces of warm water. Add an eighth teaspoon of cayenne pepper and a half teaspoon of maple syrup (optional) or a few drops of stevia to taste (especially if you had candida, are diabetic, or hypoglycemic). This recipe is taken from the Stanley Burroughs cleanse. You will drink a lot of this during the mucus and kidney and bladder cleanse.

Pure Synergy

Pure Synergy is a freeze-dried powerhouse of organically grown greens and seaweeds developed by Mitchell May, which helped him regenerate and heal muscles, bones, tendons, and ligaments after a serious car accident. It also is great for keeping the blood sugar in balance and keeping you from feeling hungry. It tastes good stirred into water. (Many greens do not taste good unless they are mixed with fruit juices.) Mix a teaspoon of this powder in eight ounces of water and drink it throughout the day (except when you are on the liver cleanse). It has one gram of fat from essential oils in it.

BATHS AND THERAPIES

Throughout the cleanse, special baths can be very beneficial (try a ginger bath to improve circulation or an Epsom salts bath to relieve tired muscles). Other baths that might feel refreshing are outlined in the Tool Kit for Choosing Rejuvenating Body Treatments and Beauty Aids in chapter 3. Try walking in sand, walking in cold water up to your knees, deep breathing, yoga, or the therapies outlined in chapter 3.

For people with chronic ailments, the cold sheet treatment is helpful, usually on the ninth night, after the liver cleanse. The cold sheet treatment, also described in chapter 3, should be done only with a responsible adult or skilled practitioner present. This treatment helps draw toxins out of the body through the skin.

SPECIAL NOTES FOR SPECIAL PEOPLE

If you are very thin, you may eat more avocados on this cleanse as well as more nut and seed sauces. (Do not eat these during the liver cleanse because you must avoid fats that day.) This cleanse will help balance your metabolism so you will be able to gain whatever weight you need to be healthy. If you are overweight, this cleanse will help you lose weight. Be very careful getting on and off the cleansing board. Ask for help if you need it.

If you have high blood pressure, consult a knowledgeable doctor about the cleanse. Some people have been able to balance their blood pressure with liquid calcium and magnesium while doing this cleanse. If you have severe hemorrhoids, let them heal before beginning the cleanse. If you have mild hemorrhoids, lubricate the hose tip well and take bioflavonoids and rutin throughout the cleanse to help tighten them up. Keep them lubricated with castor oil throughout each day. Sitz baths with baking soda may be soothing.

If you are on a medication, do not go off the medication without asking your doctor. If you have an illness or disease, consult your doctor.

If you have anorexia or bulimia, use this cleanse only with the cleansing broths or soups. Some people become addicted to cleansing the colon because they think it helps them lose weight. Such an addiction is just another form of vomiting! This cleanse is to be respected, used only as a cleanse (not during days of eating the regular nutrition program). If you have anorexia or bulimia, be honest with yourself. Use the tools in this book and consult with a trained counselor.

YOUR ATTITUDE DURING A CLEANSE

Attitude is important during the cleanse. Negativity and bitterness can actually cause the body to go through tremendous cramping both on and off the cleansing board. Before you get on the board, breathe deeply and relax. Go into a cleanse with gratitude that such a wonderful opportunity has come to you to assist your body in healing. Be joyful that you are participating in something wonderful that can add years to your life. A cleanse can also help you look better and have much more energy.

ESSENTIAL OILS, BACH FLOWER REMEDIES, COLOR, AND HEALING TONES

Oils have been used from the beginning of time and are mentioned in the Bible for their healing properties. The wise men brought frankincense and myrrh to the Christ child. Music and tones have been used for centuries to sooth and heal those in distress. The Bach flower remedies, discovered by Dr. Edward Bach in the 1930s, have successfully eased stressful emotions for over a hundred years. Color has been used since time began to bring joy to those who were sad. Our Creator gave us a soothing blue sky to gaze upon each day and colorful flowers and rainbows to make us happy.

Essential oils, Bach flower remedies, color, and healing tones are wonderful ways to nurture someone who is going through a cleanse. If cramping or nausea occur, it may help to put a little peppermint oil under the nose or to sip a bit of ginger tea. This relieves the nausea and promotes relaxation. Birch and eucalyptus oils can be rubbed into the back or on the calves of the legs if there is any pain.

If there is fear at any point during the cleanse, Rescue Remedy from the Bach flower remedies is most helpful. This oak flower remedy helps to relieve the fear of not getting well. Aspen is for vague, unknown fears for which there is no explanation.

Beautiful music and soothing tones can be very healing. While on the cleansing board, play soothing music. I also recommend a tuning fork treatment performed by someone trained in the Solfeggio scales. These frequencies help balance the nervous system and calm the emotions.

Color is also most helpful during a cleanse. Wear colors that lift your spirit, such as lavender or rose. Place colorful flowers in the room. Rest under blue or green blankets. Colors have vibratory frequencies that can be a blessing to the eyes, mind, body, and spirit.

GENERAL WHOLE BODY CLEANSE
FOR DAYS 1, 7, 9, AND 10

During the ten-day whole body cleanse, three days are focused on cleansing mucus, two on cleansing the kidney and bladder, and one on cleansing the liver. The other four days—days 1, 7, 9, and 10—are general in nature, preparing the body to receive the full benefits of the cleanse. These days are specially prepared to cleanse the whole colon and all of the tissues of the body. They are not designed to cleanse any one particular organ of the body. The purpose of these days is to allow the body to rest from an intense cleansing of specific areas, while continuing to do an overall cleansing of the colon and tissues of the entire body. On day one, you will begin the whole body cleanse, which is a general cleansing and prepares the body for days 2, 3, and 4 which are specific and focused with the nutrients to help remove mucus from the body. On days 5 and 6, after having cleansed the general lymph fluids of the body, you will then cleanse the kidneys. Day 7 is a day of rest and general cleansing with no specific areas targeted. Day 8 is specifically designed to cleanse and remove wastes from the liver. On days

9 and 10, you will be back on the regular whole body cleanse and the completion of the entire cleansing program.

General Whole Body Cleanse Daily Schedule

The following is the program you will be following for the four days of general, overall body cleansing. Remember that these days are just as important as the days targeted for specific organs because you will be cleansing the colon and all the tissues of the body. So follow these directions completely, and do not slack off, thinking these days are not so important. These days prepare the body for the special days of specific cleansing.

Here is the schedule for the four days of whole body cleansing.

6:00 A.M. Upon arising each day, take the psyllium and bentonite clay drink. (See the recipe under "Beverages During a Cleanse.")

6:30 A.M. Record your blood pressure, temperature, and weight.

7:00 A.M. Do a cleanse with 2 to 4 five-gallon buckets of warm purified, filtered, and/or distilled water. See the recipe for a whole body cleanse solution below. On day one, you may be able to finish only one to two buckets comfortably without becoming weary. If you are feeling achy or weary from lying on the board, you may stop at one to two. If you feel you can do three or four, that's great too. (See "Setting up the Bucket and Board," below.)

8:45 A.M. Do skin brushing, then take a shower. (See chapter 3 for instructions on skin brushing.)

9:00 A.M. Take supplements: four beet tablets; two Nova Scotia dulse tablets; four chlorella tablets; one fifty-milligram niacin tablet (to improve circulation); two digestive plant enzymes; one teaspoon of flaxseed oil or two capsules of flaxseed, borage, or wheat germ oil; and one tablespoon of liquid minerals that includes calcium, magnesium, and phosphorus, such as Calphonite (take with water, herbal tea, vegetable juice, or pure synergy drink). Calphonite can help tremendously with regulating high or low blood pressure.

9:15 A.M, Eat breakfast. Suggestions: (1) a bowl of cooked millet, quinoa, or brown rice, blended and served with raw almond milk or rice milk; (2) soft noncitrus fruit, such as banana and papaya with two to three tablespoons of raw almond cream; or (3) a Good Morning Health Shake; (4) Avocado Pudding (see the recipe in chapter 1).

10:30 A.M. Have a healthy drink, such as raw vegetable juice, Jensen's Vegetable Seasoning Powder mixed in warm water, or mineral whey drink with two beet tablets and two chlorella tablets.

12:00 noon. Repeat the supplements taken in the morning.

12:15 P.M. Eat lunch. Suggestions: (1) vegetable soup, blended raw soup with sesame cream (see the recipes in chapter 1); (2) raw vegetable juice soup with a baked potato; or (3) baked squashes with vegetable juice soups.

Afternoon. Rest, walk, do yoga, listen to soothing music, get a massage.

2:00 P.M. Drink herbal teas and raw vegetable juices with two beet tablets and two chlorella tablets.

3:00 P.M. Drink the psyllium and bentonite clay mixture again.

4:00 P.M. Drink herbal teas, Jensen vegetable seasoning and/or mineral whey powder—one teaspoon of each to a cup of hot water (see resources), potato peeling broth, or raw vegetable juice.

5:00 P.M. Repeat the supplements taken with breakfast and lunch.

5:15 P.M. Eat dinner. Suggestions: (1) Dr. Bieler's potassium soup, (2) butternut squash soup, (3) raw vegetable juice soup with sesame seed and sunflower seed sauce, (4) lentil soup (vegetarian), or (5) split pea soup (vegetarian).

7:00 P.M. If desired, have some broth, vegetable juice, or herbal tea. Do not eat afterward. Your body needs to rest and cleanse during the night.

9:00 P.M. Drink the psyllium and bentonite clay mixture again.

9:30 P.M. Go to bed.

Setting up the Bucket and Board

1. Sterilize the bucket and board with a hydrogen peroxide and water solution. Run water and peroxide through the tubes and tip and wash the tip well. Then run clean purified water through the tubes and tip.

2. Set up the bucket on the countertop. Place the colander in the toilet if you would like to view the material that comes out of the bowel while cleansing. Place the board with the end that has the opening for the buttocks over the toilet and the other end on the two-foot square table, stool, or chair.

3. Extend the tubing from the bucket to the end of the board over the toilet to see how much you will need. It must be loose, not stretched tight.

Cut the tubing at one end with a strong pair of kitchen scissors to the length you need. Cut the tube straight across and not at an angle.

4. Attach the tube at one end to the short extended opening at the bottom of the bucket where the tube should go. Slide the clamp used to stop the water up over the tube so that it will be near you while you are lying on the board so you can stop the flow of water at any time. Attach the other end of the tube to the two-inch piece of hard plastic provided for you. Stick the tip into the other end of the hard piece of plastic.

5. Place the tip attached to the hard piece of plastic and the tube into the hole in the colon-cleansing board just above the toilet. Tip should extend out far enough to enter the rectum about two and one half to three inches. It should never go into the rectum more than three inches because there are only five inches in the rectum to the flexure where the colon bends to go into the sigmoid or ascending colon.

6. Clamp off the tube and fill the bucket with warm filtered water. Water should be warm to the wrist, never too cold or too hot. Unclamp the tube and allow a little bit of water to flow through until it is coming out of the tip to ensure flow. Then clamp off and dry off the board where the water has come out.

7. Add nutritive ingredients to the bucket and stir well with a long spatula or spoon.

8. Lay a towel over the board. Place a pillow at the head. Have another large towel available to cover you. Put on some soothing music or something positive you'd like to listen to, or get a book that will be comforting to read.

9. Lubricate the tip.

10. Place one quarter cup of warm olive oil near the board. I recommend you place a stepping stool right beside the board where you can place the oil and a good book to read.

11. Undress (you may wear a t-shirt and socks) and sit down on the board. Then slowly lie down placing your head on the pillow and sliding your buttocks up to the opening in the board over the toilet. Sit up slightly and insert tube into rectum approximately two and a half to three inches.

12. Lie back down and cover up. Make sure you are comfortable. Your legs will be placed on each side of the end of the board over the toilet and bent, or you can stretch them out from time to time and place them

on the back of the toilet. Then, take the tube with the clamp into your hand. Unclip the clamp and allow the water to begin flowing into the rectum. Water should flow in very gently since it is flowing with gravity rather than forced pressure. When you feel like you do when you are going to have a bowel movement, use your abdominal muscles to press water and fecal matter out. This will go directly into the toilet. Then relax and let more water flow in. You should never have to stop the water flow with the clamp throughout the entire bucket of water unless you are having cramps.

13. If cramping occurs, stop the flow of water with the clamp. Breathe gently and relax. Massage the abdomen with the warm olive oil until water releases into the toilet and cramping stops. Then let the water flow into the rectum again. If cramping persists, get up from the board and add one quart of catnip tea to the water. If the bucket is still completely full, you will have to extract one quart of solution in the bucket, then add the quart of catnip tea. The quart you extracted can be added to your next bucket. Catnip tea will soothe the colon and prevent cramping.

14. To get off the board, clamp off the tube—even if the bucket is nearly empty, water will remain in the tube—gently pull the tip from your rectum, bring your legs around to the floor and carefully sit upright. Place each of your hands on the board on either side of you and slowly stand up. If you are elderly or feel you need help, keep a phone nearby so you can call for assistance.

15. You can fill each bucket yourself, or if you have a willing person to help, you may call them when you are ready to have the bucket filled (with added ingredients) each time.

16. At the end of the two to four buckets that you do each day, make sure you have evacuated all material from your bowel. Then attach the implant container with implant solution so that ingredients will go through the tip into the rectum. Instructions for this come with the implant container that comes with the board. Allow implant to flow into rectum. Some people can hold the implant inside of them indefinitely and some will expel right away. Try to hold the implant for at least fifteen minutes, if possible. If you do not have an implant container with your board, a syringe will also work. A syringe will usually hold about two ounces. To use the syringe, you will need to get off the board first.

17. When getting off the board, follow directions in step 14. You should drink your electrolyte drink while sitting on the board, before you stand up. This drink will keep you from getting dizzy.

18. If you did not use an implant cup attached to the board for your implant, it's time to use the syringe. Make sure all fecal matter is out of your colon. Fill the syringe with the implant ingredients and lie on your right side to insert. Stay there for at least fifteen minutes so the good ingredients can flow into the colon.

19. Check contents in toilet. This might sound strange to some people, but it is important to review the fecal material that comes from the bowel. It will show you what you are cleansing from the body. To check the contents, put on your gloves and carefully lift the colander out of the toilet. Place it on a strong piece of plastic on the floor. Take a stick of some type or an old long-handled spoon from your kitchen and stir through the matter. You may see worms of all shapes and colors. These include pinworm, roundworm, hookworm, tapeworm, whipworm, and liver flukes. The worms may still be moving or dead. Unfortunately, many people have one or more of these worms in their digestive tract. To get them out is wonderful, because they are the cause of much intestinal distress as well as illness. In addition, pieces that look like old black rubber tubing (this is very old matter from the lining of the colon), pieces of popcorn, undigested food, or even pennies or dimes may be in the colander. Some people find things that were swallowed during childhood. Whatever it is, be glad you are rid of it and on to better health and digestion! To view pictures of what has come from colon cleansing, see Dr. Bernard Jensen's book, *Tissue Cleansing Through Bowel Management.*

20. Clean up the board by taking a pot of water and pouring over it so that the water and any fecal matter is washed into the toilet. Flush the toilet. Pull the tip and tube out of the board. Then spray off the board on both sides with the hydrogen peroxide solution. Wipe with a damp cloth and then a dry cloth.

21. Rinse two gallons of water that contains one quart of the hydrogen peroxide solution through the bucket, tube, and tip. Detach the tip from the tube and place in a container with enough hydrogen peroxide solution to cover it. Keep the tip in the solution until the next use.

22. When the ten-day cleanse is over, sterilize the tip with the hydrogen peroxide solution, rinse well, dry, and store in a sealed plastic bag until the next time. Dry the bucket well and store it for using the following day. You may keep the tube attached to the bucket during the entire ten days. At the end of the ten days, cleanse the tube well, let it dry and store inside the bucket.

23. Store the bucket, tube, and tip (inside the sealed baggie) in a large clean plastic garbage bag. To store the board, cover it completely with a large clean garbage bag. Keep everything together in a closet until the next time.

Whole Body Cleanse Solution for Buckets

1 ounce garlic juice

1 cup celery juice, ¹/₂ cup chlorophyll, or ¹/₄ cup wheatgrass juice

1 cup to 1 quart flaxseed tea or ¹/₂ cup to 1 cup aloe vera juice 2 table-spoons Eugalan Topfer Forte powder or ¹/₄ cup Vita Biosa

4 droppersful or 8 capsules of antiparasite herbs (wormwood, black walnut, cloves)

1 cup to 1 quart catnip tea, optional

1 tablespoon bentonite clay—add to the last bucket each day

Add the ingredients to each of four five-gallon buckets of purified, filtered, and/or distilled water.

Additional nutrients and herbs may be added to the water to meet special needs. For example, catnip tea is very soothing and relieves cramps. For constipation, the larger amounts of flaxseed tea or aloe vera juice should be used. For colitis, additional flaxseed tea should be added as well as slippery elm. If fever is present, white willow bark tea should be added. Select from the teas listed later in this chapter.

MUCUS CLEANSE FOR DAYS 2, 3, AND 4

Follow the mucus cleanse program for three days—days 2, 3, and 4. Drink lots of distilled water between other recommended drinks. Rest throughout the day. Walk, get fresh air, jump on the trampoline, listen to soothing music. Smile, say your prayers, be happy!

Mucus Cleanse Daily Schedule

Some mucus, as was stated earlier, is normal for certain bodily functions. Excess mucus in the body can dwell in the head and sinus cavities, throat, lungs, bowel, and throughout the lymph channels. Mucus is a substance in which parasites may dwell. Excessive mucus can be quite uncomfortable, often causing sinus drainage, lung congestion, and coughing. Some people report having to sleep sitting up all night because they have so much mucus in their sinuses. The following cleanse is designed with foods, broths, herbal teas, and nutrients to help pull excessive mucus from the body. During these three days, you may blow a lot of mucus from your nose, cough up mucus from your lungs, or see mucus in your stools. When the cleanse is over, you will be amazed by how much better you will feel. Here is the schedule for all three days of the mucus cleanse.

6:00 A.M. Upon arising each day, take the psyllium and bentonite clay drink. (See the recipe under "Beverages During a Cleanse.")

6:30 A.M. Prepare a drink with one organic lemon and a one-inch square piece of gingerroot. Juice the lemon with the rind and the ginger. Add eight ounces of warm distilled water and one teaspoon of maple syrup or raw, organic tupelo honey or stevia to taste (if you are diabetic, hypoglycemic, or have candida). Drink it slowly.

6:45 A.M. Record your blood pressure, temperature, and weight.

7:00 A.M. Do a cleanse with four five-gallon buckets of warm, purified water and regular daily bucket ingredients. You may add one cup of mullein or fenugreek tea to the water to pull out mucus from the bowel. After the cleanse, drink an electrolyte drink before getting up from the board. Do implant either on the board (if implant cup is attached) or after you get off the board with a syringe. See the recipe for a whole body cleanse solution.

8:45 A.M. Do a skin brushing, then take a shower. (See chapter 3 for instructions on skin brushing.)

9:00 A.M. Take the same daily supplements you took for day one: four beet tablets; two Nova Scotia dulse tablets; four chlorella tablets; one fifty-milligram niacin tablet (to improve circulation); two digestive plant enzymes; one teaspoon of flaxseed oil or two capsules of flaxseed, borage, or wheat germ oil; and one tablespoon of liquid minerals that includes calcium, magnesium, and phosphorus, such as Calphonite (take with water, herbal tea, vegetable juice, or pure synergy drink). Calphonite can help tremendously with lowering high blood pressure.

9:15 A.M. Eat breakfast: twelve ounces of juice made from four ounces of celery, three ounces of parsley, two ounces of carrot, two ounces of beet, and one ounce of ginger juice with two scoops of almond cream (see recipes in chapter 1) or an avocado smoothie with the juice and pulp of one whole lemon blended in to the mixture (see recipes in chapter 1).

10:30 A.M. Drink eight ounces of warm distilled water with the juice of one whole organic lemon and one-eighth teaspoon cayenne pepper; you may add one teaspoon of Grade B organic maple syrup or several drops of stevia to taste.

12:00 noon. Repeat the supplements taken in the morning.

12:15 P.M. Eat lunch: twelve to fourteen ounces of Dr. Bieler's Potassium Soup (see recipe in chapter 1), vegetable soup, or squash soup. Add one teaspoon of flaxseed oil and one teaspoon of olive oil to the broth to move fats out of the liver.

2:00 P.M. Have a cup of mullein tea to clean mucus out of the lungs.

3:00 P.M. Drink the psyllium and bentonite clay mixture again.

3:30 P.M. Drink eight ounces of the same vegetable juice mixture recommended as a breakfast choice.

4:30 P.M. Drink eight ounces of warm distilled water with one tablespoon of raw apple cider vinegar and a little raw organic honey or stevia to taste. Sweeteners are optional.

5:00 P.M. Repeat the supplements taken with breakfast and lunch.

5:15 P.M. Eat dinner: twelve to fourteen ounces of vital potassium broth, mucus-cleansing vegetable soup (the recipe follows), or butternut squash soup. Add some vegetable broth powder, cayenne, and olive oil for seasoning.

8:00 P.M. Drink a cup of mullein tea or fenugreek tea.

Vital Potassium Broth

2 quarts distilled water

2 cups carrot tops, finely chopped or grated

2 cups celery tops, finely chopped or grated

3 cups celery stalks, finely chopped or grated

2 cups potato peelings
1 yellow onion, chopped ($^1/_2$-inch thick)
1 clove garlic, minced
1 teaspoon flaxseed oil
1 teaspoon olive oil

Bring the water to a boil. Add the vegetables and reduce the heat to simmer. Simmer for thirty minutes. Strain the mixture and add the flaxseed and olive oil. Discard the solids and drink only the broth.

Mucus-Cleansing Vegetable Soup

$^1/_2$ cup chopped onion
2 cloves minced garlic
$^1/_2$ cup chopped carrots
$^1/_2$ cup chopped string beans
$^1/_2$ cup chopped zucchini
$^1/_4$ teaspoon oregano
$^1/_2$ teaspoon basil
Pinch of cayenne pepper
$^1/_2$ teaspoon unrefined seasalt
2 tablespoons pure virgin olive oil
3 tablespoons organic tomato paste
3 tablespoons Jensen's Vegetable Seasoning
3 cups purified water

Saute vegetables in olive oil until slightly done. Bring water to a boil and add Jensen's vegetable seasoning, oregano, basil, cayenne, and tomato paste. Stir well and add vegetables. Reduce heat to simmer. Simmer for fifteen minutes. Add one tablespoon coconut oil and let simmer two minutes more. Turn off burner and add sea salt. Makes five cups.

KIDNEY AND BLADDER CLEANSE FOR DAYS 5 AND 6

This part of the cleanse is very important for people with kidney stones, uric acid crystals, frequent kidney or bladder infections, or skin problems. It is also important for people who have a history of any of these problems in the family or who would like to prevent these disorders. The urine pH should stay between 6.8 and 7.2 in the morning, between 6.8 and 8.4 right after meals, and between 6.8 to 7.2 a couple of hours after meals. Alkalization of the urine is crucial in dissolving kidney stones and uric acid crystals. Get some litmus paper and check your pH balance each day. To understand more about pH balance and to learn how to check your pH levels, see chapter 4.

Kidney and Bladder Cleanse Daily Schedule

During this cleanse, it is important to drink lots of water between recommended drinks and meals. If you have had a kidney disease at any point in your life, any types of frequent kidney or bladder infections, or kidney stones it would be best if you consult a knowledgeable natural health practitioner or doctor before and during this procedure. This cleanse often helps clear up acne or other skin ailments because the toxins are better able to pass through the kidneys rather than having to exit through the skin. It also helps clear up existing kidney or bladder infections as well as vaginal infections in women. During this cleanse, urine may appear cloudy while debris from the kidneys and bladder is being eliminated. It may even have an unpleasant odor. This is a normal part of this cleanse. If a severe pain occurs in the kidney area or if blood appears in the urine, stop the cleanse and seek medical advice immediately. If a fever occurs in the body, make the cleanse water in the buckets cooler to help cool down the body. If the fever is more than 101°F and persists more than a day, see a doctor. None of these things are meant to be frightening in any way, but cleansing old wastes from the kidneys can stir up the toxins that may be there. Some people experience a bit of fear or anxiety during a kidney cleanse. This is because cleansing the kidneys also cleanses the adrenal glands that sit on top of the kidneys. The adrenal glands are responsible for feelings of "fight or flight." This is normal and one should realize that it will pass. Practice deep breathing, go for a walk, or do some journaling to release old fears. Write yourself a letter and tell yourself that you are safe and all is well. Most people, even those who have had kidney disease, have great results with this cleanse and in addition to having clearer skin, begin to have more energy and stamina. They release old fears and feel more confident and peaceful inside.

Here is the schedule for the kidney and bladder cleanse.

6:00 A.M. Upon arising each day, test your urine pH with litmus paper.

6:15 A.M. Take the psyllium and bentonite clay drink. (See the recipe under "Beverages During a Cleanse.")

6:30 A.M. Record your blood pressure, temperature, and weight.

6:45 A.M. Drink one cup of lemon juice drink. (See the recipe under "Beverages During a Cleanse."

7:00 A.M. Do a cleanse with four five-gallon buckets of warm purified, filtered, and/or distilled water. Include the regular nutrients (see the recipe for a whole body cleanse solution). Also add one cup of kidney and bladder tea to the cleanse water (the recipe follows). After the whole body cleanse, drink the electrolyte drink and do the implant.

8:45 A.M. Do skin brushing, then shower.

9:00 A.M. Take the same supplements you took on days one and two: four beet tablets; two Nova Scotia dulse tablets; four chlorella tablets; one fifty-milligram niacin tablet (to improve circulation); two digestive plant enzymes; one teaspoon of flaxseed oil or two capsules of flaxseed, borage, or wheat germ oil; and one tablespoon of liquid minerals that includes calcium, magnesium, and phosphorus, such as Calphonite (take with water, herbal tea, vegetable juice, or pure synergy drink). Calphonite can help tremendously with lowering high blood pressure. Take it with one cup of kidney and bladder tea.

9:15 A.M. Eat breakfast: watermelon or watermelon delight (the recipe follows).

10:30 A.M. Drink two ounces of carrot juice mixed with two ounces cucumber or celery juice and four to five ounces parsley juice.

12:00 noon, Take the same supplements you took in the morning, with a cup of kidney and bladder tea.

12:15 P.M. Eat lunch: blended raw vegetable soup or Dr. Bieler's potassium soup, adding chopped garlic, broth powder, and olive oil to either one. You may have some sesame sauce or sunflower seed sauce with the soups (see recipes in chapter 1).

2:00 P.M. Drink eight to twelve ounces of organic raw apple juice or one cup of warm distilled water with one tablespoon of raw organic apple cider vinegar and one teaspoon of honey. Both of these drinks help dissolve stones.

3:00 P.M. Take the psyllium and bentonite clay drink.

4:00 P.M. Take some potato peeling broth or vital potassium broth.

5:00 P.M. Take the same supplements as at breakfast and lunch, with a cup of kidney and bladder tea.

5:15 P.M. Eat dinner. Suggestions: Dr. Bieler's potassium soup or blended raw vegetable juice soup, with lemon, garlic, ginger, or olive oil mixed in either one.

7:00 P.M. Drink kidney and bladder tea, apple juice, potato peeling broth, or apple cider vinegar drink.

9:00 P.M. Take the psyllium and bentonite clay drink.

If you have stones, soak in hot Epsom salts baths each night, rinse off, and place a warm castor oil poultice on your kidneys (see chapter 3).

Kidney and Bladder Tea

6 teaspoons juniper berries
6 teaspoons corn silk
6 teaspoons uva ursi
6 teaspoons gravel root
6 teaspoons hydrangea
3 quarts distilled water

Soak the herbs in the distilled water overnight in a stainless steel pot. (These herbs disinfect the kidneys and bladder and help dissolve stones.) In the morning, bring the whole container of water and herbs to a boil and immediately reduce the heat to simmer. Simmer the mixture, covered, for ten minutes. Let it sit another ten minutes, then strain and serve. Use this tea in the buckets of water, and drink as much as you can for two days.

Watermelon Delight

1 cup organic watermelon, chunks
1/2 cup organic watermelon seeds with pulp

Place the watermelon chunks and seeds into a blender, and blend until creamy. Strain the mixture. This thick, rich cream contains vitamin C, zinc, iron, and, protein. This is a great kidney and bladder drink!

LIVER CLEANSE FOR DAY 8

The liver cleanse should be done only after seven days of comprehensive colon cleansing. The bowel must be clean enough for the liver to dump toxins into it. In addition, it is important to realize that the liver is directly connected with feelings of passion and anger. These emotions affect the liver more than any other organ. Feelings of anger may arise during a liver cleanse. Be prepared for this! If anger arises, let it go. Then go out and hug a tree! Feel the absence of anger, fear, and judgment that a tree stands for. In addition, while you are cleansing you may release gelatinous stones that will harden after they come out. These can be green or yellowish in color due to the coloration from the bile from the liver. These stones have been stored in the gallbladder and it's wonderful to get them out. You will have much better digestion and better energy afterwards.

Do not eat any fats during this cleanse, *not one gram!* If you are not sure whether a food has fat in it, don't eat it. The only supplements allowed with this cleanse are beet tablets, chlorella tablets, and liquid minerals. Drink distilled water throughout the day. Try to drink a gallon of water before 2:00 P.M. in between meals.

Liver Cleanse Schedule

6:00 A.M. Upon arising, take the psyllium and bentonite clay drink.

6:30 A.M. Record your blood pressure, temperature, and weight.

7:00 A.M. Do a cleanse with four five-gallon buckets of warm purified, filtered, and/or distilled water with the regular daily nutrients in the buckets of water. (See the recipe for a whole body cleanse solution). Add a cup of the liver-gallbladder tea to the buckets of water (the recipe follows). After the cleanse, drink the electrolyte drink and take the implant.

8:45 A.M. Do a skin brushing, then take a shower

9:00 A.M. Take four beet tablets, two dulse tablets, four chlorella tablets, two enzymes, and one tablespoon of liquid calcium-magnesium (such as Calphonite) with one cup of liver and gallbladder cleansing tea. Do not take flaxseed oil or any other oil supplement!

9:15 A.M. Eat breakfast. Suggestions: fruits such as papaya, pears, apples, and blended bananas and melons. Steamed vegetables and raw vegetable juice.

10:30 A.M. Drink liver and gallbladder cleansing tea or a cup carrot, beet, and celery juice.

12:00 noon Take the supplements as in the morning with liver and gallbladder cleansing tea.

12:15 P.M. Eat lunch. Suggestions: baked potato with liquid aminos and steamed vegetables, including a good portion of steamed beets, vegetable soup, and blended raw vegetable juice soup with beets.

2:00 P.M. From this time forward, do not have any food or drink at all unless recommended.

6:00 P.M. Mix one tablespoon Epsom salts in one cup of warm distilled water. Drink the mixture slowly. Afterwards, have just a taste (less than one-fifth teaspoon) of raw organic honey on the tip of a teaspoon to get rid of the salty aftertaste.

8:00 P.M. Mix one tablespoon Epsom salts in one cup of warm distilled water. Drink the mixture slowly. Have a taste of honey if necessary. Massage your colon and visit the bathroom as often as necessary.

9:45 P.M. Prepare the grapefruit and olive oil drink (the recipe follows). Place this drink beside your bed. Prepare a third dose of Epsom salts in one cup of warm distilled water and place it by the bed for later also. Visit the bathroom again just to be sure.

10:00 P.M. Drink the grapefruit and olive oil mixture, and take four capsules of L-Ornithine or a passion flower-valerian root combination to help you sleep. Lie down immediately on your right side and do not move for at least thirty minutes. You should fall asleep. Set the alarm for 3:00 A.M.

3:00 A.M. Upon waking, take the dose of Epsom salts that you placed by your bed earlier. You can eat a light meal two hours later.

5:00 A.M. Eat a light meal. Suggestions: cooked millet, quinoa, or brown rice with almond milk, or a bowl of fruit with almond cream.

Love yourself and love your liver! Within the word liver is the word *live.* Once you have cleansed your liver, you will feel so much more alive! Colors will appear brighter and you will be more joyful. Cleansing the liver helps improve eyesight. Two weeks after the comprehensive cleanse, do this liver cleanse again. After a cleanse, the liver can rapidly fill back up with the toxins the body is trying to eliminate. Assist your body and your liver by cleansing it again.

Liver and Gallbladder Cleansing Tea

1 teaspoon burdrock root
1 teaspoon dandelion root

1 teaspoon yellow dock root

1 teaspoon Oregon grape root

2 teaspoons red clover blossoms

1 teaspoon Pau d'Arco

$^1/_2$ teaspoon gingerroot powder

2 quarts of distilled water

Soak the herbs in the water in a stainless steel pot overnight. In the morning, bring the entire contents of the pot to a boil, then reduce the heat to a simmer. Simmer for five minutes. Turn off the burner and let the tea steep for fifteen minutes.

Citrus and Olive Oil Drink

1 grapefruit, pink or white or 4 lemons

$^1/_2$ cup olive oil

2 quarts of distilled water

Peel the grapefruit or lemons and carefully remove all the seeds. Chop the fruit and place it in the blender with the olive oil.

KEEP A DAILY JOURNAL

Get a beautiful journal just for you—one that you really like. Record your temperature, blood pressure, and weight each day. Record your pH levels on the days you are doing the kidney and bladder cleanse. Each day record how you are feeling physically, emotionally, mentally, and spiritually. Write about your dreams. They may be trying to give you a message. Write any thoughts that occur to you. You may come to know yourself on a very intimate level. If you are searching for answers while doing this cleanse, write at the top of a page, "I now know the answer to . . . ." Write any insights or revelations that come to you. You may be surprised by what you discover! Enjoy your cleanse! It is one of the finest things you can do for your total health.

ENDING THE CLEANSE

Day 9, you should continue to follow the regular cleanse schedule after you have completed the liver cleanse and had your light meal early that day. Day 10 follows the general schedule as well and is usually the day to end the cleanse. Some people feel they would like to go one more day. Some very ill people have gone for several more weeks. Just remember to use the implants! This is crucial! If you do not use the implants, you will wash all of the friendly bacteria out of your bowel and harmful bacteria can move in, just the opposite of what you are trying to achieve. Implants will help you to have healthy bowel movements when you are finished with the cleanse.

Two Weeks after the Cleanse
After two weeks, do the liver cleanse again. This is crucial to the health of your liver.

Nutrition after the Cleanse
It is very important that you eat lightly for at least three days after a cleanse. I knew of a man at the clinic where I studied in Switzerland who ate a pizza after his cleanse! He became so ill that he had to be rushed to the hospital. He had undone all the hard work of his cleanse.

Day 1: Eat the same way you did on the general days of cleansing–days 1, 7, 9, and 10. You may have a raw vegetable salad. Chew it really well!

Day 2: Have a light breakfast such as the Avocado Pudding and continue to have salads and soups. You may add one-quarter to one-third cup brown rice or other grain during the day such as millet or quinoa.

Day 3: Have a light breakfast such as papaya with almond cream. Continue with soups and salads. You may add some fish.

Day 4 and after: Follow the meals for optimal health plans presented in chapter 1.

Supplements after the Cleanse
For at least one month after the cleanse, continue taking the supplements you took during the cleanse. These will help keep your thyroid balanced, keep your liver and gallbladder cleansed, improve your circulation, and give you the vital enzymes, trace minerals, and essential fatty acids you need. I also recommend that you add the following:

· Multivitamin/mineral supplement (follow the directions)
· One thousand milligrams of vitamin C with bioflavonoids, daily

- Two capsules of antiparasite herbal formula containing black walnut, wormwood, and cloves, two times per day with lunch and dinner
- Two capsules of lactobacillus acidophilus two times per day on an empty stomach
- 1 tablespoon of flaxseed oil per day or 2 capsules of flax and borage or wheat germ oil, twice a day.

Maintenance

Choose one day each month, such as the first Saturday, and eat foods from the general cleanse that day. Take the general cleanse the next morning with four five-gallon buckets of warm water and the added nutrients. Be sure to take the implant!

After the cleanse and maintenance program, you should feel like a whole new person with vibrant health and energy. If not, you may need a more extensive program that would require the help of a doctor, nutritionist, or natural health practitioner. In the final chapter of this book, you will see into the lives of others who have experienced this cleanse.

PART 2

Case Studies

MY FATHER-IN-LAW, Dr. Bernard Jensen, wrote a book called *Nature Has a Remedy*. In it, he included many profound stories of people who had come to his Hidden Valley Health Ranch and healed with the natural "medicines" provided by nature. These included fresh air, sunshine, exercise, pure water, time for rest, organic food from the huge gardens there, fruits from the orchards, and herbs, vitamins, and minerals he recommended. I too aspired to help people get well in these wonderful natural ways, so I studied and learned all I could from him. Now I have had the privilege of working with thousands of people as a health coach.

chapter 7 ∞

Learning from the
Lives of Others

Nature, time, and patience are three great physicians.
–H.G. Bohn

AGAIN AND AGAIN, I have been inspired by people's dedication to their intention to heal. The miracles that have occurred in many of their lives lift me up and give my own life such special meaning. Here are some of their amazing stories and the nutritional programs, supplements, teas, physical therapies, cleanses, and emotional therapies they followed in order to get well. Perhaps you will see a bit of yourself in some of these people and find pieces of information that might be helpful to you. Their names have been changed to protect their privacy.

Katherine: Healing Body and Mind
to Enable Pregnancy

Katherine was a beautiful young woman of thirty-two. She was very slim for her height. She had been happily married to a great guy for several years. During that time she had not been able to become pregnant. She had the following symptoms:

- Allergies to pollens, dust, and molds
- Sinus infections and sinus headaches
- Poor circulation, with cold hands and feet
- Hypoglycemia and a craving for sweets
- Difficulty with digestion, especially foods containing fats
- Erratic periods, with cervical dysplasia (a term used to describe the appearance of abnormal cells on the surface of the cervix, the lowest part of a

woman's uterus) diagnosed and treated at age eighteen with no recurrence.
· Suffered from tension, having been abused as a child

NUTRITIONAL PROGRAM

Katherine's nutritional program avoided dairy products, wheat flour, refined sugars, and fried foods. (She did not drink caffeine or alcohol.) She ate lots of green leafy vegetables and beets to support her liver. She limited her diet to only two fruits per day, one to two gluten-free whole grains per day, three to four servings of legumes that had been soaked overnight and cooked per week, two to three servings of soft-boiled or over-easy organic eggs per week, two to three servings of fish per week, and one to two servings of poultry per week. She properly combined proteins with vegetables and grains with vegetables and ate fruit alone.

SUPPLEMENTS

Katherine enhanced her nutrition program with propolis, echinacea, and goldenseal to relieve allergies and heal sinus infections. She took vitamin E to improve her circulation and regulate her periods. She took a full-spectrum digestive enzyme with her meals and a good multivitamin including all the B vitamins and minerals to feed and relax her nervous system. She also took essential fatty acids, including flaxseed oil and evening primrose oil, to balance her nervous system and her hormones. She took dulse tabs to feed her thyroid and improve her circulation, plus false unicorn to specifically stimulate blood flow through the pelvic area. She took vitamin C with bioflavonoids to strengthen her immune system.

TEAS

Katherine drank herbal teas—such as ginger, rosemary, catnip, cinnamon, and cloves—to improve blood and lymphatic circulation to her pelvic area. She drank oatstraw tea to support nerve function and relieve stress in her body.

CLEANSE

After three months of this program, Katherine did a colon and tissue cleanse as outlined in chapter 6, adding fenugreek and fennel teas to help remove excess mucus from her body.

EMOTIONAL THERAPIES

Katherine wanted to release any negative emotions that were stored in her body so she began to work with and practice the emotional therapies. I guided her in New Decision Therapy, a profound therapy using kinesiology to identify and release emotional trauma that may have weakened the immune system. This therapy is thoroughly presented and described by Kandis Blakely in *Your Body Remembers*. Through this therapy, Katherine was able to release a lot of tears, sadness, and pain.

RESULTS

After eighteen months of therapies, all Katherine's symptoms had disappeared and she became pregnant. Nine months later, she delivered a healthy boy weighing eight pounds and three ounces and measuring twenty-two inches long! Katherine nursed him and had plenty of milk for twenty-one months.

Jay: Healing Vertigo and Tension

Katherine's husband, Jay, was forty-two. He appeared quite fit because of his outdoor work as a firefighter, but he was about ten pounds overweight. He had the following complaints:

- Dizziness, following an on-the-job head injury
- Loss of memory
- Nervousness (his father had been in the military and had been very strict)
- A craving for sweets

NUTRITIONAL PROGRAM

Jay craved sweets. He was also tense and nervous. I asked him to follow the same nutritional program that I had prescribed for Katherine. The foods would help balance his body and it would be calming and healing for them to enjoy their meals together.

The nutritional program avoided dairy products, wheat flour, refined sugars, and fried foods. Jay was to eat lots of green leafy vegetables and beets to support his liver. He was to limit his diet to only two fruits per day, one to two gluten-free whole grains per day, three to four servings of legumes that had been soaked overnight and cooked per week, two to three servings of soft-boiled or over-easy organic eggs per week, two to three servings of fish per week, and one to two servings of poultry per week. He was also to properly combine proteins with vegetables and grains with vegetables, and eat fruit alone.

SUPPLEMENTS

Jay supplemented his nutritional program with phosphatidylserine and ginkgo biloba to feed his brain and nervous system. He took a multivitamin with all the B vitamins and minerals, including chromium picolinate to balance his blood sugar and zinc for his prostate gland. He took digestive enzymes with each meal for optimum utilization of nutrients. He also took ginger capsules to relieve his dizziness. Wild oat, lecithin, false unicorn, and pumpkin seeds increased his sperm count.

TEAS

Jay drank the same teas as Katherine—ginger, rosemary, catnip, cinnamon, and cloves—to increase circulation of his blood and lymph. He also drank ginseng tea to strengthen his reproductive organs.

CRANIAL SACRAL THERAPY

Chiropractors or massage therapists generally do cranial sacral therapy to gently balance the bones and muscles of the head and upper spine. It helps to relieve dizziness caused by injury to the head or upper spine. Jay had injured his head while on the job as a firefighter, and cranial sacral therapy eased his resultant dizziness.

EMOTIONAL THERAPIES

Jay did the New Decision Therapy with me and released tremendous amounts of stored anger.

He also wrote about his anger, then tore up the paper, and burned it. This helped him release stored up emotions as well.

CLEANSE

Jay undertook the full ten-day whole body tissue cleanse.

RESULTS

Jay released sixty gallstones during his liver cleanse and lost ten pounds. The cranial sacral therapy and ginger stopped all his dizziness. His memory improved, and he was able to relax. He and his wife had a healthy baby boy eighteen months after he started therapies, and he is a happy, loving father.

Carolyn: Relieving Depression

Carolyn was five foot seven and weighed 165 pounds. She was fifty-seven years old and suffering from severe depression. She cried easily, often feeling her life was difficult and hopeless. Having taken many medications over the years in an effort to get well, Carolyn found that after a while, the medications were no longer effective, and she needed to take them in stronger and stronger doses. She had these symptoms:

- Depression
- Excess weight
- Leg cramps
- Fibrocystic breasts
- Joint pains
- Varicose veins
- Muscle aches
- Exhaustion
- Sinus congestion

Carolyn craved and ate a lot of sweets and fried foods. She drank a lot of caffeinated drinks, including black tea, sodas, and coffee. At age thirty-five, she had had her uterus removed because of fibroid tumors.

Prior to our meeting, Carolyn had suffered a nervous breakdown due to problems with her marriage and business. Also, her son had been severely injured in motorcycle accident.

At that time, she was given the following medications:

- Lamictal for depression
- Remiron for depression
- Synthroid for depression and because she was borderline low thyroid

As she took these medications, she became swollen with fluids so she was also given the following:

· Maxide to reduce fluid and swelling
· Lodine for leg cramps

Carolyn started having terrible cramps and burning in her stomach, so she was also given:

· Tagamet and Zantac for burning stomach
· Esterase for hot flashes

She continued to try every depression medication available, each one stronger than the last. Eventually, none of them worked anymore, and she was prescribed shock therapy. Carolyn was in tears a great deal of the time and felt severely depressed. This was when she decided to try natural therapies.

NUTRITIONAL PROGRAM

Carolyn's nutritional program suggested that she avoid pasteurized dairy products, white flour, refined sugars, fried foods, pork, red meat, salt, aspartame, and caffeinated beverages. (She did not drink alcohol.) She was to eat lots of raw and steamed vegetables, no more than two fruits daily, gluten-free whole grains, soaked raw organic almonds, sunflower and pumpkin seeds, sesame butter, olive oil, salads, legumes, organic eggs, baked or broiled fish, chicken, and turkey. She was to drink raw vegetable juices daily, including carrot, beet, and celery. She was also to drink herbal teas, using stevia to sweeten them.

TEAS

Carolyn drank oatstraw tea to balance her nervous system. She also drank any other herbal teas she liked in place of the caffeinated beverages she had been drinking. Examples of these teas were lemon balm (calms nerves), peppermint (helps open up the sinuses), and ginger (promotes circulation and helps relieve joint pain). She was not taking these especially for medicinal purposes, but because she liked their flavors. However, she did receive the healing benefits outlined in chapter 2 of this book.

SUPPLEMENTS

Carolyn took St. John's wort, ginkgo biloba, phosphatidylserine (to feed her brain and nervous system), and lecithin to feed her brain and nervous system and clean her vessels. She took a multivitamin with all the Bs, minerals, and herbs for her liver, vitamin C with bioflavonoids, including rutin for her varicose veins, collagen and elastin cream for her varicose veins, calcium and magnesium to support her bones, and vitamin B for circulation. She also took an herbal tincture combination of dong quai root, wild yam root, chaste tree berry, and hops to support her hormonal levels, with L-tyrosine and ATP (adenosine triphosphate) to help relieve her depression. L-tyrosine is a building block of protein called a nonessential amino acid, which the body makes from phenylalanine, another amino acid. Essential amino acids are those we must acquire from foods. L-tyrosine is a precursor or helps to form several neurotransmitters or substances in the body that help improve nerve function. Often, L-tyrosine taken as a supplement helps improve nerve function and relieve depression. ATP, or adenosine triphosphate, within the body is the energy within a cell that helps deliver energy to all metabolic pathways in the body, making sure the body uses carbohydrates, proteins, and fats properly. Taken as a supplement, it helps ensure that nutrients are absorbed properly and helps promote energy.

PHYSICAL THERAPIES

Carolyn took Epsom salts baths to relieve her aches and pains; used castor oil poultices on her breasts (to help soften fibrocystic lumps). She also walked in fresh air and sunshine daily and practiced deep breathing.

EMOTIONAL THERAPIES

Counseling with Carolyn helped her learn to practice joy. She cut out pictures from magazines and made a poster of the things she loves to help her focus on that which brings her happiness. She read positive uplifting books.

Slowly, over several months, with the supervision of a medical doctor, Carolyn was able to come off all her medications. As she was coming off her medications, she began to have trouble sleeping and developed red itching skin around her eyes and dry skin in general. At that point we added vitamins A and D and an oil combination of flaxseed, black currant seed, pumpkin seed, and safflower. She used MSM lotion topically and switched to all natural cosmetics. She also added an herbal combination to help her relax and sleep at night, which included passion flower, valerian root, hops, and kava kava. The medical doctor on our team changed the synthroid (medication she was taking to regulate her thyroid) to the more natural Armour Thyroid for her thyroid.

RESULTS

Carolyn lost thirty pounds over a period of one year. All her dryness, redness, and itching disappeared. Her legs, joints, and muscles no longer ache, and she is able to walk two miles per day and sleep soundly at night. Blood tests show her thyroid and hormonal levels have come into balance. She divorced her husband and now, with counseling, she sold her business and moved to a new home that she loves. She is teaching her son, who had an accident, about nutrition and his health is improving. Her depression is gone completely, and she is now a very self-confident, happy lady running two creative businesses and square dancing!

Rhonda: Healing Psoriasis, Alcoholism, and Compulsive Eating

Rhonda was a sweet young woman with a beautiful spirit, but she was very sad at age thirty-four. She was dating a guy who was verbally abusive, and she was working at a job where the boss was unkind. Rhonda was five foot six and weighed 170 pounds. She had had severe psoriasis over most of her body since age twenty, and it often cracked and bled. Her very traumatic background included over a decade of sexual abuse. She was a very small child who was too terrified to tell her parents. At age thirteen, she started using coffee, cigarettes, drugs, alcohol, and food to numb her emotional pain. She took marijuana, LSD, speed, beer, vodka, and gin until she was twenty-five. At that time, she stopped the drugs but continued drinking, smoking, and overeating. Her symptoms included:

· Severe psoriasis over most of her body
· Obesity
· Chronic constipation, with a bowel movement about once a week
· Depression, drinking alcohol every night, hating her job
· Craving and eating lots of sweets
· Severe PMS and cramps with menstruation

NUTRITIONAL PROGRAM

Rhonda's nutritional program avoided soft drinks, candy, pasteurized milk, wheat-flour products, pork, red meat, and fried foods. She weaned herself from coffee, using half regular and half decaffeinated. She slowly cut down on alcohol and cigarettes. She ate raw fruits and vegetables, steamed and baked vegetables, millet, quinoa, amaranth, basmati rice, lentils, soft-boiled eggs (organic), lots of baked and broiled cold-water fish, some chicken and turkey, some natural yogurt, ground flaxseed, a few raw almonds, and sunflower, pumpkin, and sesame seeds. She ate watermelon for breakfast and fruits for snacks. (Watermelon and fruit help relieve constipation and cleanse the kidneys. In cases of chronic constipation, I often allow more than two fruits per day until constipation is resolved.)

SUPPLEMENTS

Rhonda's program included digestive enzymes, alfalfa tablets, chlorella tablets, blue-green algae, liquid calcium and magnesium, evening primrose oil, flaxseed oil, omega-3 and -6 EFAs, fish oil, vitamin B complex, vitamins A and D, a multivitamin, acidophilus, colostrum, and cascara sagrada (sparingly as needed for constipation). She tested her thyroid (see the home thyroid test on page 205). Her temperatures were consistently low so she added dulse tablets, which helped improve her metabolism.

TEAS

Rhonda drank oatstraw tea, shave grass tea (both are high in silicon good for rebuilding her skin), red clover tea (to clean her blood), and flaxseed tea (to lubricate her stools).

PHYSICAL THERAPIES

Rhonda used only natural lotions and cosmetics, and she wore only cotton clothes. She soaked in a tub of warm water with one cup of raw apple cider vinegar to relieve her itching, and rubbed cold-pressed organic sesame oil mixed with small amounts of oregano oil into her psoriasis at night. She walked one mile daily to improve circulation and help get natural vitamin D from the sun. Walking also helped her lose the pounds she needed to lose.

EMOTIONAL THERAPIES

Rhonda and I had a counseling session once a week. She worked on healing her spirit and nurturing her soul. She worked on confidence and self-esteem, and learned to find and do some things in life that were meaningful to her. She was able to release much sadness, grief, anger, and pain, and to reclaim her will to live. Rhonda eventually decided to go to Alcoholic Anonymous, and she was able to quit drinking altogether. She read the following books help keep her mind focused on healing: *Nutrition Handbook* by Dr. Bernard Jensen, *Co-Dependent No More* by Melodie Beatty, *Feeding the Hungry Heart* by Geneen Roth, *The Secret Language of Eating Disorders* by Peggy Claude Pierre.

CLEANSE

After four months of the program, Rhonda did the whole body cleanse outlined in chapter 6. She took an antiparasite herbal combination with black walnut, wormwood, and cloves. During the week of the cleanse, she cried a lot and broke up with her boyfriend, who didn't support the changes she was making. After the cleanse, she continued her healing program. Cleansing the body always brings on emotional cleansing as well.

RESULTS

Rhonda lost thirty pounds within eight months. She stopped smoking and drinking alcohol. Her skin became healthy and clear. Her periods became normal and free from pain, and she began to have daily bowel movements. She even met a wonderful man and got married! They had a beautiful wedding, and Rhonda looked like a princess. She was healthy and radiant. They moved to a new area, and Rhonda acquired a job that she loves.

Glenda: Healing Chronic Ulcerative Colitis

Glenda was a young housewife and mother of a four year old. She was thirty-four years old, five foot four, and 125 pounds. While her husband traveled a lot with his work, Glenda had taken it upon herself to manage the construction of their home, which was a tremendous undertaking. She was a perfectionist and extremely driven. She started at 5:00 A.M. every morning and drank several cups of coffee throughout the day. She ate lots of sugar, refined foods, and fried foods. She was very acidic from this type of diet as well as from stress. When she called me, she was frightened. Her symptoms included:

- Chronic ulcerative colitis
- Severe bleeding with stools
- Cramping and pain in her abdomen

NUTRITIONAL PROGRAM

Per her nutritional program, Glenda immediately removed all salt, sugar, caffeine, pasteurized milk, pork, red meat, and fried foods from her diet. She ate homemade vegetable soups, as well as steamed vegetables, including lots of different kinds of squashes. (Squashes are very soothing to the intestinal tract.) She ate salads with avocado and olive oil, blended or chewed well. She ate noncitrus fruits, including bananas, papayas, blueberries, peaches (only two fruits per day); well-cooked basmati and brown rice; lentils, potato peeling broth; yogurt; soft-boiled eggs; well-cooked millet; barley; oatmeal; baked potatoes; flaxseed and olive oil; baked and broiled fish; and chicken and turkey in small amounts.

BEVERAGES

Glenda drank raw vegetable juices with lots of cabbage, carrot, and parsley; slippery elm, white willow bark, white oak bark, flaxseed, and oatstraw teas; and purified and distilled water with liquid trace minerals added. She occasionally drank some black cherry juice to prevent anemia.

PHYSICAL THERAPIES

Glenda took daily enemas with flaxseed tea, Eugalan Topfer Forte, slippery elm, and chlorophyll for one week, then three times per week for one month, then twice a week for two weeks, then once per week.

EMOTIONAL THERAPIES

Glenda attended counseling sessions.

RESULTS

After one month following her recommended therapies, Glenda became pregnant and then lost the fetus. After five months on the healing program,

Glenda was doing well with no noticeable symptoms. After nine months, her doctor reported, "Patient is doing great." Two years after Glenda began her healing therapies, she gave birth to a healthy girl and was able to nurse her for eighteen months with plenty of milk. She still watches what she eats and drinks and is a healthy mother.

Glenda's note: "Thank you for teaching me to save my life and really live!"

Carrie: Healing Sore Throats, Nasal Discharge, and Ear Infections

Carrie was a darling little girl of five who had chronic sore throats, nasal discharge, and ear infections. She coughed so hard during the night that it was frightening her family. Carrie craved anything with sugar and dairy products, especially ice cream. Her symptoms included:

- Sore throats, coughing, thick nasal discharge, and ear infections
- No improvement after having her tonsils and adenoids removed
- A recommendation to have tubes placed in ears to drain the fluid

NUTRITIONAL PROGRAM

Carrie's nutritional program removed all dairy products and refined sugars from her diet. She switched to rice milk, rice ice cream, and rice pudding. She also ate rice pasta. She ate whole-grain cookies made from oat or rice flour and sweetened with fruit juice. She was encouraged to eat fruits, vegetables, whole grains, raw nuts, organic eggs, fish, chicken, and turkey.

SUPPLEMENTS

Carrie took a multivitamin for children; chlorella; chewable vitamin C (she used these supplements five days per week); echinacea tincture and tincture made of colloidal silver; tea tree oil; aloe vera and Swedish bitters to build her immune system and stop her sinus drainage (the tinctures were placed in apple juice). She also had mullein-garlic oil ear drops rubbed just inside her ear when symptomatic.

EMOTIONAL THERAPIES

Carrie was invited to help make cookies with rice or oat flour. She was also included in discussions about the important role of nutrition would play in helping her get well.

RESULTS

Carrie did not have to have tubes placed in her ears. She learned to tell her kindergarten teacher that she could not have milk. The frequency of her sore throats, sinus infections, earaches, coughing, and colds diminished.

Noland: Healing Cradle Cap

Noland was a precious two-year-old boy who had been nursed all his life. He was very healthy except for cradle cap on his head. His mother had tried Vaseline and sesame oil for several months and neither had helped.

PHYSICAL THERAPIES

Noland's parents put MSM drops on his scalp each day. When the drops dried, they massaged his scalp with colloidal silver herbal salve, which contains colloidal silver, goldenseal, comfrey, vitamin E, aloe vera, olive oil, and beeswax.

RESULTS

Noland's cradle cap cleared up in two days.

Joy: Healing a Wartlike Growth

Joy was seventy-four years old with lots of sparkle and a determination to be healthy. She had been through a number of emotional traumas in her life, including several unhappy marriages. Physically, she had suffered a great deal as well. At age twenty-two, she endured second- and third-degree burns from a topical medication she had been given for hemorrhoids. At forty-five, she contracted polio and could not walk. Her doctor treated her polio with stewed grapefruits, including the rinds, which he said contained natural quinine. He also used physical therapy and colored lights. After several months she was able to walk again. At age seventy, she had a cancerous growth removed from her breast and turned to wheatgrass juice and raw vegetable juices to help strengthen her body and build her immune system. For years she had a black wartlike growth on top of her head about the size of a quarter. Joy also had moles on her forehead and shoulder. Her symptoms included:

- Lifelong chronic constipation
- Trouble remembering
- Poor eyesight
- Varicose veins
- A tendency toward high cholesterol
- Anemia
- Poor circulation, with cold hands and feet
- Fungus on her feet as a result of low thyroid function
- Leg cramps
- A wartlike growth on her head, one inch in diameter
- Moles on her forehead and shoulder
- Dry skin and very dry nasal passages and vaginal tract

NUTRITIONAL PROGRAM

Joy's nutritional program avoided all dairy products and meats with hormones. She also avoided gluten, fried foods, sugars, salt, and caffeine. She ate lots of cruciferous vegetables; one to two fruits per day; basmati rice; and rice, millet, or quinoa cereal, cooked well with ground flaxseed; pumpkin; almond and sesame meal on top of the cereal; soaked and well-cooked lentils (beans were constipating for her); small amounts of raw, organic cheese; small amounts of organic yogurt; salads; steamed and baked vegetables; organic eggs; baked or broiled cold-water fish; chicken; turkey; flaxseed oil, borage oil, or evening primrose oil; and pumpkin seed, sesame, and olive oil.

BEVERAGES

Joy drank raw vegetable juices, including carrot, beet, celery, parsley, and wheatgrass juice. She also drank Pau d'Arco tea and essiac tea (which is a combination of sheep sorrel, burdock root, slippery elm bark, and rhubarb root) to strengthen her immune system; oatstraw tea to nourish her skin, hair, and fingernails; red clover tea to cleanse her blood; flaxseed tea to lubricate her stools; bilberry tea to strengthen her eyesight; and purified and distilled water with liquid ionic trace minerals (meaning minerals of the smallest size for easier absorption taken from plant sediment in the Great Salt Lake in Utah) added to build her bones and neutralize her pH. It also often helps relieve constipation because of the magnesium.

SUPPLEMENTS

Joy took coenzyme Q-10; ginkgo biloba to help her memory; dulse tablets to strengthen her thyroid; a natural iron formula that included vitamin B12; chlorella to cleanse her liver, colon, and blood; lecithin granules and A-Flow to cleanse her arteries and help lower her cholesterol; liquid calcium and magnesium to build her bones; digestive enzymes; a multivitamin/mineral complex including B complex; a tincture with milk thistle, Oregon grape, wormwood, black walnut, ginger, garlic, and fennel to detoxify her liver and kill parasites and microbials; vitamin C with bioflavonoids to strengthen her veins; and olive leaf extract to eliminate fungus.

PHYSICAL THERAPIES

Joy took Epsom salts baths; placed castor oil poultices on her breast (traditionally used to help soften scar tissue and prevent any tumorous growths from returning); did skin brushing; walked; did yoga; used a rebounder; and got massages. She soaked her feet in a solution of water and food-grade hydrogen peroxide and applied tea tree oil and bloodroot salve on her moles followed by a colloidal silver herbal salve. She placed essential oils—geranium, lavender, eucalyptus, marjoram, melaleuca—one at a time in layers on the wart on her head three times per day.

CLEANSE

Joy underwent a ten-day whole body cleanse, as outlined in chapter 6. During the cleanse, she took antiparasite herbs, fenugreek tea, and added raw salads once per day.

EMOTIONAL THERAPIES

Joy attended New Decision Therapy and Time Risk counseling sessions as part of her healing program. New Decision Therapy helps identify and release painful emotions from the past using kinesiology. Time Risk was developed by Daniele LoRito, MD, from Italy and involves emotional release work through the stimulation of specific acupressure meridians.

RESULTS

The moles dropped off Joy's forehead and shoulder. The large wart finally came off her head after six months of persistent care. It came off in layers, as it turned out to be very deep. The fungus on her toes went away; her circulation improved; her constipation was alleviated; her vision and memory greatly improved; and her blood report showed normal cholesterol levels and no anemia. At seventy-eight, Joy was running up and down stairs and feeling like she was only forty! She was truly one of the most cheerful, determined individuals I have ever met.

Corine: Healing Allergies and Stopping Excessive Menstrual Bleeding

Corine was forty-eight years old and an extremely hard worker. Her diet had never been good because she ate whatever she could on the run. Her mother had German measles when she was three months pregnant with Corine. Corine was born with poor vision, and one of her ears was deformed, though it finally grew to be normal. At eight years old, she had her tonsils removed, and her recovery was very slow. At age twenty-five, her appendix ruptured, and she suffered a major infection. She was in several car accidents. She had surgery for endometriosis four different times and eventually had her right ovary and tube removed because it was so diseased. She had severe cramping and pain with her periods. She was menstruating every two weeks. When she took estrogen and progesterone, her periods got worse, with continued bleeding. She started taking just progesterone, and the bleeding finally stopped after twenty-two days.

She also craved sweets. And she had had allergies and fatigue for years. She was allergic to pollen, molds, cats, and even live Christmas trees. Her allergies caused her to lose her voice and suffer with upper respiratory infections. Allergy medications brought some relief, but it was not lasting. Her symptoms included:

- · Allergies
- · Fatigue
- · Aching in her knees
- · Menstruation every two weeks and excessive bleeding

NUTRITIONAL PROGRAM

Corine had to change her lifestyle and follow a good nutritional program one step at the time. So we began slowly. She followed the nutritional plan outlined in chapter one as closely as possible, considering her busy schedule. She ate a poached egg for breakfast with sprouted grain toast or a fruit smoothie made with fruit and almond cream. For lunch she ate salads, vegetables, and polenta or turkey or fish. Sometimes she had sprouted grain sandwiches with mayonnaise from the health store and cucumber, tomato, avocado, and/or lentil soup. For dinner she has salad, steamed or baked vegetables, fish, chicken, turkey, or a type of vegetable soup and rice crackers. She occasionally ate rice pudding for dessert.

BEVERAGES

Corine drank purified water and herbal teas including lemon balm and chamomile to calm the nerves.

SUPPLEMENTS

Corine took a multivitamin with minerals. She also took liquid calcium and magnesium to support her bones; propolis to boost her immune system; cayenne capsules to help stop the bleeding; natural iron tablets because she had lost a lot of blood; an allergy formula with glutamic acid; pepsin and bee pollen; and digestive enzymes to ensure proper digestion.

PHYSICAL THERAPIES

Corine used an herbal cream called Complete Tissue and Bone on her knee and progesterone cream. She took Epsom salts baths to relax her muscles and put castor oil poultices on her abdomen.

CLEANSE

After about six months of following a good nutrition program, Corine followed a ten-day cleanse, including a mucus and liver cleanse. She released lots of mucus in her stools.

EMOTIONAL THERAPIES

Corine worked with prayer and meditation daily to give her strength and help her gain calm inside. She released a lot of fears including those about her sisters having multiple sclerosis. She wanted to be healthy so she could perhaps avoid this dreaded illness.

RESULTS

Corine dropped fifteen pounds and all her allergies disappeared. Her excessive bleeding stopped. She no longer needed allergy medicine or hormonal tablets.

Faye: Healing a Swollen Arm, a Hardened Breast, and Lymph Nodes

Faye was a beautiful mother of three children. She was an artist, seamstress, and housewife, and she homeschooled her children. She loved nature and horses. Faye believed in eating natural wholesome foods and served them to her family. She got sick with a flu one winter, and a lymph node swelled under her arm. After that, the swelling affected her arm to such a degree that she was unable to use her arm or hand. Her breast became hardened as well. She was determined to get well using natural methods.

NUTRITIONAL PROGRAM

Faye's nutritional program avoided all animal products and all fruit. She ate whole natural organic vegetables, nuts, seeds, gluten-free grains, and beans. Her meals consisted of steamed vegetables, soups, and broths high in potassium, blended salads, and lots of raw garlic. She soaked all nuts and seeds, and blended them before eating them, and she soaked the beans before cooking them. She washed all her vegetables well with a solution of one teaspoon of food-grade hydrogen peroxide to one quart of water. She always ate dinner before 6:00 P.M.

312 &) HEALTH IS YOUR BIRTHRIGHT

BEVERAGES

Faye drank raw vegetable juices, including carrot, beet, celery, parsley, and garlic. She drank wheatgrass juice and eight glasses of purified water per day. She also drank herbal teas, including mullein, oatstraw, and chaparral.

CLEANSE

Faye followed a whole body cleanse for six months, including a colon cleanse, mucus cleanse, and liver cleanse. She did a liver cleanse once a week. She used lots of cloves, wormwood, and black walnut in her colon cleanse water and implants. She also used a drop of liquid poke root and two drops of sheep sorrel in her implants. Poke root is considered an alterative herb, which stimulates metabolism and helps cleanse the lymph system. It contains triterpenoid saponins or substances that encourage immunity.

SUPPLEMENTS

Faye took several supplements while on her cleanse, including vitamins A and D; vitamin B complex; vitamin C; flaxseed oil; vitamin E; dulse; calcium and magnesium; ionic trace minerals; black walnut, wormwood, cloves, echinacea, and goldenseal as needed; olive leaf extract; propolis (periodically); coenzyme Q-10; acidophilus; and bifidus.

PHYSICAL THERAPIES

Faye did skin brushing daily before her bath or shower and a cold sheet treatment once a week. She also put poultices with castor oil, poke, comfrey, wheatgrass and/or blended cabbage, and sheep sorrel on her breast and arm. She walked and rested often, soaked in Epsom salts baths, soaked in baths with one cup of food-grade hydrogen peroxide, and got foot and back massages.

EMOTIONAL THERAPIES

A lot of emotional feelings emerged during Faye's healing program, including sadness, fear, and anger. She wrote about her unwanted feelings and then burned the paper in the fireplace. She prayed often and worked within herself to have faith that she would get well. She had many discussions with her family and her husband. Her husband helped her fill the buckets of water and prepare the implants each day during her cleanse, staying by her side to massage her abdomen. Everyone in her family worked together to help her get well.

RESULTS

Over time, Faye began to be able to move her fingers and hand and use her arm again. The swelling went down, and her arm, hand, fingers, and breast returned to normal. Faye began to feel well and strong again. She was able to embroider a beautiful handkerchief for me using both hands.

Marta: Healing a Cyst in the Breast

Marta was a woman in her late forties who had gone out her back door one day and fell onto a rough branch that had dropped from a tree in her yard. She felt at the time that she had somehow damaged her right breast and indeed it began to cause her pain. She went to her doctor for an exam and was told she had a cyst in that breast. (The cyst was perhaps already there and the fall caused enough pain for her to have it checked, we don't know.) A biopsy showed it was not cancerous. The doctor told her she could either have it removed or monitor it for a while. She chose to have it removed in a month. In the meantime she followed several natural therapies.

Her symptoms included:

· Benign cyst in right breast
· Pain in right breast

NUTRITIONAL PROGRAM

Marta followed healthy meal plans like those presented in chapter 1. She avoided wheat, dairy products, sugar, caffeine, salt, beef, pork, and fried foods. She ate a variety of raw and steamed vegetables, two fruits per day, whole grains including millet and quinoa, seven grain sprouted bread, raw almonds, beans, soft boiled eggs, fish, chicken, and turkey. She ate from two to four cloves of raw garlic daily and used cayenne pepper on her foods.

BEVERAGES

Marta drank lots of purified water, raw vegetable juices including carrot, celery, beet, parsley, and herbal tea that included the following herbs:

1 part red clover–helps to cleanse the blood

1 part yellow dock–helps to cleanse the liver and blood

1 part burdock–also cleanses liver

1 part Dong Quai–helps to balance hormones

1 part Pau d' Arco–helps to clean the blood and known for its tumor-reducing qualities

1 part ginger–helps circulation of the blood so that toxins can be carried out of the body

1 part juniper berries–helps the kidneys release wastes from the lymph fluid

cinnamon to taste for flavor

SUPPLEMENTS

Marta took colloidal silver, acidophilus, chlorella, and borage oil.

PHYSICAL THERAPIES

She used a poultice of poke-root or sage mixed with castor oil on the breast, placed a piece of plastic over it and then a piece of wool flannel. Each night, on top of the flannel, she placed a heating pad and kept it on low. She washed it off each morning.

EMOTIONAL THERAPIES

Marta visualized her breast healed, and prayed.

RESULTS

Marta's cyst totally disappeared and she did not have to have the surgery. She is thankful for her amazing good health.

Raymond: Lowering Cholesterol, Triglyceride, and Glucose Levels, and Healing Skin Rash and Vertigo

Raymond was thirty-six years old, five foot six, and pudgy at 165 pounds. He had a skin rash that wouldn't go away and vertigo. Every time he stood up, he felt as if the room were spinning. His dizziness had begun when he hit his head really hard on his surfboard. His blood test showed high cholesterol, high triglycerides, and high glucose levels. In his own words, he had lived the life of a party animal, eating lots of fats and sweets, and drinking alcohol. His symptoms included:

· Skin rash
· Vertigo
· A high cholesterol level, 244 (normal range: 75-220)
· High triglycerides, 290 (normal range: 40-160)
· High glucose, 128 (normal range: 60-120)

NUTRITIONAL PROGRAM

Raymond followed a nutritional plan that avoided saturated fats from pork and beef, hydrogenated fats, including margarine, and fried foods. He also avoided foods high in gluten, including wheat. He did not eat dairy products except for nonfat yogurt and cottage cheese. He avoided caffeine, alcohol, sugar, artificial sweeteners, and salt. He used stevia to sweeten his lemonade and herbal teas because stevia helps to balance the pancreas. He ate foods high in fiber, such as steamed and raw vegetables, some fruits, and whole grains with a low gluten content, such as brown rice and millet. He also ate rice bran, which is excellent for lowering cholesterol. He ate beans and lentils, broiled fish, chicken, and turkey.

BEVERAGES

Raymond drank raw vegetable juices, including carrot, celery, beet, and ginger. Carrot juice flushes fat from the bile in the liver and helps control cholesterol. Beets and beet juice act to cleanse the liver and gallbladder, and ginger helps improve circulation. He drank eight glasses of distilled water with ionic liquid trace minerals added daily. He drank oatstraw tea to improve his skin and strengthen his nervous system, and any other herbal teas desired.

SUPPLEMENTS

Raymond took apple pectin and garlic to help lower his cholesterol, A-Flow (a natural oral chelating agent that cleans arteries and lowers cholesterol), essential fatty acids (black currant seed, flaxseed, borage oil, and primrose oil), and cayenne capsules to improve his circulation and lower cholesterol. He also took a multivitamin with B-complex to strengthen his overall body and nervous system, niacin to improve blood flow to his brain, CoQ10 to improve his circulation, chromium picolinate to balance his pancreas, and silica to help heal his skin.

PHYSICAL THERAPIES

Cranial sacral therapy with atlas adjustment improved Raymond's vertigo. He also saw an ergonomics specialist to help rearrange his office and suggest types of chairs; physical therapy to learn how to walk, sit, and stand; and corrective exercises for the vertigo. He had a deep tissue massage; did skin brushing; wore cotton clothing, and used calendula cream on his skin.

RESULTS

Raymond turned his life around. He stopped partying and drinking. He changed his eating program. He did specific exercises to free himself from the vertigo and rearranged his office furniture so it would support him ergonomically. His preliminary blood test was taken in October 1997. A followup test was taken in February 1998. At the second test, his glucose level was 87, within normal range. His cholesterol had dropped from 244 to 223, and his triglycerides had come down from 290 to 198. Within another three months, his cholesterol and triglyceride levels had fallen within normal range. Raymond lost twenty pounds and felt terrific. His skin cleared up, and he was no longer troubled by dizziness.

The following is a letter from Raymond:

Hi Ellen,

Please allow me to take a moment and thank you for all your help! It's hard to describe how instrumental you and your holistic health care techniques and recommendations have been for me. The improvements to my health have been nothing short of remarkable. You truly are my holistic health care angel.

I have regularly followed the holistic supplements and dietary guidelines you recommended. Also, I followed your additional recommendations to utilize other holistic practitioners, who have provided physical therapy, corrective exercises, deep tissue massage, and atlas adjustments.

The most amazing thing was how quickly I regained my health just by adjusting my diet and taking supplements. The high vegetable diet made me feel so much better, and my incident of illness reduced dramatically. While stabilizing my diet, I also focused on resolving the reoccurring vertigo.

After all the best doctors had exhausted determining what could be wrong with me, a holistic health practitioner you recommended pinpointed the vertigo to a cervical problem in a four-hour evaluation. Following an exercise treatment program, the vertigo almost completely subsided within one month. For the next six months I followed a corrective exercise program, had cervical atlas adjustments, deep tissue massage, completely redesigned my work environment in an ergonomically sensible fashion, and utilized cervical techniques to have a cervical change that most chiropractors would say is impossible (an almost 25-degree turnaround in my cervical spine).

Through the dietary and exercise changes recommended, I have been able to achieve some remarkable results. Every phase of my life is better. I regularly take holistic herbs and supplements, follow a relatively simple diet, and exercise on a consistent basis. At thirty-eight years old, I'm in the best shape of my life. I now regularly surf, golf, run, swim, and bike as well as run a successful computer business.

The greatest achievement, which I mainly contribute to my newfound health, was last weekend, when I completed my first triathlon.

Was it easy to switch diets and completely adjust the way I exercise and work? No, it took desire and discipline. For me, it came when I was told I could likely acquire diabetes if I did not change my lifestyle. Also, walking around dizzy all the time wasn't any fun either.

Did it happen over night? No, even though I felt much better immediately, it took six months to a year before I really saw the radical changes start to take effect. Was it worth it? One hundred percent *without a doubt, it was the best commitment I've ever made. I feel at least fifteen years younger since I started utilizing holistic medicine, and I've only just begun.*

Ellen, I can't thank you enough for introducing me to holistic health as well as all your love, support, and assistance with my contin-ued health quest!

Sincerely,

Raymond

Brent: Healing Chronic Fatigue

Brent was twenty-five years old and forty pounds overweight. He had dis-abling fatigue but could not sleep at night. He was a professional golfer and was no longer able to play. His diet had been fast foods, fried foods, sweets, lots of meat (a nutritionist had put him on an all-protein diet), coffee, and some alcohol. He had low thyroid function according to the thyroid basal temperature test. His temperatures were 96.5°F to 97°F. Normal tempera-ture is 97.8°F to 98.2°F. His blood test revealed a low platelet count indi-cating a possible viral infection according the medical doctor on our team. He had felt badly since being vaccinated for influenza in his junior year of college. He often had to drag himself into my office and was so exhausted he could hardly hold his head up or pay attention.

Brent had chronic fatigue syndrome, a condition that causes exhaustion regardless of how much bed rest or sleep a person might get. Other symp-toms resemble those of viral infections or influenza, such as muscle aches, headaches, digestive disorders, sleep disturbances, swollen lymph nodes, sore throat, and even fever. Chronic fatigue syndrome is thought to be caused by the Epstein-Barr virus because the symptoms are so similar. However, a per-son can have chronic fatigue syndrome and not have Epstein-Barr.

His symptoms included:

· Overweight
· Chronic Fatigue
· Low blood platelets, possible viral infection
· Low thyroid function

NUTRITIONAL PROGRAM

Brent's nutritional program avoided fried foods, dairy products, wheat, sugar, salt, caffeine, alcohol, and pork. He ate no more than two fruits per day. He began to eat lots of steamed vegetables, raw vegetables, and salads. He cut down on beef consumption and had some fish, chicken, or turkey in his diet. For breakfast, Brent had cooked millet, quinoa, oats, or two eggs over easy with seven-grain sprouted toast. For lunch he had a large salad with olive oil dressing; a seven-grain sprouted bread sandwich with tuna, chicken, turkey, healthy mayonnaise, lettuce, tomato, and raw vegetables; tuna salad on lettuce with raw vegetables; or vegetable soup and raw vegetables. A snack was celery with sesame butter or almond butter, an apple, almonds; or rice crackers with sesame butter. Dinner was baked or broiled fish, chicken, or turkey with a salad and steamed vegetables; rice pasta with marinara sauce and a salad; or a steamed vegetable plate with beans and rice. He selected desserts from the suggestions in chapter 1.

BEVERAGES

Each day, Brent drank two ounces of wheatgrass juice; eight ounces of carrot, celery, beet, and parsley juice; eight ounces of purified water with five drops of liquid ionic trace minerals six to eight times; and eight ounces of Pau d' Arco tea two times. Chamomile tea at night.

PHYSICAL THERAPIES

Brent regularly walked outside in the sunshine and fresh air, practiced deep breathing, did a slant board exercise, and did skin brushing.

SUPPLEMENTS

Throughout his six-month recovery program, Brent took various supplements at different times to support his healing. He took EBV by Monastery of Herbs, an herbal formula known to relieve viruses, especially Epstein Barr. He also took CoQ10 to fight free radicals and improve his overall healing; a thyroid formula with kelp, zinc, and bovine thyroid to improve his thyroid function; an adrenal formula with bovine adrenal to strengthen his adrenal glands; a natural iron formula to build his blood; chlorella to cleanse his liver and colon; olive leaf to boost his immune system; acidophilus to place good bacteria into his intestinal tract; an herbal tincture with reishi, shitaki, maitake, Pau d'Arco, and echinacea extracts to boost his immune system; colostrum to boost his immune system; a multivitamin/ mineral to ensure he had all necessary nutrients; and digestive enzymes to ensure proper digestion. He also took L-tyrosine to help fight depression and fatigue; and an herbal combination with passion flower, valerian, and hops, taken with chamomile tea to help him sleep.

CLEANSE

Brent underwent a whole body cleanse as described in chapter 6. He added salads to his lunch menu. He also used flaxseed tea to cleanse his colon, fennel and fenugreek tea to cleanse his liver, oatstraw tea to support his nerves, and Pau d'Arco tea to boost his immune system during the cleanse.

RESULTS

Brent gradually began to feel better. After three months on this program, he undertook a cleanse, which was the turning point in his recovery. He began to feel much more energy. He continued the program for three more months and felt great. He lost forty pounds, and his face glowed. He truly became a whole new person who was alert, alive, and healthy! He started playing golf again and, with time, began winning tournaments.

Elsbeth: Healing from a Heart Attack

Elsbeth was a creative artist. She had gone through a traumatic divorce and lost custody of her three precious children. Afterward, she endured intense fear, stress, and emotional pain. When she was forty, her cholesterol level was over 750 and was unresponsive to any medications she tried. She suffered a terrible heart attack and damage to her heart muscle. She was unable to afford medical care and did not have the strength keep struggling with her life, so she sought rest and solitude for nine months in a rudimentary old cabin. During that time, she became very calm and began to eat simply and consciously. She chose foods from nature's table, such as mushrooms, dandelion, chamomile, and herbs from the forest. She incorporated nutritious broths, soups, and teas into her diet. She thought about her life and began to dream a new dream of what her life could become. She prayed fervently and released negative thought patterns, including fear and worry.

It was at that point that I met Elsbeth. She came to Dr. Bernard Jensen's ranch, where I worked with her to continue her healing.

Her symptoms included:

· High cholesterol over 750
· Weakened heart due to a heart attack

NUTRITIONAL PROGRAM

Elsbeth's nutritional program featured more fresh, whole, and natural foods. She drank purified water.

PHYSICAL THERAPIES

Elsbeth walked barefoot on the earth, bathing in fresh air and sunshine. She had a beautiful voice, and she sang healing songs for which she had written the lyrics.

CLEANSE

Elsbeth cleansed her colon and did a whole body cleanse.

SUPPLEMENTS

Elsbeth took various natural food supplements at different times. She included garlic and lecithin to help lower cholesterol; milk thistle to balance her liver; flaxseed oil and borage oil to provide essential fatty acids; B vitamins to strengthen her nervous system; and gymnema sylvestre to lower her insulin levels. She took vitamin E to improve her circulation; CoQ10 to fight free radicals and heal the damaged tissue in her heart; hawthorne berries to strengthen her heart; calcium, magnesium, potassium, and trace minerals to balance her heart and keep her bones strong; as well as vitamin C with bioflavonoids and silica from horsetail to strengthen her connective tissue. She took digestive plant enzymes to ensure that all the foods she ate were digested well. Elsbeth also took lots of greens, such as blue-green algae and chlorella, to cleanse her blood, colon, and liver and nourish her body.

RESULTS

Two weeks into her cleanse, Elsbeth's cholesterol dropped from 750 to 450, and within the following month, it stabilized at 200. Today she is a healthy, happy woman. She lives in a beautiful home and is teaching others about the benefits of cleansing and the power of conscious positive thinking. She is singing and recording her music.

Betsy: Healing from Chronic Kidney and Bladder Infections

Betsy was a gorgeous, talented girl of eighteen who suffered with chronic kidney and bladder infections. She was drinking a gallon of water a day to try to keep from getting sick. When she had a kidney infection, the pain was agonizing. When she took antibiotics, the infection and pain would stop, but almost as soon as she stopped the antibiotics, the infection would return.

Her symptoms included:

· Severe, painful kidney and bladder infections
· Vaginal yeast infections

NUTRITIONAL PROGRAM

Betsy improved her diet by adding lots of vegetables, whole grains, and fish. She avoided eating many sweets, fruits, processed foods, pork, and red meat. She avoided all dairy products except yogurt, and she avoided caffeine, alcohol, salt, pork, and red meat (which is high in uric acid). She ate lots of raw vegetables, such as asparagus, parsley, celery, cucumber, green leafy lettuce, watercress, and garlic. She ate some watermelon but not with other foods. She also ate steamed vegetables, brown rice, quinoa, millet, lentils, and beans. She drank cranberry juice and raw vegetable juices, including parsley, celery, and cucumber.

EMOTIONAL THERAPIES

Betsy worked on releasing emotional pain from her past. She became very conscious of her thoughts each day and was very prayerful about her healing.

SUPPLEMENTS

When she got a kidney and bladder infection, Betsy took three capsules of acidophilus three times per day on an empty stomach to help fight yeast overgrowth, and two droppers of kidney and bladder tincture (one part each juniper berry, uva ursi leaf, corn silk, burdock root and seed, and parsley leaf and root) in two ounces of water four times per day to strengthen her kidneys and bladder. She also massaged her kidneys and bladder with one part tea tree oil or oregano oil and two parts jojoba oil (the oils soak in and kill infections).

Betsy took olive leaf and propolis to help strengthen her immune system, and she drank distilled water with ionic trace minerals. She also drank kidney and bladder tea.

RESULTS

Betsy became a healthy, vibrant young woman. She is wise beyond her years. She enjoys horseback riding, camping, traveling, writing, and singing.

On Being a Champion
> *A champion is a winner,*
> *A hero . . .*
> *Someone who never gives up*
> *Even when the going gets rough.*
> *A champion is a member of a winning team . . .*
> *Someone who overcomes challenges*
> *Even when it requires creative solutions.*
> *A champion is an optimist,*
> *A hopeful spirit . . .*
> *Someone who plays the game,*
> *Even when the game is called life . . .*
> *Especially when the game is called life.*
> *There can be a champion in each of us,*
> *If we live as a winner,*
> *If we live as a member of the team,*
> *If we live with a hopeful spirit,*
> *For life.*

—*Mattie J. T. Stepanek, age 9,*
Journey through Heartsongs

September 1999

Conclusion

We can see from the courage of these wonderful people that it is entirely possible to step up and take our power back. The time is now! For if not now, when?

Spend some time in quiet reflection and get to know yourself. Learn where your weaknesses are and where your strengths are. Use the tools provided in this book to help you heal your physical body as well as your mind and soul. Love yourself! Love your life! Be all you can be!

I have a unique and beautiful friend. Her name is Jewel. She wrote the following song, which has inspired me and thousands of others around the world. Feel the meaning of the words, and it will inspire you!

Life Uncommon
> *Lend your voices only*
> *To sounds of freedom*
> *No longer lend your strength*
> *To that which you wish to be free from*
> *Fill your lives with love and bravery*
> *And you shall lead a life uncommon*

> —*Jewel*

Bibliography

Airola, Paavo, ND, PhD. *How to Get Well*. Phoenix, AZ: Health Plus Publishers, 1974.

An Introduction to Natural Health, Health Manual. St. George, UT: Tree of Light Institute, 1999.

Antol, Marie Nadine. *Healing Teas*. Garden City Park, NY: Avery Publishing Group, 1996.

Appleton, Nancy, PhD. *Lick the Sugar Habit*. Garden City Park, NY: Avery Publishing Group, 1996.

Attele, A.S., J.A. Wu, and C.S. Yuan. "Ginseng pharmacology: multiple constituents and multiple actions." *Biochem Pharmacology*, 1999;58(11):1685-1693.

Balch, James F., MD, and Phyllis A. Balch, CNC. *Prescription for Nutritional Healing*, 2nd ed. Garden City Park, NY: Avery Publishing Group, 1997.

Balch, James F., MD, and Phyllis A. Balch, CNC. *Prescription for Nutritional Healing*, 3rd ed. Garden City Park, NY: Avery Publishing Group, 2000.

Barnes, Broda O., MD, and Lawrence Galton. *Hypo-Thyroidism: The Unsuspected Illness*. New York: Harper and Row, 1976.

Batmanghelidj, F., MD. *Your Body's Many Cries for Water*. Vienna, VA: Global Health Solutions, Inc., 2001.

Benson, Herbert, MD. *The Relaxation Response*. New York: Harper Collins Publishers, 1975.

Blakely, Kandis, MFCC. *Your Body Remembers*. Mt. Shasta, CA: Atherika Productions, 1995.

Bland, Jeffrey, PhD. *Digestive Enzymes*. New Canaan, CT: Keats Publishing, Inc., 1993.

Blumenthal M., ed. *The Complete German Commission E Monographs: Therapeutic Guide to Herbal Medicines*. Boston, MA: Integrative Medicine Communications, 1998.

Bradley P., ed. *British Herbal Compendium*. Dorset, England: British Herbal Medicine Association, 1992.

Brown, Kathleen. *Herbal Teas: 101 Nourishing Blends for Daily Health and Vitality*. Pownal, VT: Storey Books, 1999.

Brown, Royden. *The World's Only Perfect Food*. Prescott, AZ: Hohm Press, 1993.

Caine, Kenneth Winston, and Brian Paul Kaufman. *Prayer, Faith and Healing*. Emmaus, PA: Rodale Press, 1999.

Carroll, Lenedra J. *The Architecture of All Abundance: Creating a Successful Life in the Material World*. Novato, CA: New World Library, 2001.

Cerny, A., and K. Schmid. "Tolerability and efficacy of valerian/lemon balm in healthy volunteers (a double-blind, placebo-controlled, multicentre study)." *Fitoterapia*. 1999; 70:221-228.

Chopra, Deepak, MD, and Simon David, MD. *Grow Younger, Live Longer*. New York: Harmony Books, 2001.

Claude Pierre, Peggy. *The Secret Language of Eating Disorders*. New York: Random House Inc., 1997.

Davis, Patricia. *Aromatherapy, An A to Z*. Essex, United Kingdom: C.W. Daniel Company Limited, 1988.

DesMaisons, Kathleen, PhD. *The Sugar Addict's Total Recovery Program*. New York: Ballantine Publishing Group, 2000.

DiGeronimo, Theresa Foy, MEd. *New Hope for People with Fibromyalgia*. Roseville, CA: Prima Publishing, 2001.

Douglass, William Campbell, MD. *The Milk of Human Kindness Is Not Pasteurized*. Marietta, GA: Last Laugh Publishers, 1985.

Dreher, Christine. *The Cleanse Cookbook*. San Diego, CA: Christine's Cleanse Corner and Gemini Services, 1998.

Dyer, Wayne W. *Inspiration: Your Ultimate Calling*. Carlsbad, CA: Hay House, Inc., 2006.

Feingold, Ben F., MD. *Why Your Child Is Hyperactive*. New York: Random House, 1975, 1996.

Ford, Debbie. *The Secret Power of the Shadow: The Power of Owning Your Whole Story*. New York: Harper Collins Publishers, Inc., 2002.

Ford, Norman. *How to Get a Good Night's Sleep*. Monroe Township, New Jersey: Barnes and Noble Books, 2000.

Gershon, Michael D., MD. *The Second Brain*. New York: Harper Collins Publishers, 1998.

Gerson, Max, MD. *A Cancer Therapy*. Bonita, CA: The Gerson Institute, 1999.

Gilbere, Gloria. *The Invisible Illness*. Topanga, CA: Freedom Press, 2002.

Goldbeck, Nikki, and David Goldbeck. *The Supermarket Handbook: Access to Whole Foods*. New York: The New American Library, 1976.

Grieve, M. *A Modern Herbal*. New York: Dover, 1971.

Guillory, Gerard, MD. *IBS: A Doctor's Plan for Chronic Digestive Troubles, the Definitive Guide to Prevention and Relief*. Point Roberts, WA: Hartley and Marks, Inc., 1991.

Haas, Elson, MD. *The Staying Healthy Shopper's Guide*. Berkeley, CA: Celestial Arts, 1999.

Hofstein, Riquette. *Grow Hair and Stop Hair Loss: A Natural, Whole-Body Approach*. Beverly Hills, CA: Riquette International, 2003.

Horne, Steven. *Dr. Mom, Dr. Dad*. St. George, UT: Tree of Light, 2005.

Hurd, Frank J., DC, MD, and Rosalie Hurd, BS. *A Good Cook ... Ten Talents*. Chisholm, MN: Dr. Frank J. and Rosalie Hurd, 1996.

Hutchens, A. *Indian Herbalogy of North America*. Boston: Shambhala Publications, 1991.

Ingrams, Dr. Cass. *The Cure Is in the Cupboard*. Buffalo Grove, IL: Knowledge House, 2001.

Jarvis, Deforrest C., MD. *Folk Medicine*. New York: Fawcett Crest, 1958.

Jensen, Bernard, DC, PhD. *Tissue Cleansing through Bowel Management.* Escondido, CA: Bernard Jensen International, 1981.

Jensen, Bernard, DC, PhD. *Bee Well, Bee Wise with Bee Pollen, Bee Propolis, Royal Jelly.* Escondido, CA: Bernard Jensen International, 1994.

Jensen, Bernard, DC, PhD. *Body Systems—Their Functions and Biochemical Therapies.* Escondido, CA: Bernard Jensen International, 1993.

Jensen, Bernard, DC, PhD. *Doctor-Patient Handbook.* Escondido, CA: Bernard Jensen International, 1976.

Jensen, Bernard, DC, PhD. *Juicing Therapy.* Lincolnwood, IL: Keats Publishing, 2000.

Jensen, Bernard, DC, PhD. *Nutrition Handbook.* Escondido, CA: Bernard Jensen International, 1993.

Jensen, Bernard, DC, PhD. *Soil and Immunity.* Escondido, CA: Bernard Jensen International, 1988.

Jensen, Bernard, DC, PhD. *Surivive . . . This Day.* Escondido, CA: Bernard Jensen International, 1976.

Jensen, Bernard, DC, PhD. *The Chemistry of Man.* Escondido, CA: Bernard Jensen International, 1983.

Jensen, Bernard, DC, PhD, and Mark Anderson. *Empty Harvest.* Garden City Park, NY: Avery Publishing Group Inc., 1990.

Jones, Marion D. *A Practical Guide to Herbal Extracts.* Kingwood, TX: Lady's Slipper Press, 2002.

Kano, Susan. *Making Peace With Food: Freeing Yourself from the Diet/Weight Obsession.* New York: Perennial Library, 1989.

Keim, John W. *Comfort for the Burned and Wounded.* Quakertown, PA: Philosophical Publishing Company, 1999.

Lake, Rhody. *Liver Cleansing Handbook.* Vancouver, Canada: Alive Books, 2000.

Lark, Susan M., MD. *The Estrogen Decision.* Los Altos, CA: Westchester Publishing Company, 1994

Ley, Beth M. *Castor Oil: Its Healing Properties.* Viejo, CA: BL Publications, 1996.

Lo Rito, Daniele, MD. *Bach Flower Massage.* Rochester, VT: Healing Arts Press, 1995.

Mader, Sylvia S. *Inquiry into Life.* Dubuque, IA: Wm. C. Brown Communications, Inc., 1994.

Matschek, Cheryl A., PhD. *Cooking for Health: Without Meat, Dairy, or Refined Sugar.* Portland, OR: Princess Publishing, 2001.

McGarey, William A., MD. *The Oil That Heals: A Physician's Success with Castor Oil Treatments.* Virginia Beach, VA: A.R.E. Press, 1993.

McIntyre, Anne. *Herbal Medicine.* Boston: Charles E. Tuttle Company, Inc., 1993.

Mehlmauer, Leonard, and Nenito Samiento. *Recipes for Better Health.* Camarillo, CA: Leonard Mehlmauer, ND, HP, 1997.

Mendelsohn, Robert S., MD. *How to Raise a Healthy Child . . . in Spite of Your Doctor.* New York: Ballantine Books, 1993.

Meyerowitz, Steve. *Power Juices, Healthy Drinks.* New York: Kensington Publishing Corp., 2000.

Millspaugh, C. *American Medicinal Plants.* New York: Dover Publications, 1974.

Mowry, D. *The Scientific Validation of Herbal Medicine.* New Canaan, CT: Keats Publishing; 1986:3-6, 57-63.

Murphy, J.J., et al. "Randomised double-blind placebo-controlled trial of feverfew in migraine prevention." *The Lancet,* ii:189-192, 1988.

Murray, Michael T., ND, and Jade Beutler, RRT, RCP. *Understanding Fats and Oils.* Encinitas, CA: Progressive Health Publishing, 1996.

Murray, Michael, ND, and Joseph Pizzorrno, ND. *Encyclopedia of Natural Medicine.* Rocklin, CA: Prima Publishing, 1990.

Naraghi, Farideh, MA, RN. *The Quintessential Recipes for Vibrant Health.* Moraga, CA: Whole Life Healing Resources, 1998.

Newall C., L. Anderson, and J. Phillipson. *Herbal Medicines: A Guide for Health-care Professionals.* London: Pharmaceutical Press, 1996.

Northrup, Christiane, MD. *Women's Bodies, Women's Wisdom.* New York: Bantam Books, 1995.

Nyholt, David. *The "Complete" Natural Health Encyclopedia.* Tofield, Alberta, Canada: Global Health Ltd., 1993.

Pal, Raj, PhD, RNC. *Hardening of the Arteries, Heart Attack, Stroke.* Anaheim, CA: Raj Pal, 1994.

Patton, Darryl. *Mountain Medicine: The Herbal Remedies of Tommie Bass.* Birmingham, AL: Natural Reader Press, 2004.

Pattrick, M., et al. "Feverfew in rheumatoid arthritis: a double-blind placebo controlled study." *Ann Rheum Dis,* 48:547-549, 1989.

Quillin, Patrick, PhD, RD, CNS. *The Diabetes Improvement Program.* North Canton, OH: The Leader Co., Inc., 1999.

Reed, Barbara, PhD. *Food, Teens, and Behavior.* Manitowoc, WI: Natural Press, 1983.

Ritchason, Jack, ND. *The Little Herb Encyclopedia.* Pleasant Grove, UT: Woodland Health Books, 1995.

Roth, Geneen. *Feeding the Hungry Heart: The Experience of Compulsive Eating.* New York: Penguin Group, 1993.

Roundtree, Bob, MD, Rachel Walton, RN, and Janet Zand, LAc, OMD. *Smart Medicine for a Healthier Child.* New York: Penguin Putnam Inc., 1994.

Santillo, Humbart, MH, ND. *Food Enzymes, The Missing Link to Radiant Health.* Prescott, AZ: Hohm Press, 1993.

Santillo, Humbart, ND. *Intuitive Eating.* Prescott, AZ: Hohm Press, 1993.

Scheer, James F., Lynne Allison, and Charlie Fox. *The Garlic Cure.* Los Angeles: Alpha Omega Press, 2002.

Selfridge, Nancy, MD, and Franklynn Peterson. *Freedom from Fibromyalgia: The 5-Week Program Proven to Conquer Pain.* New York: Three Rivers Press, 2001.

Simon, J.E., A.F. Chadwick, and L.E. Craker. *Herbs: An Indexed Bibliography.* Hamden, CT: Archon Books, 1984.

"Silver, Our Mightiest Germ Fighter." *Science Digest,* 1978.

Smith, Lendon. *Feed Your Kids Right.* New York: Bantam Doubleday Dell, 1980.

Snyder, Jacqueline T. *Beyond Common Thought: The Joy of Being You.* Issaquah, WA: Windsor House Publishers, 1990.

Solomon, Eldra Pearl, and Gloria A. Phillips. *Understanding Human Anatomy and Physiology.* Philadelphia: W.B. Saunders Company, 1987.

St. Claire, Debra. *Pocket Herbal Reference Guide.* Berkeley, CA: Ten Speed Press, 1992.

Steinman, David. *Diet for a Poisoned Planet.* New York: Crown Publishers, 1990.

Stewart, Mitchell. *Naturopathy: Understanding the Healing Power of Nature.* Columbus, OH: Grade A Publishing, 2001.

The Olive Leaf. Kent, OH: The National Life Extension Research Institute, 1999.

Thomas, John. *Young Again! How to Reverse the Aging Process.* Kelso, WA: Plexus Press, 1994.

Tierra, Lesley, LAc, AHG. *A Kid's Herb Book: For Children of All Ages.* Bandon, OR: Robert D. Reed Publishers, 2005.

Tierra, Michael CC, ND. *The Way of Herbs.* New York: Pocket Books, 1990.

Tribole, Evelyn, MS, RD, and Elyse Resch, MD, RD. *Intuitive Eating.* New York: St. Martin's Press, 1995.

Tyler, V. *The Honest Herbal: A Sensible Guide to the Use of Herbs and Related Remedies.* 3rd ed. Binghampton, NY: Pharmaceutical Products Press, 1993.

Vanderhaeghe, Lorna R., and Patrick Bouic JD, PhD. *The Immune System Cure.* New York: Kensington Publishing Corp, 1999.

Vorberg G. "Ginkgo biloba extract (GBE): A long-term study on chronic cerebral insufficiency in geriatric patients." *Clinical Trials,* 2:149-157, 1985.

Walker, N.W., DSc. *Diet and Salad* Phoenix, AZ: O'Sullivan Woodside and Company, 1983.

Walker, N.W., DSc. *Fresh Vegetables and Juices.* Prescott, AZ: Norwalk Press, 1970.

Walker, N.W., DSc. *The Natural Way to Vibrant Health.* Phoenix, AZ: O'Sullivan Woodside and Company, 1981.

Walker, N.W., DSc. *Water Can Determine Your Health!* Prescott, AZ: Norwalk Press, 1974.

Weil, Andrew, MD. *Spontaneous Healing.* New York: Ballantine Books, 1996.

Weiss, R.F., MD. *Herbal Medicine.* Beaconsfield, England; Beaconsfield Publishers LTD, 1991.

Winston, David. *Herbal Therapeutics.* Broadway, NJ: Herbal Therapeutics Research Library, 2003.

Wood, Matthew. *The Book of Herbal Wisdom: Using Plants as Medicines.* Berkeley, CA: North Atlantic Books, 1997.

Wright, J.V., MD. *Dr. Wright's Book of Nutritional Therapy.* Emmaus, PA: Rodale Press, Inc., 1979.

Resources

Alpine Products
(888) 675-2616
www.alpineairproducts.com

Alternatives Newsletter
www.drdavidwilliams.com

Aranizer Air Purifier Inquiries
(303) 550-0557

Aubrey Organics
(800) 282-7394
www.aubrey-organics.com

Bernard Jensen International
1255 Linda Vista Drive
San Marcos, CA 92078
(888) 743-1790
www.bernardjensen.org

Body Slant
www.ageeasy.com

Bragg Health Products and Books
(800) 446-1990
www.bragg.com

CC Pollen
5455 North 51st Avenue, #17
Glendale, AZ 85301
(800) 875-0096

Chopra Center
www.chopra.com

Clayton College of Natural Health
www.ccnh.edu

Cleanse Program
(808) 966-8581

Devita
www.devita.net

Dr. Christopher–Christopher's Originals
155 West 250 North
Spanish Fork, UT 84660
(801) 794-6888

Genesis Today, Inc.
(800) 916-6642
www.genesistoday.com

Hippocrates Health Institute, Florida
www.hippocratesinst.org

IIPA
(888) 682-2208
www.iridologyassn.org

Leveluk DXII Ionized Water Generator
(877) 587-7086

Lotus Lodge
(330) 878-7379

Monastery of Herbs
17438 San Fernando Mission Boulevard
Granada Hills, CA 91344
(818) 360-4871

Miessence Organic Cosmetics
www.onegrp.com

Mt. Capra Products
279 SW 9th
Chehalis, WA 98532
(800) 574-1961

Natural Path/Silver Wings
PO Box 210469
Nashville, TN 37221
(800) 952-4787

Optimum Health Institute
www.optimumhealth.org/OptimumHealth

Path To Health
1395 Cambridge Drive
Idaho Falls, ID 83401
(877) 587-7086

Riquette International
(310) 551-5253
www.riquette.com

Royal Nutrition International
1215 North Tustin Avenue
Anaheim, CA 92807
(800) 524-3727

Sanoviv
(800) 726-6848
www.sanovivi.org

Sun Chlorella
3305 Kashiwa Street
Torrance, CA 90505
(800) 829-2828

Tac-A-Wah Herbs
4260 T.R. 628
Millersburg, OH 44654

Teeccino, Inc.
(800) 498-3434
www.teeccino.com

The Synergy Company
2279 South Resource Boulevard
Moab, UT 84532
(800) 723-0277

Trace Mineral Research/White Egret
1996 West 3300 South
Ogden, UT 84401
(800) 624-7145

Tree of Light Institute
(800) 416-2887
www.treelite.com

Ultimate Concepts, Inc.
5526 West 13400 South, Suite 213
Riverton, UT 84605
(800) 682-3241

University of Natural Medicine
www.universityofnaturalmedicine.com

Vita Biosa and Light Matrix Organics
www.light-matrix.org

Vita Mix Corporation
8615 Usher Road
Cleveland, OH 44138
(800) 848-2649

Vitally Yours Rebounders
(336) 547-8191

Well Being Journal, Inc.
405 North Nevada Street
Carson City, NV 89703
(775) 887-1702
www.wellbeingjournal.com

Westbrook University
www.westbrooku.edu

Index

Printed in the United States
by Baker & Taylor Publisher Services